MEDICAL–SURGICAL NURSING CARE PLANS

MEDICAL–SURGICAL NURSING CARE PLANS

Barbara Engram

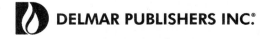

DELMAR PUBLISHERS INC.

NOTICE TO THE READER

Delmar Staff:

Associate Editor: Elisabeth F. Williams
Senior Project Editor: Christopher Chien
Editorial Production Assistant: Lori McDonald

Senior Production Supervisor: Larry Main
Design Coordinator: Karen Kunz Kemp

For information address Delmar Publishers Inc.
3 Columbia Circle Drive, Box 15-015
Albany, New York 12203-5015

COPYRIGHT © 1993
BY DELMAR PUBLISHERS INC.

Printed in the United States of America
Published simultaneously in Canada
by Nelson Canada,
a division of The Thomson Corporation

10 9 8 7 6 5 4 3 2 1 XX 99 98 97 96 95 94 93

Library of Congress Cataloging-in-Publication Data

Engram, Barbara White.
   Medical-surgical nursing care plans/Barbara Engram.
      p.   cm
   Includes bibliographical references and index.
   ISBN 0-8273-3413-3 (textbook)
   1. Nursing care plans.   I. Title.
   [DNLM: 1. Nursing Process—methods. 2. Patient Care Planning—methods—nurses's instruction.
   WY 100 E58m]
RT49.E54 1993
601'.73—dc20
DNLM/DLC
for Library of Congress

Outline

CHAPTER 12 Problems of the Reproductive System

CHAPTER 13 Problems of the Immune System

CHAPTER 14 Problems of the Integumentary System

Preface

The nursing profession is currently facing a tremendous challenge — providing quality patient care amid a shrinking budget. Increasingly, external accrediting agencies of hospitals are placing more emphasis on patient outcomes and nursing competency. In addition, the focus on quality has shifted from quality assurance to continuous quality improvement activities. Nurses can be creative in their approaches to meeting these challenges.

The purpose of this book is to provide nurses with a mechanism for assuming a proactive position in the quality movement by building quality improvement into the actual day-to-day care given. An ongoing self-monitoring system promotes continuous quality improvement. To continually improve patient care, nurses must assess and improve those processes that most affect patient outcomes. These processes are thorough assessment of the patient, correct analysis of data collected, and appropriate interventions. Thus, the nursing process constitutes the foundation from which to launch the transition from quality assurance to continuous quality improvement.

This book presents common medical problems and surgical interventions within the framework of the nursing process. The chapters are divided according to body systems to allow rapid access to information. To promote anticipatory planning, the mean length of stay is given based on the diagnostic related group classification.

Each medical-surgical entry includes in-depth description of the problem, assessment data base, nursing diagnoses with defining characteristics, patient outcome, and evaluation criteria. Nursing interventions with rationale are delineated for each nursing diagnosis.

The Assessment Data Base section outlines risk factors and common clinical manifestations based on physical examination and diagnostic evaluation of the patient. Ongoing assessments are essential to ensure desired patient outcomes. Ongoing assessments are reflected throughout the book as an essential nursing action by using the term "Monitor".

The Nursing Diagnoses sections, approved by the North American Nursing Diagnosis Association (NANDA), are used throughout the book with the exception of one — "High risk for complications". (The author introduces this proposed diagnostic category as it more appropriately reflects the nature of various collective threats to a patient's recovery.) This section contains the following parts: Related to Factors, Defining Characteristics, Patient Outcome, and Evaluation Criteria. Related to Factors refer to entities that precipitate the health threat. Defining Characteristics are those collective signs and symptoms exhibited by the patient. Only the most common factors and characteristics are listed. Additional ones may be added based on an assessment of individual patient differences. Patient Outcomes are the goals and are important clinical indicators of the effectiveness of nursing interventions. To achieve some patient outcomes, nurses must collaborate with other members of the health team. From a quality improvement perspective, collaboration may be referred to as a set of actions characterized by a shared vision and cooperation among health professionals as they come together to meet patient needs and expectations. Patient outcomes requiring collaboration have been labeled "collaborative." Time frames may be added to individualize the outcomes. Evaluation Criteria are important clinical indicators of a patient outcome.

Nursing Interventions essential to achieving each patient outcome are succinctly outlined, followed by rationale. The reader should remember that because of regional differences, the scope of nursing functions may vary.

Some key features of this book are:

- Integrative Care Plans — plans of care that should be incorporated with the primary plan to develop a comprehensive, standard plan of care for the given medical-surgical entry.

- Discharge Considerations — identifies focal areas for the nurse to begin discharge planning when the patient is first admitted to a medical/surgical unit.

- Competency Checklists — conveniently placed in the appendix and includes statements of nursing behaviors and skills essential to increasing the probability of desired patient outcomes. Competency statements and performance criteria are addressed for each body system.

- Reference list — at the end of each chapter.

- Rapid Assessment Guides — outlines essential physical assessment parameters for rapidly screening a given body system. Because diagnostic studies provide more definitive data, only those assessment parameters found to consistently yield reliable data rapidly are listed. These assessment guides are conveniently located in the appendix.

- Boxes — where appropriate to provide rapid access to essential information.

How to use this book

Nurses, nursing students, and nursing faculty will find that the major orientation of this book is practical rather than theoretical. It can be used for anticipatory planning, as well as for self-monitoring and evaluation of actual care.

Given a patient with a health alteration listed in this book, the nurse can refer to its description to obtain a brief and thorough review of the nature of the medical problem or surgery. The nurse can compare actual assessments made with those identified in this book to monitor completeness of data collection. The clinical manifestations listed for each medical problem can provide the nurse with clues about what to look for when conducting a physical examination of the patient and when examining results of diagnostic studies.

The physical assessment guides can be used alone or in conjunction with those of any facility to focus initial and ongoing assessments of a given body system. Following data collection, the nurse can refer to the defining characteristics to determine which nursing diagnosis would be best. The nurse can then incorporate the given nursing diagnosis and patient outcome into a facility-specific plan of care documents. The nurse can refer to the nursing interventions to determine specific and practical actions that must be taken to increase the probability of the desired patient outcome. To determine if the desired patient outcome was achieved, the nurse can refer to the evaluation criteria.

To determine what knowledge and skills are needed to provide safe care for a patient with a particular medical problem, the nurse may refer to the competency checklists.

C

HAPTER ONE
Problems of the Respiratory System

Respiratory Failure

Acute respiratory failure (ARF) is a life-threatening event characterized by impaired gas exchange. **Adult respiratory distress syndrome** (ARDS) is often a complication of ARF.

ARDS is a form of pulmonary edema characterized by respiratory failure. It develops when a disease process or trauma damages the alveolar-capillary membrane. Platelets aggregate at the damaged site, releasing inflammatory substances such as histamine, serotonin, and bradykinin. This causes an increase in alveolar-capillary membrane permeability, allowing blood and plasma to escape from the capillaries into the interstitial space and alveoli. Consequently, the production of surfactant declines, the alveoli collapse causing areas of atelectasis, and gas exchange becomes impaired.

A diagnosis of ARDS is made when the patient with ARF fails to show improvement despite the administration of 100 percent oxygen. The mean length of stay (LOS) for a diagnostic related group (DRG) classification of respiratory failure is 6.0 days (Lorenz, 1991).

General Medical Management

- Supplemental oxygen
- Endotracheal intubation with mechanical ventilation
- Pharmacotherapy
  — bronchodilators widen the passageways and increase air space (e.g., albuteral)
  — corticosteroids reduce alveolar membrane inflammation (e.g., prednisone, Vanceril)
  — antibiotics reduce infection
- IV therapy (either colloid or crystalloid, depending on blood chemistry analysis)

Integrative Care Plans

- Immobility
- Mechanical ventilation
- Plan of care for the primary causative factor (shock, pulmonary embolism, head injuries)

Discharge Considerations

- Follow-up care
- Medications to continue at home
- Signs and symptoms requiring medical attention

 # ASSESSMENT DATA BASE

1. History or presence of causative factors. Essentially, any condition that causes inadequate ventilation can cause ARF, for example:
   - upper airway obstruction (aspiration of foreign bodies)
   - shock
   - chronic diseases, intracranial injuries, or drugs that severely depress the central nervous system
   - diseases that damage the muscles of respiration (myasthenia gravis, polyneuritis, poliomyelitis)
   - chest injuries
   - lung diseases (pneumonia, pulmonary embolism, asthma, chronic obstructive pulmonary disease [COPD])

2. Physical examination based on assessment of the respiratory system (Appendix A) may reveal:
   - dyspnea with tachypnea
   - central nervous system changes (agitation, confusion, disorientation, panic, restlessness)
   - tachycardia
   - use of accessory muscles with breathing (flaring of nostrils, lifting of shoulders with inspiration, retraction of abdominal muscles with expiration)
   - rales, or wheezing, or both
   - changes in skin color (dusky or cyanotic)

3. Diagnostic studies:
   - Arterial blood gases (ABG) may reveal severe hypoxemia (PaO_2 below 50 mm Hg) and hypercapnia ($PaCO_2$ above 50 mm Hg).
   - Chest x ray may reveal alveolar infiltrates if ARDS develops, as well as areas of atelectasis.

4. Assess emotional response of patient and significant others to diagnosis and treatment plan.

▶ NURSING DIAGNOSIS: IMPAIRED GAS EXCHANGE

RELATED TO FACTORS: Specify causative factors (pneumonia, shock)

DEFINING CHARACTERISTICS: Dyspnea with tachypnea, cyanosis, uses accessory muscles with breathing, hypercapnia, moist cough but inability to move secretions, restlessness, wheezing, hypoxia, confusion

PATIENT OUTCOME (collaborative): Demonstrates improved ventilation

EVALUATION CRITERIA: Normal skin color, respiratory rate between 12–24 per minute, breathes without using accessory muscles, denies dyspnea, alert and responding appropriately to verbal commands, ABG within acceptable range, clear lung sounds, absence of cough

INTERVENTIONS	RATIONALE
1. Monitor: • vital signs q2h during the acute phase • respiratory status (Appendix A) q4h during acute phase, then q8h when stable • results of ABG • intake and output q4h	To evaluate effectiveness of interventions.
2. When respiratory distress is initially detected:	
a. place in sitting position and notify physician immediately.	Fuller lung expansion is attained with sitting position.
b. initiate supplemental oxygen at 4 L/min. If history of COPD is present, start oxygen at 2 L/min.	Supplemental oxygen reduces the work of breathing. Higher concentrations of oxygen to a patient with COPD reduce the hypoxic stimulus for breathing.
c. explain all procedures. Remain with patient or have someone else remain with patient.	Dyspnea and unfamiliar diagnostic and invasive treatments evoke anxiety. A high anxiety level interferes with gas exchange.
d. carry out treatments in a calm, reassuring manner.	A competent, confident caregiver helps reduce anxiety.
e. obtain ABG stat if ordered. Notify physician of results immediately.	ABG are the best determinant of pulmonary gas exchange.

INTERVENTIONS	RATIONALE
3. Maintain bedrest as ordered with head of bed elevated approximately 30 degrees if not contraindicated. Perform interventions to prevent complications of immobility while on bedrest (see page 725).	Bedrest reduces oxygen consumption by the body but also may slow down functioning of other body processes. A semi-sitting position is the best position for matching ventilation and perfusion and for reducing abdominal pressure on the diaphragm.
4. Initiate prescribed IV therapy. Administer prescribed medications and evaluate their effectiveness.	Vascular access is needed for the administration of urgent medications.
5. Notify physician of any adverse effects of medications or worsening of symptoms.	The physician will change the dose, type, or interval of the medication to control adverse reactions. A worsening of symptoms, despite treatment, often signals the beginning of complications and a need for further testing.
6. Suction as needed (prn) if the cough is not forceful enough to expel secretions. **Avoid** prolonged suctioning since this will worsen the oxygen deficit already existing.	Suctioning clears the airway.
7. Prepare for transfer to intensive care unit (ICU). Assist with insertion of an endotracheal tube and placement on a mechanical ventilator as ordered. Provide appropriate ventilator care (see page 96).	Patients with ARF require constant care and must therefore be placed in ICU. However, those requiring long-term mechanical ventilation but medically stable may be transferred to a medical/surgical unit, respiratory care unit, or intermediate care unit. Depending on the facility, the endotracheal tube may be inserted by anyone trained in advanced cardiac life support (ACLS). Mechanical ventilation supports breathing until the patient can do so independently.

▌NURSING DIAGNOSIS: HIGH RISK FOR INFECTION

RELATED TO FACTORS: Suctioning of airway, endotracheal intubation, pooling of secretions in the alveoli

DEFINING CHARACTERISTICS: Thick, foul-smelling, colored bronchial secretions; white blood count (WBC) above normal range; temperature above 98.6°F

PATIENT OUTCOME (collaborative): Absence of signs and symptoms of infection

EVALUATION CRITERIA: Temperature 98.6°F, white blood count (WBC) between 5,000-10,000/mm³ small amount of clear and white bronchial secretions without a foul odor

INTERVENTIONS	RATIONALE
1. Monitor: • temperature q4h • results of WBC • bronchial secretions for any changes in amount, thickness, color, or presence of an odor	To identify indications of progress toward or deviations from expected outcome.
2. Adhere to sterile suctioning and good handwashing technique always. Suction only if the patient cannot cough up secretions.	To protect the patient and nurse from infection.
3. Consult physician and culture secretions when an infection is suspected (large amounts of thick, foul-smelling colored secretions). Administer antibiotic as ordered and evaluate its effectiveness.	A culture helps identify the pathogenic organism so appropriate antibiotic therapy can be prescribed.

▌NURSING DIAGNOSIS: IMPAIRED PHYSICAL MOBILITY

RELATED TO FACTORS: Altered level of consciousness, activity intolerance

DEFINING CHARACTERISTICS: Somnolence; lethargy; reports weakness, fatigue, and dyspnea with minimal physical exertion; requests assistance with some aspect of activities of daily living (ADL)

PATIENT OUTCOME: Absence of complications associated with impaired physical mobility

EVALUATION CRITERIA: Skin clean and dry without odor or breakdown, absence of constipation, urine output clear and above 30 mL/hr and free of odor, lung sounds clear, resumes previous level of physical independence without reports of muscle weakness or joint stiffness

• •

INTERVENTIONS	RATIONALE
1. Monitor tolerance to activities by taking pulse rate and respiratory rate before and after activities. Pace activities to prevent fatigue.	Physical activity requires energy expenditure. An intolerance to a physical activity is evidenced by complaints of fatigue accompanied by tachycardia and tachypnea. These findings signal a need for rest.
2. See Immobility (page 725) for additional interventions.	

Cancer of the Lung

Lung cancer (bronchogenic carcinoma) is the leading cause of cancer-related deaths among both men and women in North America. Lung cancer varies according to cell type, site of origin, and rate of growth. The four primary cell types of lung cancer are **epidermoid (squamous cell) carcinoma, small-cell (oat cell) carcinoma, large-cell (undifferentiated) carcinoma,** and **adenocarcinoma.** The first three types have been found to be directly related to cigarette smoking and exposure to environmental carcinogens. Adenocarcinoma is the only lung cancer not related to cigarette smoking. It has been found to be directly related to lung scarring and fibrosis from preexisting pulmonary diseases such as tuberculosis (TB) and chronic obstructive pulmonary disease (COPD).

Squamous cell and small-cell carcinomas commonly form in the main bronchial airways. Large-cell carcinoma and adenocarcinoma commonly grow in the small peripheral bronchi and alveoli.

The prognosis varies depending on cell type and stage of the cancer. Undifferentiated large-cell and oat cell carcinomas grow rapidly and therefore have a poor prognosis. A more favorable prognosis is given to epidermoid carcinoma and adenocarcinomas because of their slow growth.

The average life span of a patient with lung cancer following initial diagnosis is 2 – 5 years. The reason for this low survival rate is that by the time lung cancer is diagnosed, it has metastasized to the lymphatics and other sites. For patients with a coexisting condition and the elderly, this time span may be shorter. Normal pulmonary system changes that occur with aging reduce a person's ability to withstand the stress associated with metastatic carcinoma.

The mean length of stay (LOS) for a diagnostic related group (DRG) classification of lung carcinoma is 6.0 days (Lorenz, 1991).

General Medical Management

• Radiation therapy
•Chemotherapy
•Surgery

Integrative Care Plans

- Cancer
- Loss
- Chemotherapy
- Radiotherapy
- Lung surgery

Discharge Considerations

- Referral to community support services (hospice, American Cancer Society, American Lung Association)
- Follow-up care
- Medications to continue at home
- Techniques of chest physiotherapy
- Signs and symptoms requiring medical attention
- Prevention of respiratory tract infection

ASSESSMENT DATA BASE

1. History or presence of risk factors:
   - chronic, heavy cigarette or cigar smoking (major risk factor)
   - exposure to environmental carcinogens (air pollution, arsenic, metal dusts, chemical fumes, radioactive dust, asbestos)
   - chronic preexisting lung diseases that have resulted in scarring and fibrosis of lung tissue
2. Physical examination based on an assessment of the respiratory system (Appendix A) and a general survey (Appendix F) may reveal any of the following signs and symptoms, depending on tumor location:
   - persistent coughing (caused by excess fluid secretion)
   - wheezing (caused by narrowing of bronchi by tumor)
   - dyspnea (caused by narrowing of airway and excess fluid secretion)
   - hemoptysis (caused by erosion of capillaries in airway)
   - increase in sputum volume with a foul odor (caused by accumulation of necrotic cells behind the airway section obstructed by tumor)
   - recurrent respiratory tract infections (retention of necrotic cells behind the obstructed section predisposes patient to infection)
   - dull chest pain, which may radiate to the shoulders and back (as tumor enlarges, it presses against nerves in pleural tissue)
   - pleural effusion (occurs when tumor disrupts lung wall)
   - hoarseness (caused by pressure of tumor against recurrent laryngeal nerve)

- dysphagia (result of pressure of tumor against esophagus)
- edema of the face, neck, and arms (may occur if tumor obstructs blood flow in superior vena cava, a condition termed superior vena cava syndrome)

   As the carcinoma spreads to other organs, additional paraneoplastic manifestations are seen.
- hypercalcemia (result of metastasis to bone) and subsequent lung calcification
- neurological changes (blurred vision, headaches, or seizures due to cerebral edema caused by metastasis to the brain)
- endocrine dysfunctions (Cushing's syndrome, gynecomastia, hyperthyroidism)
- clubbed fingers
- peripheral neuropathies
- nephrotic syndrome
- rash
- joint pain
- muscle weakness

3. Diagnostic studies:
- Chest x ray reveals lesion site.
- Sputum for cytology analysis reveals the type of cancer cells. Three early morning specimens usually are required for this test. Tumor cells that shed into bronchial secretions may be coughed up with sputum. This test is usually done for lesions that involve the bronchial wall.
- Computed tomography (CT) scans and lung tomograms reveal tumor location and size.
- Bronchoscopy may be done to obtain tissue samples for biopsy and to collect bronchial washings for tumors that develop in the bronchi.
- Needle aspiration and biopsy of lung tissue may be done if radiological examination reveals a lesion in the lung periphery.
- Radionuclide scans of other organs determine the extent of metastases (brain, liver, bone, and spleen).
- Mediastinoscopy determines if the tumor has metastasized to mediastinal lymph nodes.

4. Assess emotional response of patient and significant others to diagnosis and treatment plan (see Loss, page 733.)

NURSING DIAGNOSIS: HIGH RISK FOR ANXIETY

RELATED TO FACTORS: Knowledge deficit about illness, diagnostic studies, treatment plan, and prognosis: fear of premature death: anticipated effects of cancer and adverse effects of treatments

DEFINING CHARACTERISTICS: Requests information: verbalizes lack of understanding: verbalizes feeling nervous, afraid, or anxious: tense facial expression

PATIENT OUTCOME (collaborative): Demonstrates less anxiety

EVALUATION CRITERIA: Reports feeling less anxious or nervous: relaxed facial expression: verbalizes understanding of illness, treatment plan, and diagnostic studies

• •

INTERVENTIONS	RATIONALE
1. Provide information about: a. nature of the illness. Explain the amount of blood in sputum does not necessarily indicate the severity of illness. b. prescribed treatments, including possible side effects and how to minimize them. Explain that although temporary side effects often occur with chemotherapy (page 707) and radiotherapy (page 719), such treatments are given to shrink the tumor and control symptoms such as hemoptysis, dyspnea, chest pain, and coughing. c. diagnostic studies, including: • purpose • brief description • preparation required before test • care after test	Knowing what to expect from medical treatments can facilitate patient compliance and help reduce anxiety associated with medical treatments.
2. Maintain effective pain control.	Pain evokes anxiety, which increases the pain.
3. Include significant others in all teaching sessions and encourage their support of the patient. 4. See Loss (page 733).	A strong support system is essential to help individuals effectively cope with a chronic or terminal illness.

NURSING DIAGNOSIS: PAIN

RELATED TO FACTOR: Carcinoma of the lung

DEFINING CHARACTERISTICS: Verbalizes pain, facial grimacing, guarding behavior (shallow breathing, assuming a static position), distracting behavior (crying, moaning, restlessness)

PATIENT OUTCOME (collaborative): Demonstrates relief from pain

EVALUATION CRITERIA: Reports pain has subsided, relaxed facial expression, fuller lung expansion, increased activity level

INTERVENTIONS	RATIONALE
1. Administer prescribed analgesic prn and evaluate its effectiveness. Consult physician if the analgesic is ineffective in controlling pain.	Comfort is the priority in caring for patients with cancer. Pain control often requires using large doses of narcotic analgesics as the disease progresses. Patient addiction is not an issue in the management of cancer pain. Patients may develop a physical tolerance to the analgesic, necessitating larger doses, but they do not become addicted.
2. To minimize bone pain: • turn carefully and support all extremities. • avoid pulling on extremities. • provide a firm mattress. • reposition q2h.	Metastasis to the bone causes severe pain. With many patients, even the slightest touch can precipitate pain.
3. To minimize pleuritic chest pain: • instruct patient to splint chest with hands or pillow when coughing. • encourage patient to refrain from smoking. • provide air humidifier as ordered. • administer antitussives if prescribed.	Deep breathing and forceful coughing stretch the pleura membrane and aggravate pleuritic chest pain. Nicotine from tobacco products causes bronchial constriction and reduces motion of the cilia that line the lower respiratory tract. Moist air helps loosen pulmonary secretions. Antitussives suppress the cough center in the brain.
4. See Pain (page 700).	

NURSING DIAGNOSIS: IMPAIRED GAS EXCHANGE.

RELATED TO FACTORS: Cancer of the lung

DEFINING CHARACTERISTICS: Hemoptysis, wheezing, persistent cough, abnormal ABG, crackles/rales, dusky or cyanotic skin color, dyspnea, orthopnea, uses accessory muscles with breathing

PATIENT OUTCOME (collaborative): Demonstrates improved oxygenation

EVALUATION CRITERIA: ABG within normal limits, normal skin color, respiratory rate 12 – 24 per minute, clear lung sounds, absence of hemoptysis, no use of accessory muscles with breathing, denies dyspnea

INTERVENTIONS	RATIONALE
1. Monitor: • respiratory status (Appendix A) q8h • results of pulmonary function studies and ABG	To identify indications of progress toward or deviations from expected outcomes.
2. When dyspneic episodes occur: • administer supplemental humidified oxygen. • implement measures to reduce anxiety by helping the patient feel a sense of control. Maintain a calm, confident approach. Remain with the patient and instruct to breath slowly and deeply. • maintain an erect position.	Supplemental oxygen helps reduce the effort of breathing by increasing the amount of oxygen available to tissue. Feelings of suffocation are often expressed when dyspnea occurs. This evokes anxiety. Anxiety can be relieved if the patient feels in control and interacts with a calm, confident caregiver. An erect position allows fuller lung expansion by reducing abdominal pressure on the diaphragm.
3. Consult physician for a referral to the respiratory therapy department for nebulizer treatments or intermittent positive pressure breathing (IPPB) treatments if pulmonary congestion persists.	The respiratory therapist is a specialist in pulmonary function studies and therapeutic modalities.
4. Prepare the patient for a thoracentesis if ordered, according to facility's policy and procedures.	A thoracentesis is performed by a physician. It involves insertion of a large-bore needle into the pleural space to remove excess pleural fluid, thereby allowing better lung expansion.

INTERVENTIONS	RATIONALE
5. Prepare the patient for lung surgery if ordered.	A pneumonectomy or lobectomy may be done for localized cancers such as Stages I and II. Surgical resection is not used for Stages III and IV carcinomas or for small-cell (oat cell) carcinomas because extensive metastases has occurred by the time of diagnosis. (See page 695 for description of staging.)
6. If mobility is impaired, implement measures to prevent complication of immobility (see Immobility, page 725). 7. Adhere to universal precautions, such as handwashing and wearing gloves when contact with blood or body fluid is likely to occur, in providing patient care. Avoid placing the patient in the same room with infectious patients. Restrict caregivers with upper respiratory tract infections from contact with the patient.	Patients with cancer are immunocompromised due to the disease process and the treatment modalities (chemotherapy, radiation therapy, and in some cases radical surgery). Nosocomial infections are spread largely by healthcare workers.
8. Maintain a fluid intake of at least 2-3 liters daily, unless contraindicated.	To help liquefy pulmonary secretions and to make it easier for patient to cough and expectorate.
9. Notify physician if symptoms of respiratory distress persist or worsen.	This could signal the development of a respiratory tract infection or further lung involvement.

NURSING DIAGNOSIS: ACTIVITY INTOLERANCE

RELATED TO FACTORS: Impaired gas exchange secondary to cancer of the lung

DEFINING CHARACTERISTICS: Dyspnea, tachypnea, and reports fatigue and weakness with minimal exertion

PATIENT OUTCOME: Demonstrates tolerance to physical activities of performing routine activities of daily living (ADL)

EVALUATION CRITERIA: Denies fatigue and weakness when performing ADL, absence of dyspnea and tachypnea when performing ADL

• •

INTERVENTIONS	RATIONALE
1. Evaluate patient's response to each activity of daily living. Provide assistance with ADL as needed. Teach patient how to pace activities to avoid fatigue. Allow uninterrupted rest periods between activities.	Pacing activities can facilitate endurance. Learning how to regain a sense of control and independence with a chronic, debilitating condition helps promote self-esteem. Rest allows the body to replenish energy expended during activities.
2. Provide a warm, quiet, pain-free environment during rest periods.	To promote rest.
3. Assist patient with identifying leisure activities that require minimal energy expenditure that could be incorporated into lifestyle (reading, writing, board games, handicrafts). Explain that the key to enjoying activities without becoming extremely fatigued is frequent rest periods during the activity.	Continuing to enjoy life to the fullest extent as perceived by the individual helps facilitate coping.

• •

 # NURSING DIAGNOSIS: SLEEP PATTERN DISTURBANCE

RELATED TO FACTORS: Persistent coughing and bone or pleuritic pain

DEFINING CHARACTERISTICS: Persistent coughing during bedtime, reports inability to sleep because of persistent coughing or pain

PATIENT OUTCOME (collaborative): Demonstrates relief from insomnia

EVALUATION CRITERIA: Reports feeling rested, fewer complaints of insomnia

• •

INTERVENTIONS	RATIONALE
1. If pulmonary treatments are prescribed, arrange for treatments to be given before bedtime. Administer prescribed antitussive.	During sleep, periodic deep breathing, which expands the alveoli, does not occur as it does while awake and moving. Consequently, secretions pool in the lungs. Special pulmonary treatments help facilitate removal of pulmonary secretions. Antitussives suppress the cough control center in the brain.
2. Ensure good room ventilation. Arrange for an air humidifier if needed. Encourage use of oxygen during sleep if needed.	Fresh air kept in motion helps control dust and bacteria. Humidity between 30% and 60% prevents drying of the mucosa. Supplemental oxygen provides additional oxygen supply to body tissue.
3. Keep room free of irritating substances, such as smoke, flowers, powder, and room deodorizers.	These irritants can trigger coughing.
4. Maintain a comfortable room temperature.	A very hot or cold temperature can trigger coughing.
5. Administer prescribed analgesic before bedtime.	To control pain and promote sleep.
6. At bedtime, have patient take a warm shower or bath, then administer a backrub. To promote relaxation. 7. Assist patient to a comfortable position, usually with the head of the bed elevated about 30 degrees.	This position promotes better lung expansion.
8. Consult physician if above measures are ineffective in relieving insomnia.	A sedative or tranquilizer may be required. However, these drugs should be used with caution since they may suppress respiratory drive and contribute to further hypoxemia.

NURSING DIAGNOSIS: HIGH RISK FOR IMPAIRED HOME MAINTENANCE MANAGEMENT

RELATED TO FACTORS: Knowledge deficit about self-care on discharge, lack of adequate support system, insufficient finances

DEFINING CHARACTERISTICS: Verbalizes lack of understanding, requests assistance with financing treatments, verbalizes need for assistance with some aspect of ADL caused by lack of family resources

PATIENT OUTCOME (collaborative): Demonstrates ways to maximize pulmonary health on discharge

EVALUATION CRITERIA: Verbalizes ways to improve oxygenation, verbalizes understanding of signs and symptoms requiring medical attention, verbalizes understanding of medications prescribed for home use, performs pulmonary exercises correctly, identifies community resources that provide support services

INTERVENTIONS	RATIONALE
1. Ensure patient or significant other has in writing: • an appointment for follow-up care • instructions for self-care at home • telephone number of physician to contact if problems arise • medications to continue at home, including name, dosage, purpose, schedule, and reportable side effects	Verbal instructions may be easily forgotten.
2. Instruct the patient to: • seek medical attention if hemoptysis, increasing pain, fever, persistent cough, increasing dyspnea or shortness of breath (SOB) at rest occur • take medication as prescribed and contact physician if adverse reactions occur • avoid overexertion and take frequent rest periods throughout the day	Discharge teaching helps improve patient compliance. Cancer patients have weakened immune systems and are susceptible to infections.

INTERVENTIONS	RATIONALE
• refrain from smoking. If unable to stop independently, enroll in a stop-smoking program • avoid persons with upper respiratory tract infections and crowded confined areas, especially during the flu season. Wear a mask when unable to avoid these situations • obtain a flu vaccine annually • avoid exposure to irritating substances (heavy perfumes, flowers) • clean respiratory care equipment after each use	
3. Evaluate understanding of home care instructions. Encourage questions. Clarify any misconceptions. Have the patient demonstrate any pulmonary exercises prescribed by the respiratory therapist.	Evaluation is essential to determine the patient's or significant other's understanding of information. Failure to understand instructions is a primary cause of noncompliance.
4. Evaluate patient's need for home care assistance and financial support with prescribed therapies. Initiate a referral to the social services or discharge planning department when home care assistance or pulmonary care equipment, such as oxygen, is required. Ensure equipment has been delivered to the patient's home before patient is discharged.	Depending on the facility, these departments are responsible for making arrangements for continued care as needed by the patient. This includes contacting community organizations and agencies to ensure patient has the necessary medical assistance, support services, and financial aid needed for self-maintenance at home.

Chest Trauma

     Chest trauma may be blunt or penetrating. Blunt chest trauma may be more difficult to detect because internal organs are damaged with no obvious break in the skin. Penetrating injuries are easier to detect because there is a break in the skin and obvious bleeding.

     The mean length of stay (LOS) for a diagnostic related group (DRG) classification of chest trauma (Lorenz, 1991) without complications is 6.2 days (Lorenz, 1991). Additional days are allowed when complications occur.

     Patients experiencing life-threatening chest injuries are placed in ICU until stable. Because of the normal physiologic changes that occur with aging, the elderly and persons with coexisting chronic illnesses are at high risk for complications.

     Some common life-threatening chest injuries and their management include the following.

1. **Tension pneumothorax** develops when a puncture in the chest wall allows air to enter but not escape the pleural cavity. This trapped air causes an increase in intrapleural pressure that eventually compresses the lung causing it to collapse. In addition, mediastinal contents (heart and great vessels) shift to the unaffected side.

General Medical Management

  a. At the scene:
   - insertion of a large-bore needle into the second intercostal space midclavicular line of the affected side
   - supplemental oxygen
   - IV therapy to control shock

  b. At the hospital:
   - insertion of a chest tube with connection to a water-seal drainage system
   - measures to relieve shock

2. **Open pneumothorax** is a collapse of the lung due to rapid replacement of normal negative intrapleural pressure with positive atmospheric pressure. It is characterized by a "sucking" sound produced when the lung is suddenly punctured.

General Medical Management

a. At the scene:
  - measures to convert to a closed pneumothorax, for example, applying the hand or occlusive dressing over the opening as the patient exhales to seal it. To prevent tension, pneumothorax, the seal should be released momentarily on expiration and then reapplied. This should be done during several breathing cycles.
  - supplemental oxygen
  - IV therapy to control shock

b. At the hospital:
  - insertion of a chest tube with connection to a water-seal drainage system
  - measures to control shock
  - surgery to repair injury
  - supplemental oxygen

3. **Hemothorax** is collapse of the lung due to accumulation of blood in the pleural space.

General Medical Management

a. Insertion of a chest tube with connection to a water-seal drainage system

b. Blood transfusion by autologous (blood from the person) transfusions using an auto-transfusion device or by analogous transfusions of whole blood

c. Measures to control shock

d. Supplemental oxygen

4. **Closed pneumothorax** is collapse of the lung without an external wound.

General Medical Management

a. Supplemental oxygen

b. Insertion of a chest tube with connection to a water-seal drainage system

c. For a small pneumothorax, insertion of a Heimlich flutter valve during transportation from the scene to the emergency department

5. **Flail chest** is segmental rib fracture (two or more broken areas on the same rib) that results in paradoxical movement of the chest wall with respiration. Puncture of the lung resulting in pneumothorax is a major complication that may occur.

General Medical Management

a. Measures to stabilize the chest:
  - Place patient on affected side.
  - Apply a sandbag to affected chest wall.

b. Use of mechanical ventilation with positive end-expiratory pressure (PEEP), based on the following criteria:

- symptoms of pulmonary contusion
- shock or severe head injury
- eight or more ribs fractured
- over age 65
- history of chronic lung disease

c. Insertion of a chest tube with connection to a water-seal drainage system if tension pneumothorax is a threat

d. Supplemental oxygen

6. **Pulmonary contusion** is bruising of the lung from sudden compression caused by blunt chest trauma. Pneumonia is a major complication that may occur from plasma leakage into the interstitial space and alveoli.

General Medical Management

a. For severe respiratory distress:

- endotracheal intubation and placement on a mechanical ventilator
- fluid restriction and use of diuretics for treatment of pulmonary edema

b. For mild contusion:

- humidified oxygen
- ultrasonic mist nebulization to keep secretions loose
- postural drainage only if patient is unable to cough productively
- restricted fluid intake
- analgesics to control pain
- antibiotics as prophylaxis against pneumonia
- limited physical activity

7. **Fractured ribs** are a serious injury because underlying structures (heart, liver, spleen, lung, esophagus, diaphragm) are at risk of being damaged.

General Medical Management

a. Limited physical activity

b. Analgesics for pain

c. An elastic Velcro fastener rib belt to stabilize the fracture

8. **Cardiac contusion** is injury to the myocardium resulting from blunt chest trauma. Cardiac dysrhythmias and cardiac tamponade are major complications that can occur.

General Medical Management

a. Supplemental oxygen

b. Measures to control cardiac dysrhythmias

c. Needle aspiration if cardiac tamponade develops; if internal bleeding continues, surgery is needed

Integrative Care Plans for All Chest Traumas

- Pain
- Immobility
- Mechanical ventilation
- Shock
- Chest tubes
- IV therapy

Discharge Considerations for All Chest Traumas

- Follow-up care
- Signs and symptoms requiring medical intervention
- Wound care and manifestations of wound infection if surgery was performed
- Medications to continue at home

 # ASSESSMENT DATA BASE

1. Presence of causative factors:

   a. Tension pneumothorax — chest trauma, obstruction of a chest tube, use of excessive PEEP with mechanical ventilation, application of an occlusive dressing to a sucking chest wound without periodic release of the dressing

   b. Closed pneumothorax — puncture of the lung by fractured ribs, rupture of blebs that develop as a sequelae of COPD, puncture of the lung with invasive procedures (thoracentesis, insertion of subclavian catheter), or excessive use of PEEP with mechanical ventilation

   c. Pulmonary contusion (or cardiac contusion) — blunt chest injury from a vehicle accident or heavy fall

   d. Open pneumothorax — acts of violence (stabbings and gunshot wounds).

   e. Rib fractures, flail chest — vehicle accident or heavy fall

2. Physical examination based on a general survey (Appendix F) and an assessment of the respiratory system (Appendix A) may reveal:

   a. Pneumothorax
      - sharp chest pain on affected side with breathing
      - dyspnea with tachypnea

- use of accessory muscles with respirations (flaring of nostrils, intercostal retractions, lifting of shoulders)
- tachycardia
- diaphoresis
- absent or faint breath sounds with unequal chest wall movement on affected side
- restlessness and agitation
- trachea shift to unaffected side
- possible cyanosis
- hypertympanic sound with percussion over affected side
- shock
- cuts and bruises on the chest (if caused by traumatic injury)

b. Tension pneumothorax
- distended neck veins
- possibly subcutaneous emphysema (a gritty sensation detected by palpation over the chest wall caused by air trapping in subcutaneous tissue
- other manifestions as in closed pneumothorax

c. Hemothorax
- dullness with percussion over affected side
- other manifestations as in closed pneumothorax

d. Open pneumothorax
- observation of an open chest wound with a sucking sound
- other manifestations as in closed pneumothorax

e. Flail chest
- cyanosis
- paradoxical chest wall movement (inward movement of affected chest wall during inspiration and outward movement during expiration)

f. Fractured ribs
- tenderness and ecchymosis over affected side
- possible crepitus
- chest pain with respirations
- cuts and bruises on the chest

g. Pulmonary contusion (severe)
- dyspnea with tachypnea
- cuts and bruises on the chest
- loose cough of blood-tinged sputum
- pleuritic-type chest pain (chest pain aggravated by deep breathing)
- tachycardia

h. Cardiac contusion
- chest pain
- cuts and bruises on the chest
- irregular heart beats and tachycardia with low blood pressure

3. Diagnostic studies:
- Chest x ray confirms collapsed lung, pulmonary infiltration, or fractured ribs.
- ABG may reveal elevated $PaCO_2$ and decreased PaO_2.
- Electrocardiography (EKG, ECG) is performed to rule out myocardial injury and to identify the specific dysrhythmia if pulse is irregular.
- Cardiac enzymes may be elevated 4–6 hours after injury if the myocardium is injured.

4. Assess emotional response of patient and significant others to injury and treatments.

5. Assess for history of coexisting medical problems when the patient has stabilized, or obtain a medical history from significant others as this information is vital for anticipating potential problems.

6. Assess last date of tetanus immunization if a penetrating traumatic chest injury exits.

NURSING DIAGNOSIS: IMPAIRED GAS EXCHANGE

RELATED TO FACTORS: Chest trauma (specify type)

DEFINING CHARACTERISTICS: Dyspnea with tachypnea, cyanosis, paradoxical chest movements, diminished or absent breath sounds, rales/crackles, hemoptysis, restlessness, confusion, abnormal ABG, chest pain aggravated by deep breathing, uses accessory muscles with breathing, tracheal deviation, abnormal sounds with chest percussion (dullness, hypertympanic), ineffective cough

PATIENT OUTCOME (collaborative): Demonstrates improved oxygenation

EVALUATION CRITERIA: Normal skin color, respiratory rate 12–24 per minute, breathes without using accessory muscles, denies dyspnea, alert and responding appropriately to commands, ABG within acceptable range, clear lung sounds, absence of persistent coughing and hemoptysis, trachea midline position, denies chest pain with breathing, fuller and symmetrical chest expansion

INTERVENTIONS	RATIONALE
1. Monitor: • respiratory status (Appendix A) q2h during the acute phase, q8h when stable • intake and output q8h • results of ABG • neck and face for swelling and distention of neck veins q8h (if tension pneumothorax is present) • chest x ray reports • EKG recordings • cardiac enzyme studies • general status (Appendix F) q8h • voice sounds • position of the trachea q4h during the acute phase	To identify indications of progress toward or deviations from expected outcomes.
2. Maintain a semi-Fowler's or Fowler's position always.	Fuller lung expansion is attained in an erect position because gravity reduces abdominal pressure on the diaphragm.
3. Encourage use of an incentive spirometer q2-4h. Provide effective pain control.	The incentive spirometer aids in full expansion of the alveoli thereby preventing atelectasis. Patients often resort to shallow breathing in an effort to control pain.
4. Report swelling of the face and/or neck with a gritty, sandlike sensation on palpation. Administer oxygen as ordered.	These findings represent subcutaneous emphysema, a condition caused by extravasation of air into subcutaneous tissue. It may occur with tension pneumothorax. A high oxygen concentration hastens the absorption of air trapped in subcutaneous tissue.

INTERVENTIONS	RATIONALE

5. Notify physician immediately of the following:
  • increasing respiratory distress
  • swelling of the neck and face that interferes with breathing
  • auscultatory changes (from normal to abnormal) in chest and heart sounds
  • decreasing distal pulses accompanied by symptoms of hypovolemic shock (see Shock, page 767)
  • Beck's triad (hypotension accompanied by muffled, distant heart sounds and distended neck veins)
  • diminishing level of consciousness
  • changes in quality of voice sound from clear to hoarseness
  • trachea shift from midline position to unaffected side
  • bile-colored fluid in chest drainage system
  • increasing pain unrelieved by analgesia
Prepare the patient for prescribed therapies according to facility policy and procedures, for example, insertion of an endotracheal tube, mechanical ventilation (page 94), pericardiocentesis, insertion of a chest tube (page 75), or surgery (page 106).
	These findings signal complications and a need for urgent intervention to prevent irreversible damage. Beck's triad is a hallmark finding in cardiac tamponade, a complication associated with penetrating or blunt injury to the heart. Mechanical ventilation provides respiratory support until the patient can breath independently. Chest tubes remove air and fluid from the pleural space to allow lung reexpansion. A shift in the trachea from its normal midline position toward the affected side signals a mediastinal shift, a hallmark finding with tension pneumothorax. Gastric juices leak into the chest cavity with an esophageal tear, giving rise to bile-colored chest drainage. Surgery is required to repair torn structures.

6. Discourage smoking.	Smoking causes vasoconstriction that interferes with O_2/CO_2 exchange.
7. Report cardiac dysrhythmias to physician. Initiate facility protocol and procedures if a dysrhythmia is detected.	Cardiac dysrhythmias may signal myocardial damage or electrolyte disturbance. Persistent, untreated dysrhythmias lead to diminished cardiac output. Manifestations of mild to moderate shock are seen by increased heart rate, falling blood pressure (BP) and decreased urinary output.

INTERVENTIONS	RATIONALE
8. Consult physician for a referral to the respiratory therapist if pulmonary congestion persists. Evaluate patient's response to any special pulmonary treatments, such as nebulization or chest physiotherapy.	The respiratory therapist is a specialist in pulmonary therapeutic modalities.
9. If an elastic rib belt is used, explain that it stabilizes the rib cage. Teach and allow the patient to practice self-application of the rib belt.	Compliance is enhanced when the patient understands the therapeutic regimen.
10. Use an infusion pump to administer all IV fluids. If symptoms of pulmonary edema (page 000) develop reduce IV flow rate, restrict oral fluid intake, and consult physician immediately. Administer diuretic therapy as ordered and evaluate its effectiveness.	An infusion pump allows for better control of the infusion rate to prevent sudden fluid overload. Pulmonary edema is.a major threat to patients with chest trauma.

◣N̄URSING DIAGNOSIS: ANXIETY

RELATED TO FACTORS: Knowledge deficit about condition, diagnostic studies, treatment plan, treat of permanent disability, threat of death

DEFINING CHARACTERISTICS: Verbalizes lack of understanding, requests information, reports feeling anxious or nervous, restlessness, tense facial expression

PATIENT OUTCOME: Demonstrates less anxiety

EVALUATION CRITERIA: Reports feeling less anxious or nervous; relaxed facial expression; verbalizes understanding of condition, treatments, and diagnostic studies

INTERVENTIONS	RATIONALE

1. Provide information about:
   a. nature of the condition (after condition has stabilized)
   b. purpose of prescribed treatments
   c. diagnostic studies, including:
     • purpose
     • brief description of test
     • preparation required before test
     • care after test
	Knowing what to expect from medical treatments can facilitate patient compliance and help reduce anxiety associated with medical treatments.

2. Provide effective pain control.	Pain often evokes anxiety.
3. Help the patient identify specific fears. Correct any misconceptions. Encourage the patient to express feelings and concerns. Keep significant others informed of patient's progress. Allow them to visit and encourage their support of the patient.	Identification of specific fears helps minimize the sense of an overwhelming threat. A strong support system is essential to help individuals cope with an illness.

• •

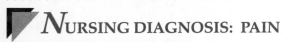

NURSING DIAGNOSIS: PAIN

RELATED TO FACTORS: Chest trauma

DEFINING CHARACTERISTICS: Verbalizes discomfort, guarding of chest, shallow respirations, moaning, facial grimacing

PATIENT OUTCOME (collaborative): Demonstrates relief from pain

EVALUATION CRITERIA: Denies pain, relaxed facial expression, fuller chest expansion, absence of moaning, fewer requests for analgesia

• •

INTERVENTIONS	RATIONALE
1. See Pain, page 700. 2. Maintain a semi-Fowler's or Fowler's position. Avoid turning to affected side (exception is a flail chest).	An erect position allows for easier lung expansion as abdominal pressure on the diaphragm is reduced by gravitational pull. Lying on affected side places strain on injured site.
3. Maintain activity limitations as ordered. Provide measures to prevent complications of immobility (page 725).	Limiting physical activity conserves energy and minimizes discomfort by reducing muscle strain.

- -

◥ NURSING DIAGNOSIS: HIGH RISK FOR INFECTION

DEFINING CHARACTERISTICS: Chest x ray reveals atelectasis, diminished breath sounds, moist cough with ineffective coughing, rales, rising temperature, increase in WBC

RELATED TO FACTORS: Retained pulmonary secretions, impaired pulmonary defense systems secondary to chest trauma, use of respiratory equipment

PATIENT OUTCOME (collaborative): Free of infection

EVALUATION CRITERIA: Temperature of 98.6°F, clear lungs via auscultation and chest x ray, denies productive cough, WBC between 5,000-10,000/mm³

- -

INTERVENTIONS	RATIONALE

1. Monitor:
  • temperature q4h
  • results of chest x ray and complete blood count (CBC) reports
  • color and consistency of sputum
  • ability to cough effectively
  • appearance of wounds
	To identify indications of progress toward or deviations from expected outcomes.

2. Administer antibiotics as ordered and evaluate their effectiveness. Notify physician if adverse effects occur. Compare all medications prescribed to prevent an adverse drug-to-drug interaction.	Antibiotics are needed to resolve an infection. They often are given prophylactically to guard against infection.

INTERVENTIONS	RATIONALE
3. Administer tetanus immune human globulin (HyperTet) as ordered if immunization history is inadequate.	Any wound resulting from a traumatic penetrating injury is considered a contaminated wound. Tetanus immunization is recommended every ten years.
4. Obtain specimens for culture (sputum or wound) and consult physician immediately if the following occur; a. pneumonia — persistent cough accompanied by chills, fever, headache, and increasing chest pain b. wound infection — redness, increased tenderness, fever, purulent drainage	Pneumonia and infection are major threats with any chest injury. Antibiotic therapy is required to resolve an infection. Appropriate antibiotic therapy is identified by a specimen culture.
5. Refrain from assigning healthcare workers with upper respiratory tract infections, such as a common cold, to chest trauma patients. Adhere always to universal precautions such as handwashing before and after care and wearing gloves when contact with blood or body fluid is likely to occur.	To prevent nosocomial infection. Healthcare workers are the most common source of nosocomial infections. Patients with chest trauma are already immunocompromised because of the injury.

NURSING DIAGNOSIS: HIGH RISK FOR IMPAIRED HOME MAINTENANCE MANAGEMENT

RELATED TO FACTORS: Knowledge deficit about self-care on discharge, insufficient finances, inadequate support systems

DEFINING CHARACTERISTICS: Verbalizes lack of understanding, requests information, may report concerns about outstanding debts or financial crisis, significant other reports inability to provide needed assistance, requests assistance in performing necessary procedures

PATIENT OUTCOME (collaborative): Demonstrates ways to manage recuperative activities on discharge

EVALUATION CRITERIA: Verbalizes understanding of discharge instructions, performs self-care activities independently and correctly, verbalizes understanding of signs and symptoms requiring medical attention, verbalizes understanding of medications prescribed for home use

• •

INTERVENTIONS	RATIONALE
1. Ensure the patient or significant other has in writing: a. an appointment for follow-up care. b. instructions for self-care at home. c. medications to continue at home, including name, purpose, dose, schedule, and reportable side effects. d. telephone number of physician to contact if problems arise.	Verbal instructions may be easily forgotten.
2. Review any prescribed activity limitations. Instruct the patient to seek medical attention if the following occur: • increasing dyspnea, recurring chest pain, fever, persistent productive cough • wound infection (redness, increased tenderness, drainage, fever)	These respiratory distress findings signal a need for further evaluation. An antibiotic is required to resolve an infection.
3. Instruct the patient to take rest periods throughout the day and to avoid overexertion. Review any instructions given by the physician. If wound care is to be performed: • provide at least a three-day supply of wound care materials. • teach proper technique for wound care and allow the patient to return the demonstration. • stress the importance of hand-washing before and after wound care.	Discharge teaching helps improve patient compliance.

INTERVENTIONS	RATIONALE
4. Ensure the patient has a prescription for an analgesic for home use.	Mild pain may continue for several days, which can be easily controlled with a nonnarcotic analgesic.
5. Evaluate understanding of home care instructions. Encourage questions. Clarify any misconceptions.	Evaluation is essential in determining the patient's or significant other's understanding of information. Failure to understand instructions and information is a primary cause of noncompliance.
6. Evaluate patient's need for financial assistance or home care assistance with prescribed therapies. Initiate a referral to social services or discharge planning department if the patient is unable to perform required self-care procedures independently, has no significant other to provide assistance, or if financial assistance is needed to purchase needed supplies and medications.	Depending on the facility, these departments make arrangements for continued care as needed by the patient. This includes contacting community organizations and agencies to ensure the patient has the necessary medical assistance, support services, and/or financial aid needed to maintain self at home.

Chronic Obstructive Pulmonary Disease

Chronic obstructive pulmonary disease (COPD) refers to conditions in which air flow through the lungs is continuously obstructed. The disease process is often a combination of two or more of the following conditions with one the primary cause and the other(s) a complication of the primary disease (Petty, 1990).

1. **Asthma** is an intermittent, reversible, diffuse airway obstruction characterized by excess mucus production, bronchospasms, and swelling of the bronchial membranes. It may be extrinsic (triggered by a specific allergen) or intrinsic (unknown etiology).

2. **Emphysema** is an irreversible lung disease that develops as a sequela of bronchiectasis or chronic bronchitis. It is characterized by hyperinflation of the alveoli, increased airway resistance, and impaired gas exchange. The diseased alveoli may rupture and collapse.

3. **Bronchitis** is characterized by inflammation of the mucosal lining of the tracheobronchial airway and excess mucus production. It may be acute or chronic. Bronchiectasis (permanent abnormal dilation of one or more large bronchi) or emphysema are major complications associated with chronic bronchitis.

Hospitalization is not required for diagnosis and treatment of COPD unless there is an exacerbation of symptoms. The mean LOS for a DRG classification of COPD is 5.9 days (Lorenz, 1991).

The major complications associated with late stage COPD are cor pulmonale and acute respiratory failure. Cor pulmonale, also called right-sided heart failure, is caused by increased pulmonary vascular resistance that occurs subsequent to chronic hypoxemia and respiratory acidosis.

General Medical Management

- Pharmacotherapy (bronchodilators, steroids, antibiotics)
- Supplemental oxygen
- Aerosol-nebulization therapy
- Chest physiotherapy with postural drainage

Integrative Care Plans

- Loss
- IV therapy
- Fluid and biochemical imbalance
- Respiratory failure

Discharge Considerations

- Medications to continue at home
- Prevention of exacerbations
- Manifestations of exacerbations requiring medical attention
- Controlled breathing techniques
- Proper use of respiratory therapy equipment
- Community resources
- Follow-up care

ASSESSMENT DATA BASE

1. History or presence of contributing factors:
   - smoking tobacco products (primary causative factor)
   - living or working in an area of heavy air pollution
   - family history of allergies
   - history of asthma during childhood

2. History or presence of factors that trigger exacerbations, such as allergens (pollen, danders, feathers, mold, dust), emotional stress, excess physical exertion, air pollutants, respiratory tract infection, or failure to take medication as prescribed.

3. Physical examination based on an assessment of the respiratory system (Appendix A) may reveal:

   a. classical manifestations of COPD:
   - increasing dyspnea (most prominent finding)
   - use of accessory muscles with breathing (retracting abdominal muscles, raising of shoulders during inspiration, flaring of nostrils)
   - diminished breath sounds
   - tachypnea
   - orthopnea

   b. symptoms consistent with the underlying disease process:
   — Asthma
   - coughing (may be productive or nonproductive) and feeling of tightness in the chest

- inspiratory and expiratory wheezing, which is often audible without a stethoscope
- flaring of nostrils with respirations
- apprehension and diaphoresis

— Bronchitis

- productive cough with grayish-white sputum, which usually occurs in the mornings and is often ignored by smokers (called "smokers cough")
- inspiratory rales (crackles) and wheezing
- shortness of breath

— Bronchitis (Late Stage)

- cyanotic appearance (due to polycythemia that occurs subsequent to chronic hypoxemia)
- a generalized bloated or puffy appearance (caused by systemic edema that occurs subsequent to cor pulmonale); clinically, these patients are commonly called "blue bloaters"

— Emphysema

- thin appearance with a "barrel-chest" (the thoracic anterior-posterior diameter is increased subsequent to hyperinflation of the lungs)
- prolonged expiratory phase

— Emphysema (Late Stage)

- hypoxemia and hypercapnia but no cyanosis; these patients are often described clinically as "pink puffers"
- clubbing of the fingers

4. Diagnostic studies:

- Arterial blood gases (ABG) show a low PaO_2 and a high $PaCO_2$.
- Chest x ray reveals hyperinflation of the lungs, cardiac enlargement, and congested lung fields.
- Pulmonary function studies show increased total lung capacity (TLC) and reserve volume (RV), decreased vital capacity (VC), and forced expiratory volume (FEV).
- CBC reveals elevated hemoglobin, hematocrit, and red blood count (RBC).
- Sputum culture is positive if infection is present.
- Immunoglobin assays indicate an elevated serum IgE (immunoglobin E) if asthma is one component of the disease.

5. Assess perception of self in having a chronic illness (see Loss, page 733).

6. Assess weight and average daily fluid and dietary intake.

◤ NURSING DIAGNOSIS: IMPAIRED GAS EXCHANGE

RELATED TO FACTORS: COPD

DEFINING CHARACTERISTICS: Dyspnea, uses accessory muscles with breathing, rales, hypoxemia, hypercapnia, dusky or cyanotic skin color, reports orthopnea, wheezing, diminished breath sounds

PATIENT OUTCOME (collaborative): Demonstrates improved oxygenation

EVALUATION CRITERIA: ABG within an acceptable range, improved skin color, respiratory rate 12-24 per minute, clear breath sounds, absence of cough, denies chest discomfort, pulse rate 60-100 beats per minute, denies dyspnea

INTERVENTIONS	RATIONALE
1. Monitor: • respiratory status (Appendix A) q4h • results of ABG • pulse oximetry values • serum theophylline level • chest x ray reports • results of sputum and pulmonary function tests	To identify indications of progress toward or deviations from expected outcome. Because permanent damage has occurred to some portion of the lung with COPD, to expect normal values for ABG is unrealistic. Most COPD patients have compensated ABG with normal pH and elevated $PaCO_2$ and HCO_2 values. They are frequently termed 50-50 people since $PaCO_2$ and $PaCO_2$ values are similar.
2. Administer prescribed medications, which may include a combination of bronchodilators, steroids, and antibiotics. Evaluate their effectiveness. Schedule medications to maintain a consistent blood level of medications.	Bronchodilators open the bronchi; steroids reduce bronchial inflammation; and antibiotics eliminate infection. The desired therapeutic effect of these medications is resolution of manifestations of respiratory distress. Maintaining a consistent blood level of prescribed medications is best to ensure maximum therapeutic effectiveness. The serum theophylline level can determine therapeutic effects of theophylline-based agents.
3. Review all prescribed medications to avoid drug-to-drug adverse interactions. Consult pharmacology references and pharmacist as needed.	Combination pharmacotherapy increases the risk of drug-to-drug adverse interactions. Adverse interactions can either potentiate the effect or inhibit the action of one agent.

INTERVENTIONS	RATIONALE
4. Consult physician if symptoms persist or worsen. Prepare for transfer to ICU and placement on a mechanical ventilator if acute respiratory failure occurs (declining mental status, severe hypoxemia, and hypercapnia).	Acute respiratory failure is a major complication associated with COPD. Mechanical ventilation is required to support respiration until the patient can do so independently.
5. Provide humidified oxygen at the prescribed flow rate usually 2 L/min.	Moisture helps loosen bronchial secretion and prevents drying of the membranes. For patients with COPD, the hypoxic drive is the stimulus to breathe. A PaO_2 of 50-70 mm Hg is needed to stimulate respirations. Too much oxygen can kill the stimulus to breathe and cause respiratory arrest. Oxygen flow rate adjustments are made according to PaO_2 and $PaCO_2$ values.
6. Maintain a Fowler's position with arms abducted and supported by pillows, or sitting and leaning forward over the overbed table.	An erect position with arms abducted and supported allows fuller lung expansion by reducing abdominal pressure on the diaphragm through gravitational force.
7. Encourage fluid intake of at least three liters daily.	To help loosen bronchial secretions and to correct dehydration.
8. Encourage deep breathing with use of an incentive spirometer q2-4h. Administer or assist the respiratory therapist with prescribed chest physiotherapy, postural drainage, and aerosol treatments as needed. If unable to cough and expel secretions effectively, perform nasotracheal suctioning.	To remove pulmonary secretions and ensure airway patency.
9. Avoid excess use of central nervous system depressants (narcotics, sedatives).	These agents suppress respiratory function.

INTERVENTIONS	RATIONALE
10. Discourage smoking.	Nicotine in tobacco products causes vaso-constriction and bronchial constriction. Also, smoke is an allergen that depresses cilia function, increases coughing, and can result in decreased $SaO_2\%$.
11. Keep the room cool.	Cool air allows for easier breathing.

◤ NURSING DIAGNOSIS: ACTIVITY INTOLERANCE

RELATED TO FACTORS: Impaired gas exchange

DEFINING CHARACTERISTICS: Reports shortness of breath (SOB), weakness, and fatigue with minimal physical exertion for ADL tachypnea with minimal physical exertion

PATIENT OUTCOME: Demonstrates increased tolerance to activities

EVALUATION CRITERIA: Fewer complaints of SOB and weakness with activities

INTERVENTIONS	RATIONALE

1. Monitor:
  • pulse and respiratory rate before and after performing ADL
  • results of ABG
	To identify indications of progress toward or deviations from expected outcomes.

2. Implement energy conservation measures:
  • Provide assistance with ADL as needed. Space activities to allow frequent periods of rest. Gradually increase activities as ABG improve and symptoms of respiratory distress begin to dissipate.
  • Provide small frequent meals with foods that can easily be chewed.
	Rest allows the body to replenish energy stores. Large meals and foods that are difficult to chew require more energy.

NURSING DIAGNOSIS: ALTERATIONS IN NUTRITION: LESS THAN BODY REQUIREMENTS

RELATED TO FACTORS: Insufficient dietary intake secondary to respiratory distress

DEFINING CHARACTERISTICS: Weight loss, decreased dietary and fluid intake, verbalizes lack of appetite, dry skin with poor turgor, concentrated urine, observation of increased respiratory rate when eating, verbalizes increased SOB when eating

PATIENT OUTCOME (collaborative): Demonstrates improved nutritional status

EVALUATION CRITERIA: No further weight loss, increased dietary and fluid intake, absence of concentrated urine, increased urinary output, moist mucous membranes, absence of dry skin

INTERVENTIONS	RATIONALE
1. Monitor: • intake and output q8h • amount of food consumed with each meal • weight weekly	To identify indications of progress toward or deviations from expected outcomes.
2. Create a pleasant, odor-free environment during meal times. • Give oral care before and after each meal. • Place trash cans out of sight. • Clean table on which meal is consumed • Do not use heavy perfumes or room deodorizers. • Chest physiotherapy and nebulization treatments are performed at least one hour before meals. • Provide receptacle for proper disposal of used tissue, which may contain foul-smelling mucus from coughing or blowing the nose.	Odors and unpleasant sights during meal time can cause anorexia. Respiratory treatments given shortly after meals can precipitate nausea and vomiting.

INTERVENTIONS	RATIONALE
3. Refer patient to a dietitian for help with meal planning if consumption of each meal continues to be less than 30%.	A dietitian is a specialist who can assist the patient with planning meals that meet the nutritional requirements for age, body build, and illness.
4. Administer prescribed IV therapy and perform appropriate maintenance and preventive measures (see IV Therapy, page 764). Encourage at least three liters of fluid daily if not receiving IV therapy.	To resolve dehydration. Patients often reduce fluid intake because of SOB.

• •

◣ *N*URSING DIAGNOSIS: HIGH RISK FOR INFECTION

RELATED TO FACTORS: Inadequate primary defenses secondary to COPD

DEFINING CHARACTERISTICS: Symptoms of respiratory distress accompanied by productive cough, reports history of frequent episodes of upper respiratory tract infections

PATIENT OUTCOME (collaborative): Absence of symptoms of infection

EVALUATION CRITERIA: Temperature 98.6°F, WBC between 5,000-10,000/mm,[3] denies productive cough

• •

INTERVENTIONS	RATIONALE
1. Monitor: • temperature q4h • results of sputum cultures • results of CBC reports, particularly WBC • color and consistency of sputum	To identify indications of progress toward or deviations from expected outcomes.
2. Administer prescribed antibiotics and evaluate their effectiveness.	Infection is the most common factor precipitating respiratory distress. Antibiotics are often prescribed as treatment and prophylaxis against infection. Patients with COPD who are on maintenance doses of corticosteroids are especially predisposed to infection.

INTERVENTIONS	RATIONALE
3. Refrain from assigning patients with upper respiratory tract infection to the same room with the COPD patient. Adhere to universal precautions such as handwashing before and after patient contact.	To prevent nosocomial infection. Hand-washing is the most important measure that healthcare workers can use to prevent nosocomial infection.
4. Obtain sputum specimens as ordered for culture, especially if the patient is expectorating creamy, green, or gray, foul-smelling sputum.	A sputum culture confirms a diagnosis of upper respiratory tract infection and identifies the causative organism so appropriate antibiotic therapy can be initiated.

• •

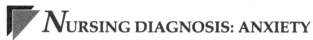

NURSING DIAGNOSIS: ANXIETY

RELATED TO FACTORS: Fear of suffocation during exacerbations, knowledge deficit about prescribed treatments and diagnostic studies

DEFINING CHARACTERISTICS: Verbalizes feelings of suffocation, tense facial expression, respiratory rate above 24 beats per minute accompanied by tachycardia and dyspnea, verbalizes fear of being alone

PATIENT OUTCOME: Demonstrates relief from anxiety

EVALUATION CRITERIA: Denies feeling a sense of suffocation, relaxed facial expression, respiratory rate 12-24 per minute, heart rate 60-100 beats per minute

• •

INTERVENTIONS	RATIONALE
1. During periods of acute respiratory distress: • Remove heavy clothing and bed covers. • Restrict the number and frequency of visitors to one at a time. • Initiate oxygen via nasal cannula at 2 L/min. • Demonstrate and encourage controlled breathing techniques. • Allow someone to remain with the patient.	These independent measures help give patient some sense of control over the condition, promote relaxation, and increase the amount of air available to the lungs.

INTERVENTIONS	RATIONALE
• Open doors and curtains. • Keep room cool. • Maintain an Fowler's position with arms supported and abducted.	

2. Avoid bombarding the patient with information and instructions when experiencing respiratory distress. Provide simple, short explanations about:
a. purpose of prescribed interventions
b. diagnostic tests, including:
  • purpose of test
  • brief description of test
  • preparation before test
  • care after test
Approach patient in a calm, reassuring manner.
	Patients retain less information when they are anxious, and too much information can increase their worry. Unfamiliar tests that may evoke discomfort often precipitate anxiety. Knowing what to expect helps reduce anxiety.

3. Use prescribed sedatives or tranquilizers sparingly.	Many patients need tranquilizers to control anxiety; however, these agents may induce respiratory failure because they suppress the respiratory center.

• •

 # NURSING DIAGNOSIS: DISTURBANCE IN SELF-CONCEPT

RELATED TO FACTORS: Loss (specify nature of loss)

DEFINING CHARACTERISTICS: Verbalizes low-self esteem, worthlessness, irritability, depression, reports self-imposed social isolation

PATIENT OUTCOME: Demonstrates adjustment to self with a chronic illness

EVALUATION CRITERIA: Participates in self-care, verbalizes ways to maintain a satisfying lifestyle in current condition

• •

INTERVENTIONS	RATIONALE
1. See Loss (page 733).	
2. Encourage participation in a community pulmonary rehabilitation program if available.	Ongoing support is essential to adaptation.

◤ NURSING DIAGNOSIS: HIGH RISK FOR NONCOMPLIANCE

RELATED TO FACTORS: Knowledge deficit about condition and self-care on discharge, depression

DEFINING CHARACTERISTICS: Verbalizes lack of understanding, requests information, uses respiratory devices incorrectly, reports frequent exacerbations, verbalizes unrealistic expectations of treatments

PATIENT OUTCOME: Demonstrates willingness to comply with treatment plan

EVALUATION CRITERIA: Verbalizes understanding of condition and self-care on discharge, reports fewer exacerbations

INTERVENTIONS	RATIONALE
1. Evaluate patient's and significant other's understanding of condition. Provide information about nature of condition based on their current understanding. Correct any misconceptions.	Compliance with the treatment plan is enhanced when patients understand the relationship between their condition and prescribed treatments.
2. If an inhaler was used at home before admission, evaluate patient's use of the device. If an inhaler is prescribed for home use, teach how to properly use and allow for a return demonstration. Instructions should include: • Shake the inhaler. • Inhale and then exhale completely. • Hold exhaled phase, insert mouthpiece, and close lips securely around mouthpiece.	Most inhalers contain a bronchodilator and are used on a scheduled basis and prn. Correct use of the inhaler is essential for the patient to completely benefit from treatment.

INTERVENTIONS	RATIONALE
• Squeeze canister to dispel mist and inhale deeply as mist comes out. • Hold inhaled mist briefly and then exhale. Emphasize that **MIST SHOULD BE INHALED, NOT SWALLOWED.**	
3. Provide discharge instructions about: a. Prevention of exacerbations: • Avoid smoking and prolonged exposure to smoke. • Avoid use of hair sprays and perfumes. • Reduce emotional stress. • Cover mouth and nose with a heavy scarf during exposure to cold, windy weather. • Avoid outdoor exercising during cold weather. • Eat a balanced high-calorie diet. • Eat small frequent meals if dyspnea is present at rest. • Avoid overexertion. Take frequent rest periods throughout the day. Conserve energy by exhaling when pushing, pulling, or exerting physical activity to move an object. • Reduce exposure to persons with respiratory infections. • Get a flu vaccine annually. • Keep respiratory equipment used at home clean. • Avoid breathing toxic chemical fumes, such as gasoline, paint, and glue.	Discharge teaching is essential to ensure patient compliance. Learning ways to control symptoms of a chronic illness provide a sense of hope and help the patient regain a sense of control over life rather than letting the illness take control.

INTERVENTIONS	RATIONALE
• Avoid exposure to known allergens that precipitate exacerbations.	
• Drink at least eight glasses daily of liquid.	
• Take medication as prescribed.	
b. Controlled breathing techniques. Encourage the patient to practice the following techniques 2–4 times daily with 6–8 breaths each time.	
• Diaphragmatic breathing — sit erect and place right hand on abdomen just beneath the xiphoid process and left hand over upper chest. Inhale and exhale slowly. During inhalation, right hand should move up while left hand remains still.	
• Pursed-lip breathing — inhale through the nose; exhale through pursed-lips.	
c. Symptoms of exacerbations and interventions:	
• Seek medical attention if condition worsens (increasing dyspnea, coughing spells worse than usual, chills, fever, increasing fatigue, discolored or foul-smelling sputum) or if medication fails to control symptoms.	
4. Ensure the patient or significant other has a written appointment for follow-up care and written instructions for self-care at home.	Verbal instructions may be easily forgotten.

INTERVENTIONS	RATIONALE
5. Provide information about medications prescribed for home use, such as name, purpose, dose, schedule, and reportable side effects.	Patients who understand their medications and their importance are usually more compliant.
6. Contact social services to arrange for placement of respiratory equipment prescribed for home use (portable oxygen, nebulizers) or home visits by a respiratory therapist if prescribed.	Social service acts as a liaison to arrange continuity of care for patients moving from the facility to home or to another health-care facility.
7. Ascertain effectiveness of current coping skills. If patient or significant other expresses continued difficulty in coping with limitations imposed by chronic illness, refer to community support groups or agencies, such as Meals-on-Wheels, American Lung Association, and Better Breathers Club.	Individuals and significant others experience a sense of loss with a chronic illness and grieve the actual or perceived loss. An ongoing support system is essential to help persons make effective adjustments to lifestyle changes imposed by chronic illness. Persons may be unaware of resources available to them.

Pulmonary Embolism

Pulmonary embolism refers to a partial or complete obstruction of one or both branches of the pulmonary artery or its tributaries. The obstructive element may be a blood clot, air, or fat globule (page 311).

The severity of signs and symptoms depends on the amount of lung tissue involved. With massive emboli, blood flow around the alveoli is impaired, leading to ventilation-perfusion imbalances evidenced by hypoxemia. Blood accumulates above the obstruction causing pulmonary hypertension that leads to right ventricular dilation and ultimately right-sided heart failure.

Pulmonary embolism is a medical emergency. One to two hours after the embolism is the most critical period with possible death occurring from complications such as pulmonary infarct (necrosis of the lung tissue) or pulmonary hypertension (increased pressure within the pulmonary artery), pulmonary hemorrhage, acute cor pulmonale with heart failure, and dysrhythmias.

The elderly are especially vulnerable to complications because of the normal changes that occur with aging in the pulmonary system (decreased lung compliance, calcification of vertebral cartilage) and cardiovascular system (narrowing of vessels, thickening of capillary walls) (Blair, 1990).

The mean LOS for a DRG classification of pulmonary embolism is 8.7 days (Lorenz, 1991).

General Medical Management

- Bedrest
- Supplemental oxygen
- Analgesics
- Pharmacotherapy:
  — thrombolytic agents such as streptokinase (Kabikinase, Streptase), alteplase (Activase, t-PA), or urokinase (Abbokinase)
  — anticoagulants such as heparin, dicumarol, or warfarin sodium

- Surgery (intracaval umbrella to filter blood clots traveling through the vena cava to right side of heart) for patients not responding to pharmacotherapy or who experience recurrent thromboemboli. This procedure prevents future emboli but does not help the present problem. The Greenfield filter or Bird's Nest filter may be implanted into the superior or inferior vena cava under local or general anesthesia. It may be inserted through a cutdown in the right jugular vein or percutaneously through a femoral vein.

Integrative Care Plans

- IV therapy
- Immobility

Discharge Considerations

- Medications to be continued at home
- Follow-up care
- Signs and symptoms of recurrence

 # ASSESSMENT DATA BASE

1. History or presence of risk factors (Handerhan, 1991) such as any condition that leads to:

   a. hypercoagulability of blood, for example, polycythemia, dehydration, cancer, oral contraceptives, pregnancy, and sickle cell anemia

   b. injury to venous endothelium, for example, long bone fractures, IV drug abuse, orthopedic surgery, venipuncture of the legs, presence of a central venous catheter or intra-arterial catheter (these catheters are primary sources of air embolism), and recent surgery

   c. venous stasis, for example, immobility, extensive burns, varicose veins, deep vein thrombophlebitis, heart failure, atrial fibrillation, and obesity

2. Physical examination based on an assessment of the respiratory (Appendix A) and cardiovascular system (Appendix G) may reveal:

   - severe chest pain on inspiration
   - warm, clammy skin or cold clammy skin depending on degree of hypoxemia
   - sudden onset of dyspnea accompanied by tachypnea
   - tachycardia
   - mild fever
   - drop in blood pressure (BP) below baseline value
   - rales/crackles, in extensive cases
   - nonproductive or productive cough of blood-tinged sputum
   - cyanosis (with total occlusion of pulmonary artery)

- jugular vein distention while in a sitting position
- petechiae on the chest, axillae, or conjunctivae (if caused by fat emboli)

   In addition, the patient often appears pale, diaphoretic, apprehensive, restless, irritable, or confused.

3. Diagnostic studies:
- CBC reveals leukocytosis.
- Arterial blood gases (ABG) reveal hypoxemia (PaO_2 less than 80 mm Hg) and respiratory alkalosis ($PaCO_2$ less than 35 mm Hg and pH greater than 7.45). Respiratory alkalosis is caused by hyperventilation.
- Prothrombin time (PT) and partial thromboplastin time (PTT) may be low if caused by a blood clot and normal if caused by air or a fat globule.
- Cardiac enzymes (CP, LDH, AST) are done to rule out myocardial infarction.
- Chest x ray may reveal infiltrates or can be normal.
- EKG is done to rule out myocardial infarction.
- Lung scan (ventilation and perfusion scans) reveal areas of hypoperfusion.
- Pulmonary angiogram provides the most definitive evidence of pulmonary emboli. Although not routinely performed, a pulmonary angiogram may be done if other radiological studies prove inconclusive and when vena cava interruption is planned. The procedure is performed in the same manner as a right-sided heart catheterization.

4. Assess emotional response to condition.

◢ NURSING DIAGNOSIS: IMPAIRED GAS EXCHANGE

RELATED TO FACTORS: Pulmonary embolism

DEFINING CHARACTERISTICS: Dyspnea; chest pain with inspiration; hemoptysis; persistent cough; crackles /rales; tachycardia accompanied by falling blood pressure, warm or cold, clammy, pale skin; and abnormal ABG

PATIENT OUTCOME (collaborative): Demonstrates improved oxygenation

EVALUATION CRITERIA: Absence of chest pain and hemoptysis, heart rate 60-100 beats per minute, blood pressure 90/60-140/90 mm Hg, respiratory rate 12-24 per minute, normal skin color, clear breath sounds, ABG within normal range

INTERVENTIONS	RATIONALE
1. During the acute phase, monitor: • results of ABGs • vital signs q2h • respiratory function (Appendix A) q2h, then q8h when stable • EKG tracings • coagulation studies, such as PTT and PT	To identify indications of progress toward or deviations from expected outcomes.
2. When symptoms of respiratory distress are detected: a. Place in a semi-Fowler's or Fowler's position immediately. Obtain vital signs and consult physician immediately. b. Start 100% oxygen using a non-rebreathing mask at 15 L/min and maintain bedrest. If history of COPD, initiate oxygen at 2–4 L/min. c. If an IV infusion is not in place, initiate one with 5% in dextrose water (D-5-W), or 0.9% normal saline solution if history of diabetes mellitus. Initiate maintenance and preventive activities for IV therapy (page 764). d. Prepare for transfer to ICU as ordered. Attach to ECG monitor and obtain rhythm strip after in ICU. e. Request all prescribed diagnostic studies stat until a diagnosis is confirmed. Notify physician immediately of test results .	Continuous monitoring is necessary to evaluate effectiveness of interventions. An erect position facilitates breathing by reducing abdominal pressure on the diaphragm. Supplemental oxygen provides additional oxygen to tissue deprived of oxygen. Excess oxygen in a patient with COPD can precipitate respiratory arrest. A nonrebreathing mask helps prevent further hypercapnia. Vascular access is needed for administering urgent medications. Cardiac dysrhythmias are a major complication associated with pulmonary embolism. Prompt intervention is essential to minimize life- threatening complications. Diagnostic studies are done stat as the patient's condition could deteriorate rapidly, depending on the extent of the infarct.

INTERVENTIONS	RATIONALE
3. Administer prescribed medication, such as thrombolytic agents and anticoagulants. Before administering thrombolytic therapy, ascertain the presence of any contraindications to thrombolytic therapy such as recent surgery, endocarditis, or cerebrovascular accident within the last two months. Consult pharmacology reference and pharmacist as needed about all prescribed medications to avoid a drug-to-drug adverse interaction. Consult physician if PTT exceeds control range or unusual bleeding occurs, such as petechiae, ecchymosis, bleeding gums, or nosebleeds. Initiate protective measures while on thrombolytic or anticoagulant therapy (page 399).	Thrombolytic agents are given to dissolve blood clots. Anticoagulants prevent the formation of new clots. Bleeding is the major adverse reaction associated with using these agents.
4. Consult physician if signs and symptoms worsen. Prepare for vena caval filter insertion or embolectomy as ordered.	This could indicate the beginning of complications, such as right-sided heart failure. Patients who experience recurrent pulmonary embolism or who do not respond to pharmacotherapy often benefit from insertion of a vena caval filter.
5. Perform preventive measures for the at-risk patient: • Administer aspirin or low-dose heparin therapy, as prescribed. • Range-of-motion exercises q2h for immobile patients and early ambulation for surgical patients. • Apply antiembolism stockings or sequential pneumatic compression stockings as prescribed. • Provide adequate hydration, at least 2–3 liters of fluid daily if not contraindicated. • Discourage crossing the legs.	Aspirin and heparin help prevent clot formation. Exercise stimulates circulation thereby preventing venous stasis. Antiembolic stockings stimulate circulation by compressing leg muscles, thus preventing venous stasis. Sequential pneumatic compression stockings are plastic thigh-high stockings with Velcro closures that are wrapped around the legs and connected to a machine that automatically inflates and deflates the stockings intermittently to prevent venous stasis. Fluids help reduce the blood viscosity. Crossing the legs promotes venous stasis.

●●●●●●●●●●●●●●●●●●●●●●●●●●●●●●

◣ Nursing Diagnosis: Anxiety

RELATED TO FACTORS: Feelings of suffocation; threat of impending death; knowledge deficit about condition, diagnostic studies, and treatment plan

DEFINING CHARACTERISTICS: Tense facial expression, tense posture, shaking voice, verbalizes fear of being alone, and reports feeling sense of impending doom

PATIENT OUTCOME (collaborative): Demonstrates less anxiety

EVALUATION CRITERIA: Relaxed facial expression; respiratory rate 12-24 per minute; reports feeling less nervous; verbalizes understanding of condition, diagnostic studies, and therapeutic plan

●●●●●●●●●●●●●●●●●●●●●●●●●●●●●●

INTERVENTIONS	RATIONALE
1. When symptoms of respiratory distress occur suddenly: • remain with the patient and have someone else notify the physician immediately. • maintain a calm, confident approach. Encourage slow deep breaths.	The presence of a competent, calm care-giver helps reduce the fear of being alone. Chest pain and difficulty breathing provoke anxiety. Tachypnea is often an outcome of anxiety, which results in reduced O_2 intake and excess loss of CO_2. Controlled breathing can help decrease anxiety.
2. Administer prescribed analgesic (morphine sulfate) and evaluate its effectiveness.	To help relieve chest pain and reduce anxiety.
3. Consult physician if analgesic fails to control chest pain.	Persistent pain could signal recurring pulmonary infarcts.
4. During the acute phase, give short, simple explanations about all treatments and procedures. When pain and respiratory distress have resolved, provide detailed information including: a. nature of the condition b. purpose of prescribed treatments c. prescribed diagnostic studies: • purpose • brief description of test • preparation required before test • care after test	Knowing what to expect helps reduce anxiety. Pain and respiratory distress interfere with learning.

NURSING DIAGNOSIS: HIGH RISK FOR IMPAIRED HOME MAINTENANCE MANAGEMENT

RELATED TO FACTORS: Knowledge deficit about self-care on discharge, inadequate support system

DEFINING CHARACTERISTICS: Requests information, verbalizes lack of understanding, reports lack of finances or transportation to meet medical needs

PATIENT OUTCOME (collaborative): Demonstrates willingness to comply with therapeutic plan

EVALUATION CRITERIA: Verbalizes understanding of self-care plan on discharge, identifies community resources to help meet medical needs

INTERVENTIONS	RATIONALE

1. Prepare the patient for discharge:
 	
  a. Ensure the patient or significant other has a written appointment for follow-up care and written instructions for self-care at home.
 	
  b. Provide information about medications prescribed for home use, such as name, purpose, dose, schedule, and reportable side effects.
 	
  c. Teach the patient signs and symptoms of recurrence of the condition. Instruct to seek medical attention if condition recurs.
	Verbal instructions may be easily forgotten. Discharge teaching helps ensure patient compliance.

2. Evaluate need for financial assistance or assistance with ADL. Consult social services or discharge planning department to arrange for assistance with medical support at home as needed.	These departments are liaisons that ensure continuity of care as needed on discharge home or to an extended care facility.

INTERVENTIONS	RATIONALE
3. If a vena cava filter was inserted, instruct the patient to avoid contact sports and jogging. Remind the patient that the risk of developing another embolus is still high, but that the filter reduces the risk of pulmonary embolism. (See Acute Peripheral Arterial Thrombosis, page 342, for further discharge instructions if a femoral site is used.)	Discharge instructions are essential to safe home care. With normal daily activities, the filter is less likely to migrate.

Status Asthmaticus

Status asthmaticus is a life-threatening emergency. It is a severe asthma attack that lasts longer than the usual attack and is unresponsive to usual drug therapy.

During an asthma attack, increased airway resistance due to bronchospasms, increased mucus, and inflammation of the bronchial lining occur. These pathological changes cause partial airway obstruction that interferes with oxygen intake. If left untreated, the patient can develop pulmonary hypertension, cardiac arrhythmias, and drift into a coma.

Because the patient is in acute respiratory distress, hospitalization is required. The mean LOS for a DRG classification of status asthmaticus is 5.9 days (Lorenz, 1991).

General Medical Management

a. Pharmacotherapy:
  - epinephrine (Adrenalin) 1/1000 or terbutaline, aminophylline (given as a continuous infusion after the epinephrine)
  - corticosteroids
b. Aerosol-nebulization treatments, which may consist of a mucolytic agent or beta-adrenergic agent
c. Mechanical ventilation if acute respiratory failure occurs

Integrative Care Plans

- IV therapy
- Loss

Discharge Considerations

- Medications to continue at home
- Use of respiratory therapy equipment
- Follow-up care
- Prevention of asthmatic attacks
- Signs and symptoms requiring medical attention

ASSESSMENT DATA BASE

1. History of exposure to factors that commonly trigger asthmatic attacks:

   - emotional stress
   - upper respiratory tract infection
   - allergens
   - failure to take prescribed medication for asthma

2. Physical examination based on an assessment of the respiratory system (Appendix A) may reveal symptoms of acute respiratory distress:

   - audible wheezing without the aid of a stethoscope
   - labored respirations
   - orthopnea
   - use of accessory muscles with breathing (flaring of nostrils, sternal retraction, raising shoulders with inspiration)
   - dehydration
   - cyanosis
   - pulsus paradoxus (drop in systolic BP of 10 mm Hg with respirations)
   - restlessness
   - tachycardia
   - diaphoresis
   - fatigue
   - apprehension

3. Diagnostic studies:

   - ABG reveal hypocapnia ($PaCO_2$ less than 35 mm Hg) due to ventilation-perfusion deficits. Later the $PaCO_2$ rises above normal as airway resistance increases.
   - CBC reveals elevated eosinophil level.
   - Pulmonary function studies show decreased forced vital capacity (FVC).
   - Sputum specimen is collected for culture and sensitivity tests to rule out infection and to identify the appropriate antimicrobial to resolve the infection if present.
   - Chest x ray reveals alveoli distention.

4. Inquire about medications currently being taken and when the last dose was taken.

NURSING DIAGNOSIS: IMPAIRED GAS EXCHANGE

RELATED TO FACTORS: Persistent asthmatic attack

DEFINING CHARACTERISTICS: Severe dyspnea and wheezing, cyanosis, orthopnea, uses accessory muscles with breathing

PATIENT OUTCOME (collaborative): Demonstrates improved ventilation

EVALUATION CRITERIA: Respiratory rate 12–24 per minute, clear breath sounds, pulse rate 60–100 beats per minute, normal skin color, denies dyspnea, ABG within normal limits

INTERVENTIONS	RATIONALE
1. Monitor: • respiratory status (Appendix A) q4h • serum theophylline reports • ABG reports • pulse oximetry • results of chest x rays, pulmonary function studies, and sputum analysis • intake and output	To identify indications of progress toward or deviations from expected outcomes.
2. Maintain a Fowler's position.	An erect position allows fuller lung expansion.
3. Initiate prescribed IV therapy. Perform maintenance and preventive activities (page 764).	To allow for rapid rehydration and to have vascular access for rapid administration of urgent medications. Most patients are dehydrated when they seek medical attention.
4. Start oxygen via nasal cannula at 4 L/min initially, then adjust according to PaO_2.	Supplemental oxygen reduces the work of breathing.

INTERVENTIONS	RATIONALE
5. Administer prescribed medications, which may include epinephrine or terbutaline, aminophylline, and corticosteroids. Evaluate their effectiveness. Consult physician if an adverse reaction occurs. Review all prescribed medications to avoid drug-to-drug adverse interactions. Consult pharmacology reference and pharmacist as needed.	Epinephrine or terbutaline halt the allergic reaction and dilate bronchioles by counteracting the activity of histamine. Aminophylline dilates the bronchioles by stimulating increased production of a chemical that inhibits bronchial muscle contriction. Corticosteroids help reduce inflammation of the bronchial mucosal lining.
6. Hold medication and consult physician if signs of theophylline toxicity occur, (nausea and vomiting, abdominal distention, serum theophylline level above normal range).	The physician will decrease the dosage to correct toxicity.
7. Encourage use of the incentive spirometer q2h.	To facilitate deep breathing thereby preventing atelectasis.
8. Ensure that pulmonary treatments (chest physiotherapy, aerosol therapy) are provided as prescribed. Arrange for additional aerosol treatments if respiratory distress occurs between prescribed intervals.	These treatments help loosen bronchial secretions.
9. Consult physician if symptoms persist after one hour of therapy or if condition worsens (crossover point where $PaCO_2$ exceeds the PaO_2 is reached, apnea occurs, mental status declines, or patient is on verge of collapsing from exhaustion due to arduous effort of breathing).	These findings indicate a need for endotracheal intubation and placement on a mechanical ventilator.

● ●

◤ NURSING DIAGNOSIS: ANXIETY

RELATED TO FACTORS: Fear of suffocation secondary to severe respiratory distress, knowledge deficit about diagnostic studies and treatment plan

DEFINING CHARACTERISTICS: Verbalizes feeling of suffocation, apprehension, tense facial expression, verbalizes difficulty breathing

PATIENT OUTCOME: Demonstrates less anxiety

EVALUATION CRITERIA: Relaxed facial expression, respiratory rate 12–24 per minute, reports feeling less nervous and afraid

● ●

INTERVENTIONS	RATIONALE
1. Remain with the patient or have someone else remain with the patient until respiratory distress begins to lessen. Maintain a calm, confident approach.	Anxiety is reduced when the patient perceives that caregiver is competent.
2. Restrict visitors until respiratory distress begins to resolve.	Visitors may be a source of stress.
3. Use short, simple directives when giving information or instructions, for example, "sit up," "breath slow and deep." Explain the purpose of all prescribed treatments. Provide information about prescribed diagnostic studies including: • purpose • brief description of test • preparation required before test • care after test	A high anxiety level inhibits learning. A knowledge of what to expect helps control anxiety.

● ●

◤ NURSING INTERVENTION: HIGH RISK FOR NONCOMPLIANCE

RELATED TO FACTORS: Knowledge deficit about condition and self-care upon discharge

DEFINING CHARACTERISTICS: Verbalizes lack of understanding, requests information, reports repeated hospitalizations for same condition

PATIENT OUTCOME: Demonstrates willingness to comply with therapeutic plan

EVALUATION CRITERIA: Verbalizes understanding of condition and self-care activities on discharge, demonstrates correct use of respiratory devices

• •

INTERVENTIONS	RATIONALE
1. When respiratory distress has subsided, evaluate patient's understanding of the condition. Correct any misconceptions. Emphasize that attacks can be controlled with proper use of prescribed medication and avoidance of factors that trigger attacks.	Compliance can be enhanced when patient understands condition and significance of therapies.
2. Evaluate the patient's use of the inhaler if one has been prescribed for home use before admission.	Improper use of an inhaler can reduce the amount of bronchodilator delivered to the bronchioles.
3. On discharge: a. Instruct the patient to: • seek medical attention if signs of respiratory tract infection occur (persistent coughing, increase wheezing and dyspnea, unresponsive to medication, nasal congestion, runny nose) • seek ways to reduce emotional stress • avoid exposure to allergens that trigger attacks • use prescribed inhaler when dyspnea and tightness in chest first occur to prevent worsening of symptoms, and seek medical attention if medication fails to halt symptoms • take medication as prescribed	Learning self-care measures to control symptoms of a chronic illness fosters independence. Verbal instructions may be easily forgotten.

INTERVENTIONS	RATIONALE
b. Teach the patient about all prescribed medication, such as name, purpose, dosage, schedule, and reportable side effects. c. Provide a written appointment for follow-up care and written instructions for self-care at home.	
4. Evaluate patient's and significant other's feelings about the condition. Allow them to express feelings about having a chronic condition.	Verbalizing feelings helps foster adaptation to a chronic condition.

*P*neumonia

Pneumonia is an inflammatory process of the lung parenchyma. It occurs as a result of invasion by an infectious agent or condition that alters the resistance of the tracheobronchial lining so normal endogenous flora become pathogenic on entering the airway.

Pneumonia may be classified according to:

1. Causative agent:
   a. protozoan (Pneumocystis Carinii) bacterial, viral, or fungal pneumonia (if due to an infectious agent)
   b. aspiration pneumonia — caused by aspiration of gastric content, food, or liquids
   c. radiation pneumonia — caused by radiation therapy for cancers involving structures of the upper torso such as (breast, lung, or esophagus)
   d. hypostatic pneumonia — associated with prolonged immobility
   e. inhalation pneumonia — inhalation of toxic gases, smoke, and chemicals

2. Area of the lung affected:
   a. lobar pneumonia — one or more lobes involved
   b. bronchopneumonia — pneumonia process originates in bronchi and then spreads to adjacent lung tissue

The pneumonia process interferes with ventilation. After the causative agent reaches the alveoli, an inflammatory reaction occurs, causing edema and extravasation of serous fluid into the alveoli. The exudate provides a culture medium for further bacterial growth. Alveolar-capillary membranes become occluded, thus preventing passage of oxygen into perialveolar capillaries in some parts of the lungs. Hypoxemia develops.

Hospitalization is usually required to treat pneumonia. The mean LOS for a DRG classification of pneumonia is 9.2 days (Lorenz, 1991).

The major complications associated with pneumonia are lung abscess, pleural effusion, empyema, respiratory failure, pericarditis, meningitis, and atelectasis. Elderly patients are at increased risk for these complications because of the normal pulmonary system changes that occur with aging (decreased lung tissue compliance, decreased coughing efficiency, and reduced chest expansion resulting from calcification of vertebral cartilage) (Caruthers, 1990).

General Medical Management

- Pharmacotherapy:
  - — antibiotics (given intravenously)
  - — expectorants
  - — antipyretics
  - — analgesics
- Oxygen therapy and aerosol nebulization
- Chest physiotherapy with postural drainage

Integrative Care Plans

- IV therapy
- Immobility

Discharge Considerations

- Medications to continue at home
- Signs and symptoms of recurrence
- Prevention of recurrence
- Follow-up care

*A*SSESSMENT DATA BASE

1. History or presence of risk factors:
   - chronic obstructive pulmonary disease
   - chronic smoking
   - prolonged physical immobility
   - continuous gastric tube feedings
   - immunosuppressive drugs (chemotherapy, corticosteroids)
   - debilitating diseases (AIDS, cancer)
   - inhaling or aspirating irritating substances
   - continuous exposure to severe air pollution
   - endotracheal or tracheostomy tube
   - depressed level of consciousness (stupor, lethargic, semicomatose, comatose)

2. Physical examination based on an assessment of the respiratory system (Appendix A) and general survey (Appendix F) may reveal a combination of the following, depending on the causative agent and the mechanism of lung invasion:
   - high fever and chills (onset may be sudden or insidious)
   - pleuritic chest pain

- tachypnea and tachycardia
- rales
- nonproductive cough initially, which progresses to a productive cough of mucoid, purulent, rusty, brown, yellow, green, or blood-tinged sputum, often foul smelling
- dyspnea
- malaise and weakness
- dusky or cyanotic skin color
- intermittent diaphoresis as fever decreases and increases
- a 24- to 48-hour period of headache, myalgia, and malaise followed by fever, a pulse-temperature dissociation (a relatively slow pulse with a high fever. Normally, the pulse increases as the temperature rises). These are classical findings with Legionella pneumonia, viral pneumonia, and mycoplasma pneumonia.

3. Inquire about a recent upper respiratory infection (URI) (sore throat, nasal congestion, sneezing, low-grade fever).

4. Diagnostic studies:
   - CBC reveals elevated WBC with pneumococcal, Legionella, klebsiella, staphylococcal, and Haemophilus influenzae pneumonias. It will be normal with mycoplasma and viral pneumonias.
   - Chest x ray shows lobar consolidation with pneumococcal, Legionella, klebsiella, and Hemophilus influenzae pneumonias. Patchy infiltrates often seen with mycoplasma, viral, and staphylococcal pneumonias.
   - Sputum culture reveals bacteria type and is negative for viral pneumonias.
   - Blood culture is positive if the pneumonia is acquired by the hematogenous route (Staphylococcus aureus).
   - Gram stain of sputum is positive for infections caused by gram-negative or gram-positive bacteria.
   - Cold agglutinins and complement fixation are done for viral studies.
   - Arterial blood gases (ABG) reveal hypoxemia (PaO_2 less than 80 mm Hg) and possibly hypocapnia ($PaCO_2$ less than 35 mm Hg).
   - Pulmonary function tests (PFT) show reduced forced vital capacity (FVC).
   - Bronchoscopy.

5. Assess emotional response to condition.

NURSING DIAGNOSIS: IMPAIRED GAS EXCHANGE

RELATED TO FACTORS: Pneumonia

DEFINING CHARACTERISTICS: Persistent, productive cough, dyspnea, tachypnea, rales, abnormal ABG, dusky or cyanotic skin color, diminished breath sounds, abnormal PFT, low incentive spirometer tidal volumes

PATIENT OUTCOME (collaborative): Demonstrates improved ventilation

EVALUATION CRITERIA: Clear breath sounds, ABG within normal limits, normal skin color, respiratory rate 12–24 per minute, pulse rate 60–100 beats per minute, absence of cough, increased volumes of inhaled air on incentive spirometer

INTERVENTIONS	RATIONALE
1. Monitor: • respiratory status (Appendix A) q8h • vital signs q4h • results of ABG, chest x rays, and PFT	To identify indications of progress toward or deviations from expected outcomes.
2. Administer prescribed expectorant and evaluate its effectiveness. Review all prescribed medications to avoid drug-to-drug adverse interactions. Schedule medication to achieve maximum therapeutic effectiveness.	Expectorants help loosen secretions so they are coughed up and expelled.
3. Encourage at least 2–3 liters of fluid daily.	To help loosen secretions. Fluids also aid in the distribution of medications within the body.
4. Suction prn if the patient has congested lungs but a poor or absent cough reflex or diminished level of consciousness.	Suctioning clears the airway.
5. Discourage smoking.	Nicotine causes airway constriction.
6. Maintain a semi-Fowler's or Fowler's position.	An erect position allows fuller lung expansion by reducing abdominal pressure against the diaphragm.

INTERVENTIONS	RATIONALE
7. Administer supplemental oxygen as prescribed. Adjust flow rate according to ABG as ordered. If the patient must be transported off the unit, provide a portable oxygen tank. If a face mask is used for oxygen delivery and the patient becomes increasingly agitated with its presence, consult respiratory therapist for a nasal cannula.	Supplemental oxygen reduces the work of breathing by making more oxygen available to the cells. Although higher concentrations of oxygen can be delivered by a face mask, it often evokes feelings of suffocation in patients, especially those in respiratory distress.
8. Depending on facility policy and procedures, administer or arrange for respiratory therapy treatments as prescribed. Consult respiratory therapist and physician for additional aerosol treatments if respiratory distress occurs between scheduled treatments.	The respiratory therapist is a specialist in respiratory care and usually performs all prescribed respiratory function studies and treatments in most facilities (nebulization, postural drainage and percussion). Aerosol treatments involve using bronchodilators and mucolytic agents to help relieve respiratory distress.
9. Consult physician if respiratory symptoms persist or worsen.	This could signal the beginning of complications.
10. Adhere to universal or specific protective care precautions (wearing a mask if on respiratory precautions, or wearing gloves when handling body secretions or blood). Provide the patient with a trash receptacle or attach a paper bag to the bedrail for proper disposal of tissue.	To prevent the spread of the disease.
11. Maintain adequate pain control if patient verbalizes pleuritic pain especially before deep breathing exercises. Monitor the patient closely when administering sedatives or narcotics. Avoid use of these agents if respiratory rate is 12 per minute or less. Evaluate effectiveness of prescribed analgesic.	Patients restrict thoracic expansion to control pleuritic pain. This contributes to hypoventilation and atelectasis. Respiratory depression is a major adverse reaction associated with narcotics and sedatives.

INTERVENTIONS	RATIONALE
12. Encourage deep breathing q2h with an incentive spirometer. Document patient's progress.	Deep breathing expands the alveoli to prevent atelectasis. The incentive spirometer promotes deep breathing and provides an objective measurement of the patient's progress.

 # NURSING DIAGNOSIS: HIGH RISK FOR FLUID VOLUME DEFICIT

RELATED TO FACTORS: Fever, diaphoresis, and diminished oral intake secondary to the pneumonia process

DEFINING CHARACTERISTICS: Verbalizes thirst, hypernatremia, dry mucous membranes, concentrated urine, poor skin turgor, daily weight loss, rapid weak pulse, falling blood pressure.

PATIENT OUTCOME (collaborative): Demonstrates improved fluid and electrolyte status

EVALUATION CRITERIA: Urinary output greater than 30 mL/hr, urine specific gravity 1.005–1.025, serum sodium within normal limits, moist mucous membranes, good skin turgor, no further weight loss, fewer reports of thirst

INTERVENTIONS	RATIONALE
1. Monitor: • intake and output q8h • weight daily • results of urinalysis and serum electrolyte reports • condition of skin and mucous membranes daily	To identify indications of progress toward or deviations from expected outcomes.

INTERVENTIONS	RATIONALE
2. Administer prescribed IV therapy and perform maintenance and preventive measures (see Intravenous Therapy, page 764).	During the acute phase, patients are often too weak and dyspneic to orally ingest sufficient fluids to maintain adequate hydration. Fluid needs are increased in the presence of fever. With fever, water loss increases because of: • excess sweating, which occurs when fever resolves • increased evaporation, which occurs as a result of peripheral vasodilation. This is a compensatory mechanism used by the body to cool itself.
3. Offer liquids orally at least q2h. Encourage clear liquids with some caloric value.	Fluids enhance medication distribution throughout the body and also help reduce fever. Clear liquids are less likely to increase mucus. Calories help guard against weight loss.
4. Consult physician if symptoms of fluid deficit persist or worsen.	This could signal the need for increased fluids or the beginning of complications.

NURSING DIAGNOSIS: ACTIVITY INTOLERANCE

RELATED TO FACTORS: Impaired gas exchange secondary to pneumonia

DEFINING CHARACTERISTICS: Verbalizes dyspnea and fatigue with minimal exertion; diaphoresis, tachypnea, and tachycardia with minimal exertion

PATIENT OUTCOME: Demonstrates increased tolerance to activities

EVALUATION CRITERIA: Performs ADL and walks longer distances without experiencing SOB, dyspnea, or fatigue

INTERVENTIONS	RATIONALE
1. Monitor pulse and respiratory rates before and after activities.	To identify indications of progress toward or deviations from expected outcomes.
2. Cease the activity if pulse and respiratory rates increase greatly and the patient reports SOB, fatigue, or dyspnea. Increase activities gradually to tolerance.	These symptoms signal activity intolerance. Oxygen consumption increases with physical exertion. Endurance can be extended when activities are paced to allow periods of rest.
3. Provide assistance with ADL as needed. Allow uninterrupted rest periods between activities.	To conserve energy.
4. Maintain oxygen therapy during activities. Initiate measures to prevent complications of immobility if bedrest is prescribed (see Immobility, page 725).	Physical activity increases oxygen demands and further stresses an already compromised system. All systems slow down with prolonged periods of physical inactivity. Specific nursing actions can minimize the complications of immobility.
5. Consult physician if dyspnea at rest persists or worsens.	This could signal the beginning of complications, especially respiratory failure.

• •

 NURSING DIAGNOSIS: ALTERATIONS IN COMFORT: PLEURITIC CHEST PAIN AND FEVER

RELATED TO FACTORS: Pneumonia

DEFINING CHARACTERISTICS: Verbalizes chest pain aggravated by breathing or coughing, auscultation of a pleural rub; chest x ray confirms pleuritis; temperature above 98.6°F, intermittent periods of diaphoresis; WBC above 10,000/mm^3; positive sputum cultures

PATIENT OUTCOME (collaborative): Demonstrates relief from discomfort

EVALUATION CRITERIA: Denies pleuritic chest pain, relaxed facial expression, temperature 98.6°F, negative sputum cultures, WBC between 5,000-10,000/mm^3

• •

INTERVENTIONS	RATIONALE
1. Monitor: • temperature q4h • WBC results • results of sputum cultures	To identify indications of progress toward or deviations from expected outcomes.
2. Administer prescribed analgesic for pleuritic chest pain prn and evaluate its effectiveness. Consult physician if analgesic is ineffective in controlling pain.	Analgesics help control pain by blocking the pain pathways. Severe pleuritic chest pain often requires narcotic analgesics to achieve effective pain control. Pain unresponsive to analgesia requires further investigation as it may signal the beginning of complications.
3. Administer prescribed antibiotic and evaluate its effectiveness. Review all prescribed medications to avoid drug-to-drug adverse interactions. Schedule antibiotics to maintain a consistent blood level of the medication.	Antibiotics are needed to resolve an infection. Maximum therapeutic effectiveness is attained when a consistent blood level of the medication is maintained. The risk of drug-to-drug adverse interaction increases with multiple pharmacotherapy. A drug-to-drug adverse interaction reduces the therapeutic effectiveness of one or both medications.
4. Consult physician for persistent fever and adverse reactions (rash, gastrointestinal (GI) disturbances, decreased urinary output, decreased hearing, increased fatigue).	These symptoms signal antibiotic toxicity and a need for withdrawing the medication.
5. Provide comfort measures such as a backrub, dry linen following diaphoresis, warm liquids, quiet environment with lights dimmed, mild sedative (if prescribed), and application of moisturizer to lips and skin.	These measures promote relaxation. A moisturizer helps prevent drying and cracking of lips and skin.

INTERVENTIONS	RATIONALE

6. Initiate measures to relieve fever:
  • cool bath
  • light top covers (maintain enough top covering to prevent shivering)
  • administer prescribed antipyretic
  • increase fluid intake
	Cool water applied to the body and light covering allow for heat loss through conduction and evaporation. Antipyretics control fever by readjusting the hypothalmic thermostat. Fluids help prevent dehydration from increased cell metabolism. Shivering generates more body heat.

7. Consult physician if pain or fever persists or worsens.	This may signal the development of complications.

 NURSING DIAGNOSIS: ALTERATIONS IN NUTRITION: LESS THAN BODY REQUIREMENTS

RELATED TO FACTORS: Increased body metabolism and decreased appetite secondary to fever

DEFINING CHARACTERISTICS: Verbalizes anorexia, consumes less than 40% of meals, weight loss, verbalizes weakness

EXPECTED OUTCOME (collaborative): Demonstrates adequate nutritional intake to meet metabolic needs

EVALUATION CRITERIA: Increased dietary intake, no further weight loss, verbalizes feeling of well-being

INTERVENTIONS	RATIONALE

1. Monitor:
  • percentage of food consumed with each meal
  • weight daily
  • results of serum studies such as total protein, albumin, and osmolarity
	To identify indications of progress toward or deviations from expected outcome.

2. Provide oral care at least q4h, if expectorating copious amounts of foul-smelling sputum. Keep room free of odors.	An unpleasant taste or smell can interfere with appetite.

INTERVENTIONS	RATIONALE
3. Refer to dietitian for assistance in selecting foods of choice that meet nutritional requirements during a febrile illness.	A dietitian is a nutritional specialist and can assist the patient in selecting foods to meet caloric and nutritional needs based on illness, age, weight, and height. Moreover, patients are more likely to consume meals that consist of their choice of foods.
4. Encourage intake of high-protein, high-calorie foods. Consult physician about vitamin supplements and other nutritional supplements (Jevity, Ensure, Isocal, Pulmocare) if dietary intake continues to be less than 30% of each meal. If weight loss continues, dietary intake continues to decline, and serum studies reveal a negative nitrogen balance, suggest a calorie count and possibly continuous enteral feeding through a nasogastric (N/G) tube or total parenteral nutrition (TPN).	Fever increases metabolism. An adequate intake of protein, vitamins, minerals, and calories is essential for anabolic activity and synthesis of antibodies. A calorie count determines the need for TPN. TPN provides calories and all essential amino acids and vitamins. In addition, essential fatty acids also can be given.
5. Provide small frequent feedings with foods that are easy to chew if severe dyspnea is present.	Small feedings require less energy.

- -

NURSING DIAGNOSIS: ANXIETY

RELATED TO FACTORS: Knowledge deficit about condition, diagnostic studies, and treatment plan

DEFINING CHARACTERISTICS: Verbalizes lack of understanding; reports feeling nervous, anxious, or afraid

PATIENT OUTCOME: Demonstrates less anxiety

EVALUATION CRITERIA: Fewer reports of feeling anxious, afraid, or nervous; verbalizes understanding of condition, diagnostic studies, and treatment plan

- -

INTERVENTIONS	RATIONALE
1. See Nursing Diagnosis: Anxiety (page 52).	

NURSING DIAGNOSIS: HIGH RISK FOR IMPAIRED HOME MAINTENANCE MANAGEMENT

RELATED TO FACTORS: Knowledge deficit about self-care on discharge, lack of adequate support system or financial resources

DEFINING CHARACTERISTICS: Requests information, requests assistance with financing medical care

PATIENT OUTCOME: Demonstrates willingness to comply with therapeutic program

EVALUATION CRITERIA: Verbalizes understanding of self-care on discharge, identifies available support systems and means for financing medical care

INTERVENTIONS	RATIONALE
1. Provide information about prevention of the spread of infection (covering mouth when coughing or sneezing, properly disposing of soiled tissue.	Most pneumonias are caused by airborne pathogens.
2. Encourage annual flu vaccinations for persons at risk (the elderly, persons who have a chronic cardio-vascular or respiratory disease, or persons taking immunosuppressant drugs).	A flu vaccination helps prevent various strains of pneumonia. A weakened immune system increases susceptibility to infections.
3. Ensure the patient or significant other has a written appointment for follow-up care and written instructions for self-care at home.	Verbal instructions may be easily forgotten.

INTERVENTIONS	RATIONALE
4. Instruct the patient to: • seek medical attention if symptoms of pneumonia recur. • take medication prescribed for home use as ordered. Provide information about medications prescribed for home use, such as, name, purpose, dose, schedule, and reportable side effects. • gradually increase activity to avoid fatigue. • avoid chilling and exposure to others with upper respiratory tract infections or viruses. • maintain resistance to infection with proper nutrition and adequate fluid intake, at least eight glasses of fluid daily.	Pneumonia does not imply immunity but places the person at increased risk for recurrent infections. Discharge teaching helps foster patient compliance.

Chest Tubes

The primary purpose of a chest tube is to drain air, fluid, or both from the thoracic cavity. For treatment of pulmonary conditions, the tube is inserted into the pleural space (space between the viscera and parietal pleura) to reestablish normal negative intrapleural pressure. With cardiac surgery, the tube(s) is placed into the pericardium or mediastinum below the sterneotomy incision.

A chest tube may be placed before closure of the incision during lung or cardiac surgery, or at the bedside as urgent treatment to relieve pneumothorax or hemothorax. A portable chest x ray is taken immediately following insertion to confirm placement. Serial x rays are taken to evaluate reexpansion of the lung.

The tube location depends on the substance to be drained. Because air rises to the top, a tube inserted into the anterior chest at the 2nd or 3rd intercostal space midclavicular line is used to drain air. A tube placed lower in the chest just posterior to the midaxillary line at the 4th or 5th intercostal space is used to drain fluid. A patient may have tubes inserted in both locations when both air and fluid must be removed.

To insert the chest tube, the physician makes a small incision at the appropriate site after injecting a local anesthetic, such a lidocaine. The tube is inserted using a trocar and then sutured to the skin proximal to the insertion site to prevent dislodgment. To create an airtight seal, a petrolatum dressing is applied around the insertion site and then covered with a dry sterile dressing. Adhesive tape is applied to create an occlusive secure dressing. The tube is connected to a water-seal drainage system (Atrium, Pleur-evac, Sentinel seal, Thora-klex, or Thora-seal III). Thora-klex is also available as a waterless drainage system.

The chest drainage system may consist of a one-bottle or a 3-chamber system when large amounts of fluid and air must be drained. If two chest tubes have been inserted, they may be connected to the same water-seal drainage system using a "Y" connector.

The nurse follows facility protocol and procedures when assisting the physician with bedside insertion of a chest tube.

The major complications associated with a chest tube are tension pneumothorax because of blockage of the tube and subcutaneous emphysema because of air trapping in subcutaneous tissue.

For assessments before insertion of the chest tube, see the specific condition being treated. This plan focuses on care after insertion of the chest tube. It is important to remember that when a patient has an intrusive device attached to the body, the nurse must make ongoing assessments of both the patient and the device.

Integrative Care Plans

- Immobility
- Pain
- Plan of care for the specific condition being treated

Discharge Considerations

- See the plan of care for the specific condition being treated

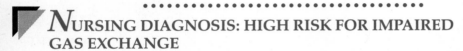

NURSING DIAGNOSIS: HIGH RISK FOR IMPAIRED GAS EXCHANGE

RELATED TO FACTOR: Possible tension pneumothorax occurring secondary to blockage of chest tube

DEFINING CHARACTERISTICS: Heavy, bloody drainage from the chest tube; large amount of clots observed in chest drainage; rapid, shallow breathing; significant changes in vital signs, skin color, and mucous membranes

PATIENT OUTCOME (collaborative): Demonstrates adequate oxygenation

EVALUATION CRITERIA: Clear breath sounds bilaterally, ABG return to normal range, denies dyspnea, respiratory rate 12–24 per minute, trachea remains midline, symmetrical chest expansion with breathing

INTERVENTIONS	RATIONALE

1. Monitor:
  • respiratory status (Appendix A) q1h for first eight hours, then q4h if stable
  • q2–4h for presence of pain
  • results of chest x ray and ABG reports
	To identify indications of progress toward or deviations from expected outcome.

INTERVENTIONS	RATIONALE
2. Monitor the chest drainage system each time the patient is assessed. • Inspect tubing connections, color, and amount of drainage, and water level. • Look for fluid fluctuation in the drainage tubing as patient inhales and exhales. • Ensure collection bottle is secure to prevent accidental breakage.	To ensure proper functioning (see Table 1-1).
3. Ensure tubing connections are securely taped. Intervene according to specific findings (see Table 1–1).	Taping the connections helps prevent accidental disconnection. To reduce the risk of complications, it is important to differentiate findings that indicate normal functioning from those that indicate malfunctioning.
4. Keep two tubing clamps or rubber-tipped hemostats at the bedside always. **Avoid** clamping the tube unless: a. instructed to do so by physician b. collection bottle is accidentally broken c. collection bottle is being changed If clamping of the tube is prescribed, release the tube immediately if the patient shows signs of respiratory distress (dyspnea, tachypnea, tachycardia, shallow respirations). Then report findings to physician.	Hemostats clamp the tubing to prevent loss of negative intrapleural pressure when there is a break in the system. A clamped chest tube, when the lung has not fully reexpanded, can lead to tension pneumothorax evidenced by respiratory distress.
5. Keep a bottle of sterile water at the bedside at all times to refill the water-seal chamber prn and to provide a water-seal chamber if the collection system is accidentally broken. Add water to the collection chamber prn to maintain the desired level, usually 20 cm.	Water acts as a seal, allowing air to leave the pleural cavity, and preventing its reentry. This water seal is important for recreating negative pressure in the pleural cavity, which facilitates lung reexpansion.

INTERVENTIONS	RATIONALE
6. Record the amount and color of the drainage in the collection chamber q8h. **Do not empty the collection system to measure output**. Instead, mark the level of output on the write-on surface of the drainage unit prn and at the end of each shift.	The chest drainage system is a closed and disposable unit. Frequent disruption increases the risk of infection and recurrent pneumothorax.
7. Consult physician if large amounts of red and bloody drainage accumulate within a short period. Obtain a hemoglobin and hematocrit immediately and prepare for autotransfusion or surgery if prescribed.	Excess bleeding signals hemothorax. Excess blood loss could lead to hypovolemic shock.
8. Keep the tubing free of kinks. **Avoid** routine stripping and milking of the chest tube. Coil extra tubing on the bed to avoid having dependent loops between patient and the drainage chamber.	A kink in the tubing and routine milking and stripping of the tube can lead to a tension pneumothorax or cause fragile lung tissue to be sucked into the tube. Fluid accumulating in dependent loops can block the tube, thus increasing the risk of a tension pneumothorax.
9. Keep the drainage apparatus always below the level of the patient.	Water from the water-seal chamber could be sucked into the chest during inspiration if the chamber is placed at chest level or above it.
10. Encourage use of the incentive spirometer q2h. Maintain effective pain control.	To enhance deep breathing, thus preventing atelectasis. Individuals often resort to shallow breathing to minimize pain.
11. If wall suction is connected to the drainage system and the patient requires transportation off the unit to a diagnostic area within the hospital, do not clamp off the suction tubing connector. Leave it open.	To prevent tension pneumothorax.

INTERVENTIONS	RATIONALE
12. Assist physician with removal of the tube when the chest x ray indicates the lung has reexpanded. • Check facility protocol and procedures and collect necessary supplies. • Assess respiratory status (Appendix A).	Two persons are needed for removal of a chest tube. The physician removes the tube and pulls the purse string suture while the nurse applies a petrolatum dressing. An assessment of respiratory function before the tube is removed provides baseline values.
13. Change the drainage system when the collection chamber is full or if the unit has a crack. Follow appropriate steps to change the unit and maintain strict aseptic technique. • Set up new unit and fill appropriate chamber with sterile water. • Clamp chest tube close to chest wall. • Disconnect old tubing and quickly connect new tubing. Remove clamp and instruct patient to breath normally. • Reapply tape to tubing connections to ensure an airtight connection.	A full system prevents further drainage of air and fluid from the pleural cavity. Aseptic technique helps prevent bacteria from entering the pleural cavity.
14. Consult physician immediately if signs of respiratory distress persist or worsen.	This could indicate tube blockage and a need for further radiologic assessment.

NURSING DIAGNOSIS: ALTERATIONS IN COMFORT: PAIN

RELATED TO FACTORS: Chest tube insertion

DEFINING CHARACTERISTICS: Verbalizes discomfort, tense facial expression, moaning, crying, tense posture

PATIENT OUTCOME (collaborative): Demonstrates relief from discomfort

EVALUATION CRITERIA: Relaxed facial expression, denies discomfort, fewer requests for analgesia, increased inspiratory volume on incentive spirometer

INTERVENTIONS	RATIONALE
1. See care plan on Pain (page 700).	
2. Reposition from a back-lying to a lateral position on **Unaffected side** q2h. **Avoid** placement on affected side.	Lying on affected side is extremely painful and interferes with lung reexpansion.
3. Assist with ADL and ambulation as needed.	To guard against injury.

● ●

NURSING DIAGNOSIS: HIGH RISK FOR INFECTION

RELATED TO FACTORS: Invasive procedure

DEFINING CHARACTERISTICS: Chest tube insertion

PATIENT OUTCOME (collaborative): Demonstrates absence of signs of infection

EVALUATION CRITERIA: Temperature 98.6°F; WBC between 5,000–10,000/mm^3; wound heals after removing chest tube

● ●

INTERVENTIONS	RATIONALE

1. Monitor:
  • CBC reports, particularly WBC
  • appearance of wound with dressing changes
  • temperature q4h
  • appearance of dressing on each shift
	To identify indications of progress toward or deviations from expected outcomes.

INTERVENTIONS	RATIONALE
2. Administer prescribed antibiotics and evaluate their effectiveness. Schedule prescribed medications so a consistent blood level of the medication is maintained. Consult pharmacology references and the pharmacist as needed to avoid drug-to-drug adverse interactions, especially when several medications are prescribed.	Antibiotics often are given as a prophylaxis against infection. Maximum therapeutic effectiveness can best be ensured when a consistent blood level of the agent is maintained and drug-to-drug adverse interactions are prevented. Some medications, when given concurrently, counteract or potentiate the effect of the other.
3. Adhere to universal precautions and strict aseptic technique (hand-washing, wearing gloves, and wearing goggles if contact with body fluids or blood is likely to occur) when performing dressing changes, obtaining a specimen from the drainage unit, or changing the drainage system.	To prevent nosocomial infections.
4. Consult physician if the following occur: • temperature 101°F and above • WBC above 10,000/mm^3 • redness, increased tenderness, and drainage from the wound Follow manufacturer's directions for obtaining a culture specimen from the chest drainage unit.	These findings signal an infection. A culture helps identify the causative organism so appropriate antibiotic therapy can be prescribed. Most chest drainage units have sampling ports. Aseptic technique reduces the risk of nosocomial infection.
5. Reinforce the chest dressing if it becomes loose. If the dressing becomes wet with drainage, apply a new dressing using sterile technique, with the assistance of another caregiver.	An occlusive, airtight dressing must be maintained over the chest tube insertion site to prevent the lung from recollapsing and to reduce the development of subcutaneous emphysema (air trapping in subcutaneous tissue).

Laryngectomy

A **laryngectomy** is performed as treatment for cancer of the larynx. The type of laryngectomy performed varies depending on the extent of the cancer. In addition, the kind of problems a patient faces postlaryngectomy may also vary to some extent depending on the type of laryngectomy performed.

1. **Total laryngectomy** results in loss of voice and a permanent tracheostomy stoma. There is no danger of aspiration of oral feedings because the trachea is no longer connected to the aerodigestive tract. A radical neck dissection is performed with this type of laryngectomy. It involves removal of lymphatic vessels, lymph nodes in the neck, sternocleidomastoid muscle, internal jugular vein, spinal accessory nerve, submandibular salivary gland, and a small portion of the parotid gland (Sawyer, 1990). A skin graft is required. The patient will experience numbness and drooping of the shoulder on the operative side.

2. **Supraglottic** or **horizontal laryngectomy** increases the risk of aspiration of oral feedings since the epiglottis is removed. The voice remains normal, and there is no alteration of the airway.

3. **Vertical** or **hemilaryngectomy** results in permanent hoarseness. There is no danger of aspiration and no alteration of the airway.

4. **Laryngofissure** with partial laryngectomy results in mild hoarseness. There is no danger of aspiration and no alteration of the airway.

The major complications postlaryngectomy are hematoma formation, infection, and salivary fistula. A salivary fistula may occur when a pharyngeal suture ruptures and allows saliva to drain into surrounding tissue. This type fistula usually closes within a few weeks to months depending on its size. The mean LOS for a DRG classification of laryngectomy without complications or comorbid condition is 7.0 days (Lorenz, 1991).

Integrative Care Plans

- Loss
- Preoperative and postoperative care
- Pain
- Radiation therapy (if the patient has had radiation therapy preoperatively)

Discharge Considerations

- Voice rehabilitation
- Community support groups
- Tracheal stoma care
- Tube feedings (if radical neck dissection is performed)
- Follow-up care
- Caloric requirements
- Mouth care
- Activity restrictions

THE PREOPERATIVE PERIOD

 # ASSESSMENT DATA BASE

1. Physical examination based on a general survey (Appendix F) may reveal common manifestations of cancer of the larynx:
   - persistent hoarseness (the earliest symptom)
   - persistent cough
   - dysphagia
   - sensation of a lump in the throat
   - persistent sore throat
   - burning sensation after drinking hot liquids
   - painful Adam's apple
   - enlarged cervical lymph nodes

2. Diagnostic studies:
   - Computerized tomography (CT) scan and barium swallow may reveal the presence of a mass.
   - Laryngoscopy allows for direct viewing of the tumor and direct tissue sampling for biopsy to confirm the diagnosis.

3. See Preoperative and Postoperative Care (page 738).

NURSING DIAGNOSIS: ANXIETY

RELATED TO FACTORS: Knowledge deficit about preoperative and postoperative events, fear of disfigurement

DEFINING CHARACTERISTICS: Verbalizes a specific concern, feelings of inadequacy, or apprehension; requests information; verbalizes lack of understanding

PATIENT OUTCOME: Demonstrates relief from anxiety

EVALUATION CRITERIA: Verbalizes feelings and concerns openly, reports feeling less anxious or afraid, verbalizes understanding of preoperative and postoperative events, verbalizes awareness of need to adapt to physical changes

INTERVENTIONS	RATIONALE
1. See Preoperative and Postoperative Care (page 738).	
2. If a total laryngectomy is to be performed, consult patient and physician about having a member of the Lost Chord Club visit. Arrange for a speech therapist to discuss alternative methods of voice rehabilitation (esophageal speech, artificial larynx, and voice prosthesis). Postpone visits from these resource persons until later in the postoperative period if the patient prefers.	Knowing what to expect and seeing a successful outcome help reduce anxiety and provide hope in reestablishing a new lifestyle.
3. Let the patient know that postoperatively: • one or two days may be spent in the ICU before returning to a regular medical/surgical unit. • a nasogastric tube may be in place. Tube feedings are necessary several weeks after discharge until the incision heals and the ability to swallow has been regained (if a radical neck dissection has been performed). • an artificial airway (either a tracheostomy or laryngectomy tube) may be in place until swelling has subsided. • a tracheostomy cuff or T-tube is attached to the artificial airway to provide humidified oxygen or compressed air.	A knowledge of what to expect from surgical interventions helps reduce anxiety and allows the patient to think of realistic goals.

INTERVENTIONS	RATIONALE
4. If a horizontal or supraglottic laryngectomy is to be performed, teach and have the patient practice how to swallow: • Sit and lean forward with head flexed when eating. • Place a small amount of food at the back of the throat. • Inhale deeply and hold. (This pulls the vocal cords together and closes the entrance of the trachea.) • Swallow using a gulping motion. • Cough and then swallow again to ensure no food is left in the throat. Explain that food aspirated into the trachea causes coughing and that suction equipment is available for use if needed. Reassure the patient that with continued practice consuming foods without aspirating can be mastered. Let the patient know that discomfort with swallowing is experienced until swelling subsides and that pain medication are available to relieve discomfort.	Since the epiglottis is removed with this type of laryngectomy, aspiration of oral feedings is a major problem. Learning how to adapt to physiological changes can be frustrating and cause anxiety. Continual practice helps facilitate learning and adjustment to change.
5. Explain method of communication that will be used postoperatively, such as use of a writing pad or magic slate, until voice rehabilitation is begun. Reassure the patient that after the artificial airway is removed, the ability to produce speech will again be possible with voice rehabilitation, although the sound quality may be changed. Let the patient know that a speech therapist will begin voice rehabilitation after swelling has subsided.	The ability to communicate fosters a sense of security and is essential for functioning as an independent person.
6. Allow the patient to express feelings about surgical outcomes.	Verbalizing feelings helps foster an awareness of reality.

THE POSTOPERATIVE PERIOD

 ## ASSESSMENT DATA BASE:

1. Assess airway patency. **This is a priority.**
2. See Preoperative and Postoperative Care (page 738).
3. Before receiving the patient, ensure the following are at the bedside:
   - extra tracheostomy tube and tracheostomy setup
   - suction equipment
   - humidification system
   - magic slate or writing pad

NURSING DIAGNOSIS: HIGH RISK FOR INEFFECTIVE AIRWAY CLEARANCE

RELATED TO FACTORS: Laryngectomy

DEFINING CHARACTERISTICS: Artificial airway in place (tracheostomy or laryngectomy tube), possibly a permanent tracheal stoma, ineffective coughing with gurgling respirations

PATIENT OUTCOME: Airway remains patent

EVALUATION CRITERIA: Clear breath sounds, respiratory rate 12-24 per minute, normal skin color

INTERVENTIONS	RATIONALE
1. Keep head of bed always elevated at least 30 degrees.	An erect position enhances breathing by reducing pressure against the diaphragm from abdominal pressure.
2. Allow to cough up secretions and wipe airway opening with a tissue. If unable to cough up secretions, suction prn using aseptic technique. Provide a mirror and teach oral and tracheal suctioning.	Suctioning removes secretions and helps keep the airway patent. Self-care fosters independence.
3. Provide care for the tracheostomy or laryngectomy tube q4h according to facility protocol and procedures.	To remove any encrusted material and maintain patency.

INTERVENTIONS	RATIONALE
4. Keep warm humidification applied to the artificial airway.	Moist warm air helps prevent drying of the mucosal lining of the trachea.
5. If oral feedings are started while a cuffed tracheostomy tube is in place, inflate the cuff before feeding. Deflate the cuff afterward if no nausea is experienced.	Inflating the cuff prevents food from entering the trachea.

NURSING DIAGNOSIS: ALTERATION IN COMFORT: PAIN

RELATED TO FACTORS: Tissue trauma secondary to laryngectomy

DEFINING CHARACTERISTICS: Communicates incisional pain and/or pain with swallowing (frowning, placing hand over neck, written request for pain medication, refuses oral feeding)

PATIENT OUTCOME (collaborative): Demonstrates relief from pain

EVALUATION CRITERIA: Positive nod of the head or written statement "yes" when asked if pain is relieved, relaxed posture and facial expression, increased oral intake

INTERVENTIONS	RATIONALE
1. See Pain (page 700).	
2. Administer prescribed oral care q2h.	To relieve sore throat and control breath odor.
3. For headache, administer prescribed analgesic prn and keep head of bed always elevated.	Headaches may be related to postoperative edema due to removal of lymphatic vessels and internal jugular vein. An erect position allows for gravity drainage of fluid and helps decrease pressure.
4. Support the arm and shoulder on the operative side, especially if a radical neck dissection was performed.	To reduce tension on the incision. Skin grafting is performed with a radical neck dissection.

● ●

▶ NURSING DIAGNOSIS: HIGH RISK FOR ALTERATIONS IN NUTRITION: LESS THAN BODY REQUIREMENTS

RELATED TO FACTORS: Impaired swallowing secondary to laryngectomy

DEFINING CHARACTERISTICS: Reports loss of taste and smell, coughing excessively after swallowing, weight loss, refuses oral feedings

PATIENT OUTCOME (collaborative): Demonstrates adequate nutritional intake

EVALUATION CRITERIA: Stable weight, increased oral intake

● ●

INTERVENTIONS	RATIONALE
1. Monitor: • weight weekly • percentage of food consumed at each meal, when oral feedings are allowed	To identify indications of progress toward or deviations from expected outcomes.
2. Administer prescribed tube feeding through N/G tube at scheduled intervals. Teach the patient how to self-administer tube feedings.	Supplemental feedings via an alternative route are necessary to provide adequate nutrition for wound healing until oral feeding can be tolerated. Self-care fosters independence.
3. When oral feedings allowed, offer soft, easily chewable foods such as mashed potatoes, rice, and so on. Consult dietitian about appropriate food choices if patient's oral intake is less than 30%.	To reduce swallowing discomfort. A dietitian is a nutritional specialist who can evaluate the patient's nutritional needs and plan a diet consistent with the patient's needs relative to current condition.
4. Perform measures to relieve xerostomia (dry mouth). • Provide hard, sour candy to suck on if not contraindicated. • Encourage use of artificial saliva (Salivart, XeroLube, Moi-stir). • Instruct dietary department to place a lemon on the plate for each meal. • Instruct patient to moisten mouth with a liquid before placing food in mouth. • Moisten dry foods with sauces or gravy.	An extremely dry mouth impairs swallowing. These measures help increase moisture within the mouth.

INTERVENTIONS	RATIONALE
5. Administer prescribed antiemetics prn.	To control nausea and prevent vomiting.
6. When oral feedings are allowed, remain with the patient during each meal. Review swallowing technique to minimize aspiration. Allow to consume meals alone when able to consume oral foods without coughing.	Difficulty swallowing and coughing triggered by oral feedings can provoke anxiety. A competent caregiver who acts quickly when aspiration occurs fosters reassurance, reduces anxiety, and thereby allows the patient to concentrate on swallowing appropriately.
7. Consult physician if excessive coughing with oral feedings persists.	N/G tube feedings may need to be restarted.

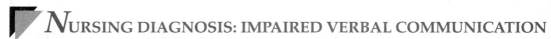

NURSING DIAGNOSIS: IMPAIRED VERBAL COMMUNICATION

RELATED TO FACTORS: Laryngectomy

DEFINING CHARACTERISTICS: Presence of an artificial airway

PATIENT OUTCOME (collaborative): Demonstrates ability to communicate personal needs

EVALUATION CRITERIA: Relaxed facial expression with communication, uses writing pad without showing frustration

INTERVENTIONS	RATIONALE
1. Place the patient in a room close to the nurses' station. Keep call bell within reach at all times. Place a notice (for example, "laryngectomy" or "can't talk") on the intercom system at the nurses' station to alert staff of the need to go to the patient's room when the call light is signaled. Also, post a sign above the patient's bed to alert other healthcare personnel of the patient's inability to talk.	Safety can be enhanced and frustration minimized when the patient is able to communicate needs.

INTERVENTIONS	RATIONALE
2. Keep a magic slate, picture cards, or writing pad and pencil at the bedside.	This allows the patient to communicate needs.
3. If a speech therapist did not visit during the preoperative period, make arrangements for a speech therapist to visit to discuss plans for speech rehabilitation.	A speech therapist is a specialist in speech rehabilitation. Speech rehabilitation is an important part of teaching the total laryngectomy patient how to resume an independent lifestyle.
4. Inform significant others of technique patient is using to communicate needs.	To foster maintenance of relationships with significant others.

● ●

NURSING DIAGNOSIS: HIGH RISK FOR COMPLICATIONS: BLEEDING, SALIVARY FISTULA, INFECTION

RELATED TO FACTORS: Laryngectomy

DEFINING CHARACTERISTICS: Has neck incision accompanied by tracheal stoma and possibly a skin graft

PATIENT OUTCOME (collaborative): Demonstrates no manifestations of complications

EVALUATION CRITERIA: Absence of wound infection, hemorrhage, and salivary fistula

● ●

INTERVENTIONS	RATIONALE
1. Monitor: • intake and output q8h • vital signs q4h • appearance of the wound q8h • amount and color of drainage from the wound drainage device q8h	To identify indications of progress toward or deviations from expected outcome.

INTERVENTIONS	RATIONALE
2. Consult physician if large amounts of red drainage accumulate in the wound drainage device within one hour. Expect a small to moderate amount of serosanguineous drainage (less than 75 mL) the first 24 hours, with drainage decreasing each day.	Continuous bright red drainage signals hemorrhage.
3. Consult physician if the following occur: • signs of hematoma formation (swelling) • development of a salivary fistula (redness, swelling, increased warmth, fever, and increased tenderness of the skin near suture line)	These complications delay wound healing.
4. Change dressings prn using aseptic technique. Consult physician if signs of wound infection occur that include redness, purulent drainage, foul breath odor, increased tenderness, fever. Administer prescribed antibiotics and evaluate their effectiveness.	A clean, dry dressing is less likely to promote bacterial growth. Aseptic technique helps prevent wound infection. Antibiotics are needed to resolve an infection.
5. If a salivary fistula develops, administer continuous moist compresses and continue tube feedings as prescribed.	N/G tube feedings are continued until the fistula heals because food will leak out through the fistula.

NURSING DIAGNOSIS: DISTURBANCE IN SELF-CONCEPT: BODY IMAGE

RELATED TO FACTORS: Change in voice quality, scaring, and possible disfigurement secondary to laryngectomy

DEFINING CHARACTERISTICS: Refuses to participate in self-care activities; communicates low self-esteem, helplessness, hopelessness, or powerlessness; refuses visits from friends; communicates fear of being rejected by others

PATIENT OUTCOME (collaborative): Demonstrates acceptance of self in current situation

EVALUATION CRITERIA: Participates in self-care, communicates ways to incorporate restrictions imposed by a laryngectomy into current lifestyle, maintains open communication with significant others

INTERVENTIONS	RATIONALE
1. See Loss (page 733).	
2. Provide a mirror for the patient to see self. Remind the patient that initial appearance will be distorted until the incisions heal and swelling subsides. Encourage the patient to express feelings about self.	Expressing feelings associated with surgery that permanently alters one's physical appearance facilitates coping. Advance preparation helps minimize the distress of disfigurement.
3. If the patient desires, arrange for a visit by someone who has had the same surgery. Refer the patient and significant others to community support groups (Lost Chord Club, American Cancer Society).	Ongoing support is essential to psychosocial rehabilitation and physical rehabilitation.
4. Begin exercises of the neck and arms; start by allowing the patient to participate in own hygienic care as much as possible. After the sutures have been removed, encourage flexion, extension, and rotation exercises of the neck and shoulder. Initiate a referral to a physical therapist for additional muscle strengthening exercises as prescribed.	Exercises are essential for preventing contractures. A physical therapist is a rehabilitation specialist who can evaluate and prescribe a muscle strengthening program consistent with the patient's health potential.

NURSING DIAGNOSIS: HIGH RISK FOR IMPAIRED HOME MAINTENANCE MANAGEMENT

RELATED TO FACTORS: Knowledge deficit about self-care following a laryngectomy, inadequate support system, insufficient finances

DEFINING CHARACTERISTICS: Communicates lack of understanding, requests information, significant others may request assistance in meeting the patient's physical needs

PATIENT OUTCOME (collaborative): Demonstrates ability to manage adaptive tasks related to current health challenge at home

EVALUATION CRITERIA: Performs stomal self-care, significant other available and can perform required health maintenance tasks safely, suctions self, administers own tube feedings, communicates understanding of the need for follow-up care

• •

INTERVENTIONS	RATIONALE
1. Evaluate the patient's and significant other's ability to perform self-care. Instruct the patient to stand in front of a mirror when doing wound care. Teach and allow return demonstration for the following: a. tracheal stoma care (Table 1-2) b. exercises of the neck and shoulder, which should be done after the incision heals, for example, flexion, rotation, abduction, extension, and adduction c. care of incisions and graft sites using a clean technique for dressing changes, for example, handwashing before and after wound care, applying clean dressings without contaminating the surface placed next to the wound d. self-administration of tube feedings (if discharged with a nasogastric tube) If patient and significant other are unable to perform required maintenance skills, contact social services or discharge planning department to make arrangements for visits by a home health care nurse.	Self-care fosters independence. These departments are responsible for ensuring continuity of care for patients who require assistance in achieving recovery or rehabilitation goals on discharge.

INTERVENTIONS	RATIONALE
2. Instruct the patient and significant other to contact physician for: • signs of wound infection (redness, swelling, increased tenderness) • signs of upper respiratory tract infection (change in color and consistency of stomal secretions accompanied by a foul smell, increased amounts of stomal secretions)	Antibiotics are required to resolve infections. If left untreated, wound healing is impaired.
3.Ensure the patient or significant other: a. has a written appointment for follow-up visits and written instructions for self-care activities at home b. knows the name, purpose, dosage, schedule, and reportable side effects of prescribed medication c. has sufficient supplies (at least five days) to perform required stomal care d. knows where to purchase additional supplies for tracheostomy care and wound care e. has a list of community support groups f. understands how to prepare required diet	Verbal instructions can be easily forgotten. Discharge teaching helps ensure patient compliance.

INTERVENTIONS	RATIONALE
4. Refer the patient and significant other to the dietitian for assistance in planning high-calorie, high-protein meals.	A dietitian is a specialist who can provide correct instructions on selecting foods that help meet the patient's nutritional needs according to age and illness. Following extensive surgery, metabolism is increased. A coexisting illness, such as metastatic cancer, is associated with increased metabolism. Protein and vitamin C are essential for wound healing.
5. Ensure humidification equipment has been delivered to the patient's home before discharge.	A continued source of humidification is needed throughout the recuperative period and periodically thereafter to keep the tracheal lining moist and to aid in healing. Anxiety associated with home management of adaptive tasks related to altered body image can be minimized by having the necessary equipment and supplies readily available.

Mechanical Ventilation

Mechanical ventilation is used to promote alveolar ventilation and thereby reduce the strain of breathing for patients experiencing respiratory failure. Ventilators are classified according to the manner in which they terminate the inspiratory phase:

1. **Volume-cycled** terminates the inspiratory phase after delivering a preset volume of gas. This is the most common type used for adults and children.
2. **Pressure-cycled** terminates the inspiratory phase after delivering a preset pressure.
3. **Time-cycled** terminates the inspiratory phase after a preset time.

Based on results of ABG and the underlying disease process, the physician prescribes the ventilator settings, for example FIO_2 (fraction of inspired oxygen), V_T (tidal volume), and the ventilation mode and rate. The respiratory therapist performs certain bedside pulmonary function tests prn and maintains the ventilator. The nurse monitors the patient's response to therapy and maintains the patient's airway.

Ventilation mode refers to how the patient receives breaths from the ventilator, based on the quality and amount of patient initiated breaths.

The three most commonly used ventilation modes are:

1. **Assist/control** in which the patient initiates breaths and breathes at a higher rate than the preset minimum number of breaths. Each breath delivered is at the tidal volume.
2. **Intermittent mandatory ventilation** (IMV) in which a preset number of mechanical breaths are delivered but the patient breathes spontaneously between without ventilator assistance and at different tidal volumes.
3. **Syncronized intermittent mandatory ventilation** (SIMV) in which the ventilator senses the patient's initiated breath and synchronizes preset breaths with the patient's breath.

IMV and SIMV are used in the weaning process.

When the patient demonstrates the ability to resume independent breathing, the ventilator is discontinued. Parameters indicating this readiness include absence of manifestations of respiratory failure and fluid overload, vital signs within normal limits (WNL), and absence of nutritional deficiencies and biochemical imbalances. To wean the patient, the number of mechanically assisted breaths per minute is gradually reduced. This allows the patient to begin increasing the breathing effort until breathing can be done without ventilator assistance.

Throughout this process, the patient's vital signs, ABG, vital capacity, tidal volume, and inspiratory force are monitored.

Depending on the disease process, the physician may prescribe additional ventilator settings such as:

a. **Positive end-expiratory pressure** (PEEP) that allows a preset amount of air-pressure to remain in the patient's lungs at the end of expiration to keep the alveoli inflated. Tension pneumothorax is the major complication associated with PEEP.

b. **Continuous positive airway pressure** (CPAP) can only be used with patients who have spontaneous respirations. The ventilator provides a continuous flow of airway pressure without delivering a preset volume of air.

To determine the patient's readiness for weaning, the respiratory therapist may assess the following pulmonary function parameters:

a. Minute volume (V_E) — normal value is 10 L/min. It is determined by multiplying the tidal volume by the respiratory rate. It reflects the amount of air inhaled and exhaled with normal breathing in one minute.

b. Respiratory rate — normal range is 12–24 breaths per minute.

c. Tidal volume (V_T) — a value greater than 6.6 mL/kg of ideal body weight is considered normal. It reflects the volume of air inhaled or exhaled with a normal breath.

d. Vital capacity (VC) — normal value is 10–15 mL/kg of body weight or two times the tidal volume. It reflects the amount of air exhaled forcibly after a maximum inhalation.

In caring for the patient on a ventilator, the nurse must assess both the machine and the patient. The nurse also must know what action to take if an alarm on the ventilator is activated. The first priority in assessment is always the patient.

The mean LOS for a DRG of mechanical ventilation is 9.8 days (Lorenz, 1992). When mechanical ventilation is initiated for acute respiratory failure, the patient is placed in ICU. However, patients who require long-term ventilatory support but are medically stable may be cared for in an extended care facility or on a regular medical/surgical unit.

Integrative Care Plans

- IV therapy
- Immobility
- Plan of care for the specific underlying disorder

Discharge Considerations

- See plan of care for the specific underlying disorder

 # *A*SSESSMENT DATA BASE

1. Assess respiratory function (Appendix A).
2. Assess patient's and significant other's response to mechanical ventilation.

●●●●●●●●●●●●●●●●●●●●●●●●●●●●●●

NURSING DIAGNOSIS: IMPAIRED GAS EXCHANGE

RELATED TO FACTORS: Ventilation perfusion imbalance secondary to (specify underlying disease process)

DEFINING CHARACTERISTICS: Gurgling respirations, poor or absent cough effort, hypoxemia, hypercapnia, cyanosis, depressed level of consciousness

PATIENT OUTCOME (collaborative): Demonstrates adequate oxygenation

EVALUATION CRITERIA: ABG within normal limits, normal skin color, pulmonary function parameters within normal limits, clear breath sounds, symmetrical chest expansion

●●●●●●●●●●●●●●●●●●●●●●●●●●●●●●

INTERVENTIONS

RATIONALE

INTERVENTIONS	RATIONALE

1. Assist respiratory therapist, nurse anesthetist, or physician with insertion of the (endotracheal ET) tube and placement on the mechanical ventilator:
 	
• Gather equipment per facility protocol and procedures.
 	
• Notify respiratory therapist of the need for mechanical ventilation.
 	
• If possible, before the procedure explain to patient and significant other:
  a. purpose of intubation
  b. speaking will temporarily be impossible while ET tube is in place
  c. method of communication
 	
• Place patient in a supine position.
 	
• Ensure suction equipment is functioning and ready for use. Suction prn as ET is being inserted.
 	
• Administer sedation as prescribed by the physician if patient is combative.
	Mechanical ventilation is considered urgent treatment. Brief, clear explanations during urgent care procedures help minimize anxiety. The patient must have an artificial airway, either an ET tube or tracheostomy, to be connected to a ventilator. The nurse, physician, and respiratory therapist work as a team to ensure the patient receives optimal ventilation. A chest x-ray helps confirm correct placement of the ET tube.

INTERVENTIONS	RATIONALE
• Immediately after ET tube has been inserted, auscultate breath sounds bilaterally. Ventilate patient with an AMBU bag until ventilator is ready. • Obtain a portable chest x ray, as prescribed.	
2. After placement on the ventilator, monitor: • respiratory function (Appendix A) q1–2h When assessing respiratory rate, count the patient's respiration and document both the respiratory rate set by the ventilator and the patient's independent respiratory rate. The patient's spontaneous breaths will be shallow, whereas machine assisted breaths will be deep. • results of ABG • pulse oximetry (if used to monitor oxygen saturation continuously) • pressures q1h if hemodynamic monitoring devices are in place, for example, pulmonary artery catheter, intra-arterial line • results of chest x ray studies • all ventilator tubing q2h to ensure freedom from kinks and absence of condensation build up • ventilator settings q2-4h to ensure they are set according to physician's orders • tidal volume when the patient initiates a spontaneous breath	To identify indications of progress toward or deviations from expected outcome.

INTERVENTIONS	RATIONALE
3. Suction prn. Intervene appropriately when a ventilator alarm is activated (see Table 1–3).	To maintain airway patency. The ventilator has alarms that signal when the patient is not receiving preset pressures. Prompt action is essential to ensure the patient receives full benefit of the ventilator.
4. Notify physician immediately if breath sounds become absent, accompanied by asymmetrical chest expansion and increased restlessness. Obtain a portable chest x ray and ABG stat as ordered.	These symptoms may signal tension pneumothorax, a major complication most likely to occur with PEEP and CPAP. It occurs when ventilator pressures are too high. A chest x ray confirms this finding. Tension pneumothorax is considered a life-threatening emergency.
5. Keep an Ambu bag at the bedside at all times.	For use when ventilator failure occurs.

NURSING DIAGNOSIS: ANXIETY

RELATED TO FACTORS: Fear of being unable to speak, fear of some aspect of mechanical ventilation (specify)

DEFINING CHARACTERISTICS: Increased respiratory rate that continually activates the pressure alarm on the ventilator, restlessness, attempts to pull out the artificial airway, tense facial expression, constantly uses call bell, may verbalize fears before being intubated

PATIENT OUTCOME (collaborative): Demonstrates less anxiety

EVALUATION CRITERIA: Respiratory rate 12–24 per minute, relaxed facial expression, less frequent use of call bell, follows verbal instructions without physical resistance, less frequent signaling of ventilator high-pressure alarm

INTERVENTIONS	RATIONALE
1. Administer prescribed analgesic, sedative, or paralyzing agent prn when the alert patient becomes restless and continually activates the high-pressure alarm on the ventilator.	To prevent the patient from fighting the ventilator.

INTERVENTIONS	RATIONALE
2. Consult physician if prescribed medication is ineffective in controlling restlessness.	This could signal a need for further assessment such as ABG to determine if an acid-base imablance is present.
3. Explain all procedures in a calm, confident manner. Reassure the patient that a competent caregiver is always close. Remind the patient that the artificial airway temporarily prevents speaking. Keep writing pad and pencil or magic slate at bedside for the patient's use.	A knowledge of what to expect helps reduce anxiety. Patients feel comfortable and reassured that their caregiver is competent by a controlled, confident approach.
4. Apply wrist restraints and explain rationale. Follow facility protocol and procedures regarding use of restraints.	To prevent the patient from accidentally dislodging the artificial airway.
5. If not already informed, explain to significant others what to expect before entering the ICU to visit the patient. Encourage their support of the patient through visitation.	To reduce their anxiety and to build a strong support system for the patient.
6. Inform the patient and significant others about the ventilator alarms. Attend promptly to ventilator alarms.	Sudden unexpected strange noise can evoke anxiety.
7. Provide a quiet environment free of distraction between ongoing assessments and care.	Inadequate rest can be a source of irritability and restlessness.

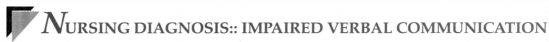

NURSING DIAGNOSIS:: IMPAIRED VERBAL COMMUNICATION

RELATED TO FACTORS: Placement of an artificial air for mechanical ventilation

DEFINING CHARACTERISTICS: Endotracheal tube or tracheostomy tube in place and attached to a mechanical ventilator

PATIENT OUTCOME: Demonstrates less frustration with communication of needs

EVALUATION CRITERIA: Absence of frustration and a relaxed facial expression when using writing pad or magic slate

INTERVENTIONS | RATIONALE

INTERVENTIONS	RATIONALE
1. Provide a writing pad and pencil or magic slate.	To allow written communication of needs.
2. Keep call bell within the patient's reach if patient is alert and oriented. If the patient is on a medical/surgical unit, flag the Kardex and the intercom system as "ventilator patient" or "unable to talk" to alert staff of the need to go to the patient's room when the call light is signaled.	To provide a means for the patient to signal for assistance when needed.

NURSING DIAGNOSIS: HIGH RISK FOR IMPAIRMENT OF SKIN INTEGRITY

RELATED TO FACTORS: Prolonged use of endotracheal tube, bedrest

DEFINING CHARACTERISTICS: Presence of endotracheal tube longer than three days, redness at corner of mouth, dry cracked lips and tongue, reddened bony prominences

PATIENT OUTCOME: Skin remains intact

EVALUATION CRITERIA: Pink, moist oral mucosa and lips; absence of redness at corner of mouth; no skin breakdown over bony prominences

INTERVENTIONS | RATIONALE

INTERVENTIONS	RATIONALE
1. Remove the tape and move the ET tube to the opposite side of the mouth each day. Have another person hold the tube in place while it is being retaped.	To relieve pressure from the corner of the mouth. Two persons are needed to perform this task to reduce the risk of dislodging the ET tube.
2. Record the number on the side of the ET tube that appears at the patient's lip line each day.	To determine if the tube has become dislodged.

INTERVENTIONS	RATIONALE
3. Apply a water soluble lubricant to the lips q2h. Provide oral care according to facility protocol q2-4h.	To provide lubrication.
4. Use the minimum air leak technique to maintain cuff pressure in the ET tube or tracheostomy. That is, release air completely from the cuff, then slowly inflate the cuff with air until no leak is detected (evidenced by patient returning the preset tidal volume).	This technique helps ensure a cuff pressure less than 30 mm Hg thus preventing tracheal necrosis.
5. See Immobility (page 725) for additional measures.	

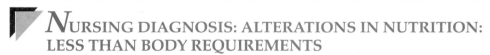

NURSING DIAGNOSIS: ALTERATIONS IN NUTRITION: LESS THAN BODY REQUIREMENTS

RELATED TO FACTORS: Inability to consume oral feedings secondary to placement of an artificial airway, depressed level of consciousness

DEFINING CHARACTERISTICS: Oral ET tube in place, serum chemistry studies show negative nitrogen balance, documented inadequate caloric intake

PATIENT OUTCOME (collaborative): Demonstrates adequate nutritional status

EVALUATION CRITERIA: Serum chemistry studies WNL, weight remains stable

INTERVENTIONS	RATIONALE
1. Monitor: • results of serum chemistry studies, especially the blood urea nitrogen (BUN) and serum sodium • weight at least twice weekly • abdomen q8h (bowel sounds, size, tenderness)	To identify indications of progress toward or deviations from expected outcome. An elevated BUN in the presence of an adequate urinary output and elevated serum sodium signal dehydration and malnutrition.

INTERVENTIONS	RATIONALE
2. Insert N/G tube as prescribed or administer prescribed parenteral feedings, such as total parenteral nutrition (TPN) or peripheral parenteral nutrition (PPN) (see Total Parenteral Nutrition, page 220). If the patient's $PaCO_2$ is persistently elevated, provide low-carbohydrate feedings. Consult dietitian about appropriate diet relative to serum chemistry studies.	Nutritional support is essential for tissue repair and for strengthening the immune system. The end products of carbohydrate metabolism are water and carbon dioxide. The dietitian is a specialist who can evaluate the patient's nutritional status and plan an appropriate diet relative to the patient's current illness.
3. Consult physician if bowel sounds are diminished or absent accompanied by abdominal distention. Withhold tube feedings.	These findings signal paralytic ileus and a need for gastric decompression.

NURSING DIAGNOSIS: HIGH RISK FOR INFECTION

RELATED TO FACTORS: Suctioning of the airway, presence of an artificial airway

DEFINING CHARACTERISTICS: Rising temperature and WBC; alterations in the color, consistency, smell, and volume of tracheal secretions

PATIENT OUTCOME (collaborative): Demonstrates absence of infection

EVALUATION CRITERIA: Temperature 98.6°F, WBC between 5,000-10,000/mm³, negative sputum cultures

INTERVENTIONS	RATIONALE
1. Monitor: • CBC reports, especially WBC • temperature q4h • tracheal secretions for changes in color, consistency, smell, and amount	To identify indications of progress toward or deviations from expected outcome.

INTERVENTIONS	RATIONALE
2. Obtain a tracheal specimen for culture if secretions change color are accompanied by foul odor, and are tenacious and copious. Administer antibiotic as prescribed and evaluate its effectiveness.	A culture helps identify the causative organism so appropriate antibiotics can be prescribed. Antibiotics are needed to resolve infections.
3. Adhere to universal precautions and aseptic technique when suctioning.	To prevent nosocomial infections for self and patient.
4. If a tracheostomy is in place, perform care according to facility protocol and procedures.	To reduce the probability of infection.

NURSING DIAGNOSIS: HIGH RISK FOR DECREASED CARDIAC OUTPUT

RELATED TO FACTORS: Use of PEEP with mechanical ventilation

DEFINING CHARACTERISTICS: Cardiac dysrhythmias, tachycardia, falling BP, increased restlessness, weight gain, edema, rales, diminished peripheral pulses, serum sodium below normal, abnormal hemodynamic parameters such as elevated central venous pressure (CVP) and pulmonary artery pressure and low cardiac output

PATIENT OUTCOME (collaborative): Demonstrates adequate cardiac output

EVALUATION CRITERIA: Stable weight, urine output approximates fluid intake, clear breath sounds, absence of edema, heart rate 60–100 beats per minute, hemodynamic pressures WNL, serum sodium WNL

INTERVENTIONS	RATIONALE
1. See Congestive Heart Failure (page 462).	Decreased cardiac output may occur abruptly with mechanical ventilation changes, especially with PEEP and changes in tidal volume. As a result of these changes, venous return to the heart is decreased and cardiac output falls.

Lung Surgery

Resection of the lung involves removal of an entire lung (pneumonectomy) or removal of a portion of a lung (segmental resection, lobectomy, or wedge resection). If metastases has occurred within the mediastinum, a radical pneumonectomy may be performed, which involves resection of mediastinal lymph nodes, resection of a portion of the chest wall or diaphragm, or removal of the parietal pleura.

A pneumonectomy is commonly performed through a posterolateral incision at the 5th intercostal space. Drainage tubes are generally not used because:

1. They would drain the fluid from the empty space, thus precipitating a mediastinal shift.

2. They would be a source of infection.

To prevent mediastinal shift and eliminate dead space postpneumonectomy, air and approximately three liters of fluid are allowed to accumulate in the pleural space. The space, previously occupied by the lung, fills with serosanguineous fluid and eventually solidifies in 1–7 months.

Chest tubes are often inserted and connected to a water-seal drainage system following a lobectomy, wedge resection, or segmental resection.

Potential complications postlung surgery are:

a. respiratory insufficiency mainly caused by atelectasis, restriction of the chest wall due to incisional pain, mediastinal shift, and retention of secretions due to ineffective coughing

b. bronchopleural fistula as a result of rupture of the bronchial stump suture. Infection and trauma from deep nasotracheal suctioning are the primary causative factors.

c. infection

d. hemorrhage

e. pulmonary edema because the remaining lung has to accommodate the cardiac output that was previously handled by two lungs

The mean LOS for a DRG classification of major chest procedures without complications is 11.5 days (Lorenz, 1991). The elderly are particularly prone to postoperative complications because of the normal pulmonary system changes that occur with aging (decreased vital capacity and coughing efficiency due to decreased lung tissue compliance, calcification of vertebral cartilage causing reduced chest expansion) (Blair, 1990).

106

Integrative Care Plans

- Loss
- Preoperative and postoperative care
- IV therapy
- Fluid and biochemical imbalances
- Immobility

Discharge Considerations

- Follow-up care
- Medications to continue at home
- Signs and symptoms requiring medical attention
- Activity restrictions
- Wound care

THE PREOPERATIVE PERIOD

 # ASSESSMENT DATA BASE

1. History or presence of disorders requiring lung surgery:
   - pulmonary lesions, such as lung abscess, bronchiectasis, extensive unilateral tuberculosis (common indications for a segmental resection, wedge resection, or a lobectomy)
   - bronchogenic carcinoma (chief indication for a pneumonectomy or lobectomy)
2. Physical examination based on an assessment of the respiratory system (Appendix A) and general survey (Appendix F) to establish baseline values.
3. Assess the patient's and significant other's feelings about the surgery.

NURSING DIAGNOSIS: HIGH RISK FOR ANXIETY

RELATED TO FACTORS: Knowledge deficit about preoperative and postoperative events, fear of some aspect of surgery

DEFINING CHARACTERISTICS: Verbalizes lack of understanding, requests information, verbalizes fear of some aspect of surgery or its outcomes

PATIENT OUTCOME: Demonstrates less anxiety

EVALUATION CRITERIA: Verbalizes understanding of preoperative and postoperative events, fewer reports of feeling anxious or afraid, reports feeling less nervous

INTERVENTIONS	RATIONALE
1. See Preoperative and Postoperative Care (page 738).	
2. Let the patient know that 2-4 days are spent in an ICU postoperatively because of the acute physiological changes that occur after lung surgery and that the following intrusive devices may be in place: • Swan-Ganz catheter or multilumen central venous pressure (CVP) catheter to monitor hemodynamic status • an intra-arterial line to monitor bood pressure (BP) and obtain blood samples for repeat ABGs analysis • Foley catheter for monitoring urinary output	Compliance is enhanced and anxiety reduced when patients understand what to expect when undergoing surgery.
3. Teach and have the patient practice: • deep breathing • splinting the chest when coughing: a. Place your hands anteriorly and posteriorly over the patient's chest wall on operative side. b. Apply firm pressure as patient coughs.	Practicing these activities before surgery helps facilitate a smoother recovery after surgery.

THE POSTOPERATIVE PERIOD

 *A*SSESSMENT DATA BASE

1. Physical examination based on a routine postoperative assessment (Appendix L). Postpneumonectomy expect to find:
   • asymmetrical chest expansion with breathing
   • a temporary rise in pulmonary artery (PA) and right ventricular pressures during the immediate postoperative period, with a gradual return to normal range

- an increase in vital capacity and total lung capacity of the remaining lung resulting from hyperventilation (increase in the rate and depth of breathing) as it compensates for loss of the other lung and meets the oxygen needs of the body
- narrowing of the intercostal spaces on the operative side caused by elevation of the diaphragm. This change contributes to reduced compliance of the remaining lung and affects the patient's exercise tolerance. Consequently, the remaining lung has to work harder to accommodate the cardiac output normally handled by two lungs.

2. Assess position of the trachea and the point of maximal impulse (PMI) of the heart. The trachea should be in its normal midline position and the PMI palpated at the 5th intercostal space, left midclavicular line.

3. See Preoperative and Postoperative Care (page 738) for additional assessments.

NURSING DIAGNOSIS: HIGH RISK FOR IMPAIRED GAS EXCHANGE

RELATED TO FACTORS: Postpneumonectomy complications such as respiratory insufficiency, bronchopleural fistula, pulmonary edema

DEFINING CHARACTERISTICS: Abnormal ABG and pulmonary function tests (PFT), cyanosis, tachycardia accompanied by tachypnea, increasing dyspnea, rales

PATIENT OUTCOME (collaborative): Demonstrates adequate oxygenation

EVALUATION CRITERIA: Respiratory rate 12-24 per minute, pulse rate 60-100 beats per minute, normal skin color, ABG and PFT within acceptable range, denies dyspnea, clear breath sounds

INTERVENTIONS

1. Monitor:
   - pulse oximetry
   - results of ABG, PFT, and chest x ray reports
   - respiratory status (Appendix A) and position of the trachea and PMI q2h x 48 hours, then q4h x 48 hours, then q8h when stable
   - hemodynamic status qh (PA pressure, CVP)
   - vital signs q1-2h
   - intake and output q8h

RATIONALE

To identify indications of progress toward or deviations from expected outcome.

INTERVENTIONS	RATIONALE
2. Encourage deep breathing with use of the incentive spirometer q2h.	To open the alveoli, thus preventing atelectasis.
3. Reposition q2h by tilting to the operative side or placing in a back-lying position. **Avoid positioning the patient on the nonoperative side for long periods.** Maintain a semi-Fowler's or Fowler's position always.	Placing the patient on the nonoperative side restricts full expansion of the remaining lung. An erect position allows fuller lung expansion by reducing abdominal pressure against the diaphragm.
4. Assist the respiratory therapist as needed with prescribed pulmonary treatments if pulmonary congestion occurs.	The respiratory therapist is a specialist in respiratory care and generally performs all prescribed respiratory treatments such as nebulization, postural drainage, and percussion.
5. Discourage smoking.	Smoking causes vasoconstriction that interferes with O_2/CO_2 exchange.
6. Administer supplemental oxygen at the prescribed flow rate. Adjust, as ordered, according to oximetry and/or ABG to maintain oxygen saturation above 90%.	Supplemental oxygen increases the amount of oxygen available to tissue.
7. Consult physician immediately and obtain ABG stat if the following occur: • confusion in a previously alert and oriented patient • restlessness accompanied by tachycardia and tachypnea	These findings could signal hypoxia. ABG can best diagnose this oxygen deficit if oximetry is not in place.
8. Consult physician immediately and obtain prescribed diagnostic studies (portable chest x ray and ABG) stat if signs and symptoms of complications are detected. Prepare for return to surgery if indicated: a. hemorrhage — hypotension accompanied by tachycardia, tachypnea, weak thready pulse, cool clammy pale skin,	Although these complications are rare, they can be fatal. Hemorrhage often is the result of a slipped ligature on a bronchial artery. Bronchopleural fistula is the result of a slipped ligature on the bronchial stump. This can occur with too vigorous endotracheal suctioning using a rigid suction catheter. A chest x ray is most diagnostic. Surgery is required to resolve these complications.

INTERVENTIONS	RATIONALE
diminished loss of consciousness (LOC), diminished breath sounds, and tracheal deviation b. bronchopleural fistula — subcutaneous emphysema (a gritty, sandlike sensation palpated over the skin near the operative site), dyspnea, productive cough of serosanguineous fluid, and change in mental status	
9. If a bronchopleural fistula is suspected, immediately place the patient in a Fowler's position.	Proper positioning is essential to prevent "drowning" in the fluid.
10. Consult physician immediately, if signs of tracheal deviation or if a shift in the PMI of the heart toward the nonoperative side occur. Obtain a portable chest x ray stat as ordered.	These findings signal mediastinal shift. A shift of mediastinal contents (heart and remaining lung) interferes with full expansion of the remaining lung, thereby predisposing patient to atelectasis. A chest x ray confirms mediastinal shift.
11. Institute aggressive pulmonary toileting qh if fever occurs during the first 24–48 hours. Suggest ultrasonic nebulizer treatments if breath sounds indicate congestion.	Fever within the first 48 hours postoperatively signals atelectasis.
12. **Avoid** deep vigorous nasotracheal or endotracheal suctioning. If unable to cough up secretions, use gentle suctioning with a soft-tip rubber suction catheter.	To avoid perforating the sutures on the bronchial stump following a pneumonectomy.
13. Consult physician if PA pressure or CVP rises above the normal limit, coupled with a drop in urinary output, hypertension, tachycardia, and pulmonary rales. Reduce fluid intake and administer bronchodilators and diuretics as ordered. Maintain a semi-Fowler's position.	These findings signal fluid overload. Increased intravascular volume leads to increased pressure. A fluid overload places additional strain on the remaining lung, which now must handle the circulating volume for two lungs. An erect position reduces venous return. A persistently high PA pressure can lead to pulmonary hypertension and ultimately cor pulmonale.

Nursing Diagnosis: HIGH RISK FOR INFECTION

RELATED TO FACTORS: Surgical incision, retained pulmonary secretions, reduced immunity secondary to radiation therapy or chemotherapy

DEFINING CHARACTERISTICS: WBC above 10,000/mm^3; temperature above 99°F; redness, increased tenderness, purulent drainage from incision

PATIENT OUTCOME (collaborative): Absence of infection

EVALUATION CRITERIA: Temperature 98.6°F, WBC between 5,000-10,000/mm^3, wound heals

INTERVENTIONS	RATIONALE
1. See Preoperative and Postoperative Care (page 738).	
2. Provide emesis basin, tissue, and receptacle for proper disposal of tissue if the patient expectorates copious amounts of secretions. Adhere to universal precautions when handling blood or body secretions.	To prevent nosocomial infections.

Nursing Diagnosis: PAIN

RELATED TO FACTORS: Surgical incision

DEFINING CHARACTERISTICS: Reports pain, tense facial expression, moaning, guarding behavior

PATIENT OUTCOME (collaborative): Demonstrates relief from pain

EVALUATION CRITERIA: Denies pain, relaxed facial expression, absence of moaning

INTERVENTIONS	RATIONALE
1. See Pain (page 700).	

NURSING DIAGNOSIS: ACTIVITY INTOLERANCE

RELATED TO FACTORS: Reduced lung capacity secondary to lung surgery

DEFINING CHARACTERISTICS: Reports shortness of breath and fatigue with minimal exertion, sustained increased respiration and pulse rate at rest following minimal exertion

PATIENT OUTCOME: Demonstrates increased tolerance to physical activities

EVALUATION CRITERIA: Performs ADL without reporting shortness of breath, fatigue, or weakness, respiratory rate and pulse rate return to normal limits within one minute after cessation of physical activity

INTERVENTIONS	RATIONALE
1. Check pulse and respiratory rate before and after activity. Monitor for signs and symptoms of activity intolerance with ambulation and when performing ADL, for example, diaphoresis, complaints of fatigue, and SOB with exertion, sustained increase in respiration and pulse rate at rest following a physical activity. Discontinue the activity and allow rest if these symptoms occur.	These findings indicate intolerance to the physical activity.
2. Allow uninterrupted rest periods between activities. Increase physical activities gradually.	Rest helps restore body energy.
3. Assist with planning leisure activities that require minimal energy expenditure (reading, writing, board games, handicrafts).	Leisure activities help relieve boredom. Sustained inactivity can lead to boredom that accentuates feelings of fatigue.
4. Provide a warm, quiet, pain-free environment during rest periods.	To promote rest.
5. Ensure adequate pain control.	Patients often restrict their movements in an attempt to control pain. Activities are better tolerated when pain free.
6. Notify physician if signs and symptoms of activity intolerance persist or worsen.	This could signal the beginning of complications (page 106).

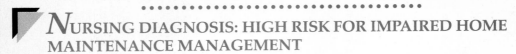

NURSING DIAGNOSIS: HIGH RISK FOR IMPAIRED HOME MAINTENANCE MANAGEMENT

RELATED TO FACTORS: Knowledge deficit about self-care on discharge, insufficient finances, inadequate support system

DEFINING CHARACTERISTICS: Verbalizes lack of understanding, requests information, reports inability to manage self-care activities, reports lack of adequate support system

PATIENT OUTCOME (collaborative): Demonstrates ability to meet home care needs on discharge

EVALUATION CRITERIA: Verbalizes understanding of instructions, performs self-care procedures correctly, verbalizes availability of community resources that can provide assistance as needed

INTERVENTIONS	RATIONALE
1. Ensure the patient or significant other has: • written appointment for follow-up care and written instructions for self-care activities at home • list of medications for home use, including name, dosage, schedule, purpose, and reportable side effects	Verbal instructions may be easily forgotten.
2. Evaluate patient's need for an analgesic. Let the patient know that some discomfort and numbness might continue for several weeks until the wound has completely healed. Ensure the patient has a prescription for a mild analgesic.	To make the recovery period more comfortable.
3. If discharged with a dressing in place, ensure the patient can perform wound care. Teach the patient and significant other aseptic technique for wound care and arrange a return demonstration. Provide at least a one week supply of wound care supplies.	The best method to evaluate a psychomotor skill is to have the learner return the demonstration.

ALARM/POSSIBLE CAUSES	ACTION
2. Low pressure alarm goes off frequently. Possibly due to: a. leak in system (possible crack in tubing, tubing disconnected, leak in balloon around airway)	Reconnect tubing. Aspirate air from cuff and compare findings with initial amount used to establish a minimal occlusive seal. Notify respiratory therapist and physician of a significant difference. Artificial airway will require changing if cuff develops a leak.
3. Tidal volume alarm goes off frequently. Possibly due to: a. absence of spontaneous breathing with SIMV b. increased stiffing of lungs c. additional causes are same as those for high and low pressure alarms	Check level at which bellow rises to compare with preset tidal volume. Follow same actions as for high and low pressure alarms.

BIBLIOGRAPHY

Benedict, S. (1989). The suffering associated with lung cancer. **Cancer Nursing, 12,** 34–40.

Bevan, N.E. (1990). Nursing care of the patient with a unilateral lung injury. **Critical Care Nurse, 10,** 85–88.

Blair, G., & Sharpe, L.D. (1989). Nutrition support in respiratory disorders. **Nutrition and Clinical Practice, 4L,** 173–175.

Blair, K.A. (1990). Aging: Physiological aspects and clinical implications. **Nurse Practitioner, 15,** 14–16, 18, 23, 26–28.

Caruthers, D.D. (1990). Infectious pneumonia in the elderly. **American Journal of Nursing, 90,** 56–60.

Crowe, M., & Ultrino, C. (1990). Psychosocial implications of lung cancer. **Journal of Practical Nursing, 40,** 36–68.

Fennelly, K.P., & Stulbarg, M.S. (1991). Chronic bronchitis: Breath sounds, chest status, and comprehensive treatment. **Consultant, 31,** 75–78, 83–44, 88–90.

Friday, G.A. (1990). Guiding the "difficult" asthmatic. **Emergency Medicine, 22,** 130–131, 135, 139–140.

Geisman, L.K. (1989). Advances in weaning from mechanical ventilation. **Critical Care, 1,** 697–705.

Holcomb, S. S. (1991). Pulmonary Embolism: Preventing a Disaster. **RN, 54,** 52–59.

Hubmayr, R.D. (1990). Physiologic approach to mechanical ventilation. **Critical Care Medicine, 18,** 103–13.

Lorenz, E.W. (1992). **1992 St. Anthony's DRG Working Guidebook.** Alexandria: St. Anthony Publishing Company.

Markowitz, S.M. (1990). Pneumococcal pneumonia: Recognizing and treating this persistent disease. **Postgraduate Medicine, 88,** 33–36, 39–47, 101–102.

Maunder, R.J., & Hudson, L.D. (1990). Pharmacologic strategies for treating the adult respiratory distress syndrome. **Respiratory Care, 35,** 241–246.

North American Nursing Diagnosis Association (1990). **Taxonomy I.** St. Louis: North American Nursing Diagnosis Association.

Petty, T.L. (1990). Chronic obstructive pulmonary disease — Can we do better? **Chest, 97,** 2S–5S.

Ramsey, K.M. (1990). Viral pneumonias: A diagnostic and therapeutic challenge. **Postgraduate Medicine, 88,** 49–50, 53–6, 101–102.

Richardson, J.L., Graham, J.W., & Shelton, D.R. (1989). Social environment and adjustment after laryngectomy. **Health and Social Work, 14,** 283–292.

Roberts, S.L. (1990). High-permeability pulmonary edema: nursing assessment, diagnosis, and interventions. **Heart Lung, 19,** 287–300.

Rostad, M. (1990). Advances in the nursing management of patients with lung cancer. **Nursing Clinics of North America, 25,** 393–403.

Rumbak, M.J. (1991). Modern management of acute asthma. **Hospital Medicine, 5,** 41–52.

Sawyer, D.L., & Bruya, M.A. (1990). Care of the patient having radical neck surgery or permanent laryngostomy: A nursing diagnostic approach. **Focus On Critical Care, 17,** 166–73.

Shanies, H.M. (1990). Mechanical ventilation: Anticipating complications. **Emergency Medicine, 22,** 108, 111–114.

Stiesmeyer, J.K. (1991). What triggers a ventilator alarm? **American Journal of Nursing, 91,** 60–64.

Vaughn, P., & Brooks, C. Jr. (1990). Adult respiratory distress syndrome: A complication of shock. **Critical Care Nursing Clinics of North America, 2,** 235–253.

C

HAPTER TWO
Problems of the Urinary System

Urinary Tract Infection

Urinary tract infection (UTI) is a general term that refers to a bacterial infection in the urinary tract. Any of several bacteria can be the causative organism. An upper UTI is located in the ureters or the kidney, while a lower UTI is located in the urethra or bladder. The infection can originate anywhere in the urinary tract and spread to adjacent areas. Untreated urinary tract infections can result in renal failure.

There are three main sources of entry for the bacteria that cause urinary tract infection. The most common source is through the meatus, resulting in an ascending infection. Descending infections originate in blood or lymph and often result in pyelonephritis — infection in the kidney. This is the most serious UTI because it often leads to renal failure (Conway, 1989).

UTI occurs most frequently in adult women and increase in incidence with age and sexual activity. Although the reason is not clearly understood, it is thought that women are more susceptible to infection than men because of a shorter urethra and the absence of antimicrobial substances such as those found in seminal fluid.

Types of UTIs are:
- urethritis — urethra
- cystitis — bladder
- ureteritis — ureter
- pyelonephritis — kidney

Hospitalization for lower urinary tract infections is not usually required unless intravenous antibiotic therapy is instituted. Nosocomial UTIs can prolong hospital stay. Descending infections in the upper tract often require hospitalization for intravenous antibiotic therapy. The mean length of stay (LOS) for a diagnostic related group (DRG) classification of UTI 4.9 days (Lorenz, 1991).

General Medical Management

- Pharmacotherapy:
  - antibiotics

Integrative Care Plans

• IV therapy

Discharge Considerations

• Medications prescribed for home use
• Follow-up care
• Prevention of recurrences

 # ASSESSMENT DATA BASE

1. History or presence of risk factors:
   • history of previous UTI
   • obstruction in urinary tract
2. Presence of factors that predispose patient to a nosocomial (hospital acquired) infection:
   • Foley catheter in place
   • prolonged immobility
   • incontinence
3. Assess for clinical manifestations of UTI:
   • urgency
   • frequency
   • dysuria
   • foul-smelling urine
   • pain—usually suprapubic in lower UTI and flank pain in upper UTI (percuss the costovertebral area to assess flank tenderness)
   • fever, especially with upper UTI
4. Diagnostic studies:
   • Urinalysis (UA) shows bacteriuria, white blood cells, and WBC casts with kidney involvement.
   • Urine culture identifies the causative organism.
   • Antibody-coated bacteria test for the presence of antibody-coated bacteria is indicative of pyelonephritis.
   • Kidney, ureter, and bladder (KUB) x ray identifies gross structural anomalies.
   • Intravenous pyelogram (IVP) identifies inflammatory changes or structural abnormalities.
5. Assess the patient's feelings about the treatment and the therapy outcome. Concerns for women often focus on fear of recurrence, which causes avoidance of sexual activity. The pain and fatigue associated with infection can affect job performance and activities of daily living (ADL).

Nursing Diagnosis: Pain

RELATED TO FACTORS: Urinary tract infection

DEFINING CHARACTERISTICS: Verbalizes burning-type pain with voiding, verbalizes flank pain that increases in intensity with percussion of flank area

PATIENT OUTCOME (collaborative): Demonstrates absence of pain

EVALUATION CRITERIA: Denies pain with voiding, denies pain with percussion of flank area

INTERVENTIONS	RATIONALE
1. Monitor: a. urine output for changes in color, smell, and voiding pattern b. intake and output q8h c. results of repeat UA tests	To identify indications of progress toward or deviations from expected outcomes.
2. Consult physician if: • previously clear amber–yellow urine appears reddish, burnt orange, smokey, or cloudy • pattern of voiding changes, for example, frequent voiding of small quantities, hesitancy, postvoiding dribbling • pain persists or worsens	These findings can signal further tissue injury and a need for more extensive testing, such as radiological studies, if not previously performed.
3. Administer prescribed analgesic prn and evaluate its effectiveness.	Analgesics block the pain pathway, thus reducing pain.
4. If frequency is a problem, ensure access to the bathroom, bedside commode, or bedpan. Encourage the patient to void whenever the desire is felt.	Frequent voiding reduces stasis of urine in the bladder and discourages the bacterial growth.
5. Administer prescribed antibiotic. Make a variety of fluids available, including fresh water at the bedside. Force fluids, up to 2400 mL/day.	The resulting increased urine output facilitates frequent voiding and helps flush the urinary tract.

NURSING DIAGNOSIS: HIGH RISK FOR INFECTION

RELATED TO FACTORS: Presence of nosocomial risk factors

DEFINING CHARACTERISTICS: Incontinence, prolonged immobility, indwelling catheter

PATIENT OUTCOME: Demonstrates absence of nosocomial urinary tract infection

EVALUATION CRITERIA: Voids clear urine without discomfort, UA within normal limits, urine culture shows no new bacteria

INTERVENTIONS	RATIONALE
1. Provide perineal care with soap and water every shift. If the patient is incontinent, wash the perineal area as soon as possible.	To prevent contamination of the urethra.
2. If an indwelling catheter is in place, provide catheter care twice a day (as part of the morning bath and at bedtime) and after each bowel movement.	The catheter provides a route for bacteria to enter the bladder and ascend in the urinary tract.
3. Adhere to universal precautions (handwashing before and after direct contact, wearing gloves) when contact with the body fluid or blood is likely to occur (giving perineal care or catheter care, emptying the urinary drainage bag, collecting a urine specimen). Maintain strict asepsis when catheterizing and when obtaining a urine specimen from an indwelling catheter.	To prevent cross contamination.
4. Unless contraindicated, reposition the immobile patient every two hours and encourage a fluid intake of at least 2400 mL/day. Assist with ambulation as needed.	To prevent stasis of urine.

INTERVENTIONS	RATIONALE
5. Initiate measures to maintain an acid urine: • Increase intake of cranberry juice. • Administer prescribed urine-acidifying medication.	An acid urine inhibits bacterial growth. Because large quantities of cranberry juice are required to achieve and maintain an acid urine, the increased fluid intake rather than the juice may account for the effect in treating UTI.

NURSING DIAGNOSIS: HIGH RISK FOR NONCOMPLIANCE

RELATED TO FACTORS: Knowledge deficit about condition, diagnostic studies, treatment, and self-care at home

DEFINING CHARACTERISTICS: Questions need to complete antibiotic therapy as prescribed if no longer symptomatic, reports history of recurrence of UTIs, requests information, verbalizes lack of understanding

PATIENT OUTCOME: Demonstrates willingness to comply with therapeutic plan

EVALUATION CRITERIA: Verbalizes understanding of condition, diagnostic studies, treatment plan, and preventive self-care measures

INTERVENTIONS	RATIONALE
1. Provide information about: a. source of infection b. measures to prevent spread or recurrence c. prescribed antibiotics, including name, purpose, dose, schedule, and reportable side effects d. diagnostic studies, including: • purpose • brief description • preparation required before test • care after test	Knowing what to expect lessens anxiety and helps foster patient compliance with the therapeutic plan.

INTERVENTIONS	RATIONALE
2. Ensure the patient or significant other has a written appointment for follow-up care and written instructions for preventive measures.	Verbal instructions may be easily forgotten.
3. Instruct the patient to take all of the antibiotic as prescribed, to drink at least eight glasses of fluid daily, especially water and cranberry juice, and to notify physician immediately if an infection is suspected.	Patients often stop taking their medication when symptoms have subsided. Fluids help flush the kidneys. The pyruvic acid of cranberry juice helps keep the urine acid. An acid environment helps prevent bacterial growth. Early detection allows for initiation of antibiotic therapy before the infection becomes widespread.
4. Advise females at risk for reinfection to: • urinate when the need is felt and after sexual intercourse • wipe from front to back after a bowel movement • avoid using bubble bath and strongly perfumed soaps • wear cotton rather than nylon underwear	To keep the lower tract free of bacteria. Proper cleansing after toileting avoids contaminating the urethra. Some soaps can cause perineal irritation. Cotton clothing allows better air circulation to permit drying of the perineal area.
5. Allow the patient to express feelings and concerns about the therapeutic plan.	To detect clues indicative of possible noncompliance and to foster acceptance of the therapeutic plan.

Glomerulonephritis

Glomerulonephritis (also called nephritic syndrome) may be acute, in which case the person may recover full kidney function, or chronic, which is characterized by a slow, insidious, progressive loss of renal function ultimately leading to end-stage renal disease. It can take 30 years for the renal damage to reach end-stage. At this point, some type of intervention such as dialysis or renal transplant is needed to sustain life. The elderly are especially at high risk for developing end-stage renal disease because of the normal physiological changes that occur in the kidney with the aging process (decreased number of renal nephrons) (Blair, 1990).

Glomerulonephritis is a syndrome characterized by inflammation of the glomeruli following exposure to some antigen that may be endogenous (such as a circulating thyroglobulin) or exogenous (infectious agent or coexisting systemic disease process). The host (kidneys) recognizes the antigen as foreign and begins to produce antibodies against it. This inflammatory response leads to a cascade of pathophysiological alterations, including decreased glomerular filtration rate (GFR), increased permeability of the glomerular capillary wall to plasma proteins (primarily albumin) and RBCs, and abnormal retention of sodium and water that suppresses the production of renin and aldosterone (Glassock, 1988).

A variety of glomerulopathies exist, each with different clinical presentations. Thus, the disease is classified according to morphology, etiology, pathogenesis, clinical syndrome, or a combination thereof. Each type of acute glomerulopathy may lead to manifestations of renal failure within three months of onset. It is then termed rapidly progressive glomerulonephritis, necessitating different initial medical interventions.

This discussion focuses on acute postinfectious glomerulonephritis. This glomerulonephritis generally follows a group A beta-hemolytic streptococcal pharyngeal or skin infection. Also, it may be caused by other bacterial, viral, protozoal, and fungal infections.

The immunopathologic findings associated with acute postinfectious glomerulonephritis include accumulation of immunoglobulins (mainly IgG), fibrin, and complement components (mainly C_3) along the glomerular capillary wall (Glassock, 1988). As a result, the surface area for filtration is reduced, leading to a decreased GFR. Urinary output falls and becomes concentrated.

Normally, the glomerular capillary wall acts as a barrier to plasma proteins, excluding molecules of a certain size and isoelectric charge from the ultrafiltrate. In acute glomerulonephritis, the anionic constituents (responsible for maintaining a charge-selective barrier) of the glomerular basement membrane are lost. In response, the pores of the capillary membrane enlarge, permitting large molecules (such as protein) to readily pass into the urine (proteinuria).

Protein loss leads to a decreased plasma oncotic pressure. Glomerular capillary pressure increases as a result of basement membrane blockage, and the Bowman's space form deposits of circulating antigen-antibody complement. These changes trigger increased tubular sodium and water retention and suppression of renin and aldosterone production. The clinical outcomes are circulatory congestion (edema, hypertension, pulmonary edema), hyperkalemia, and hyperchloremic renal tubular acidosis (Glassock, 1988).

The mean LOS for a DRG classification of glomerulonephritis is 4.9 days, and 4.3 days for nephrotic syndrome (Lorenz, 1991).

General Medical Management

- Dietary modifications:
  - restriction of fluid and sodium
  - protein restriction if BUN is severely elevated
- Pharmacotherapy:
  - immunosuppressive therapy such as cytotoxic agents and steroids for rapid progressive glomerulonephritis
  - diuretics, particularly the loop diuretics such as furosemide (Lasix), and Bumex
  - dialysis, for end-stage renal disease

Integrative Care Plans

- Loss (if end-stage renal disease develops)
- Fluid and biochemical imbalance
- IV therapy
- Dialysis (if end-stage renal disease develops)

Discharge Considerations

- Follow-up care
- Medications to continue at home
- Signs and symptoms requiring medical attention
- Measures to prevent repeat urinary tract infections

 # ASSESSMENT DATA BASE

1. History or presence of risk factors:
   - immune complex diseases such as systemic lupus erythematosus and scleroderma
   - exposure to nephrotoxic drugs or substances such as antimicrobials, anti-inflammatory agents, chemotherapeutic agents, contrast media, pesticides, illicit drugs, or heavy metals.
   - previous skin or throat infections with beta-hemolytic streptococcus or hepatitis

2. Physical examination based on a general survey (Appendix F) may reveal:
   - hematuria
   - edema—commonly appears on the face (periorbital) and legs but also may appear as ascites, pulmonary edema, or pleural effusion
   - hypertension
   - decreased urine output with decreased specific gravity
   - dark (tea-colored) urine
   - weight gain due to fluid retention
   - headache, irritability, or mild alterations in mentation due to hypertension

3. Diagnostic studies:
   - Urinalysis (UA) shows gross hematuria, protein, dysmorphic (misshapen) RBCs, leukocytes, and hyaline casts. The presence of dysmorphic RBCs indicates the bleeding originated in the glomeruli.
   - Glomerular filtration rate (GFR) is reduced. Creatinine clearance in the urine is used as a measure of GFR. A 24-hour urine specimen is collected. A blood sample for serum creatinine is also collected about halfway through the collection of urine.
   - Blood urea nitrogen (BUN) and serum creatinine are elevated when renal function begins to decline. This is a consistent finding with rapid progressive glomerulonephritis.
   - Intravenous pyelogram (IVP) reveals abnormalities in the collecting system of the kidney. Caution must be exercised if severe renal damage is present because the dye can be retained and cause additional kidney damage.
   - Renal biopsy accurately diagnoses the specific type of glomerulonephritis and the extent of damage. Diffuse endocapillary proliferative glomerulonephritis is the underlying pathological lesion.
   - Random urine specimen for protein electrophoresis identifies the type of protein being excreted in the urine.
   - Antistreptolysin O (ASO) titer is elevated, indicating recent exposure to a streptococcal infection.
   - Complement levels show decreased levels of C_3.
   - A 24-hour urine collection detects the amount and type of protein being excreted.
   - Serum electrolytes reveal elevated sodium and elevated or normal potassium and chloride.
   - Serum albumin and total protein may be normal or slightly low (because of hemodilution). With massive proteinuria, the levels are significantly lower.

4. Assess the patient's understanding of the treatment and the prognosis. Concerns often center on the possibility of progression of renal damage.

NURSING DIAGNOSIS: ALTERATION IN FLUID VOLUME: EXCESS

RELATED TO FACTORS: Glomerular capillary damage secondary to an inflammatory process, intrarenal defect resulting in decreased glomerular filtration and abnormal sodium retention

DEFINING CHARACTERISTICS: Edema, hypertension, significant drop in urinary output compared with fluid intake, elevated BP, weight gain, hypernatremia

PATIENT OUTCOME (collaborative): Demonstrates fluid and biochemical equilibrium

EVALUATION CRITERIA: BP between 90/60 - 140/90 mmHg, absence of peripheral edema, serum sodium within normal range, decreased weight

INTERVENTIONS	RATIONALE
1. Monitor: • trends of urine specific gravity and proteinuria • intake and output q2–4h • results of serum laboratory reports: electrolytes, BUN, creatinine, albumin • general status (Appendix F) q8h • weight daily (same scale, same time, same amount of clothing)	To identify indications of progress toward or deviations from expected outcome.
2. Administer prescribed loop diuretic and evaluate its effectiveness: resolution of edema, clear lung sounds, lower BP, increased urinary output, decreasing weight, serum sodium within normal range.	Hypertension in acute glomerulonephritis is volume rather than renin dependent. Diuretics rid the body of excess fluid. Hyponatremia, hypokalemia, and hypochoremic metabolic acidosis may develop with aggressive diuretic therapy.
3. Notify physician of findings signaling progressive renal insufficiency that include rising BUN and serum creatinine, and continual low or decline in urinary output accompanied by change in mentation. Administer prescribed medications (cytotoxic agents such as Cytoxan or corticosteroids such as prednisone) to prevent further	Initial treatment for rapid progressive glomerulonephritis is immunosuppressive agents. Prompt treatment is required to avert end-stage renal disease. Cytotoxic agents inhibit the deposition of immune complex in the glomeruli, while corticosteroids reduce inflammation in the glomeruli.

INTERVENTIONS	RATIONALE
glomeruli damage if rapid progressive glomerulonephritis develops. Evaluate their effectiveness. Schedule medications to achieve maximum therapeutic effectiveness and avoid drug-to-drug adverse interactions. Consult pharmacology reference or pharmacist as needed.	
4. Consult physician if manifestations of fluid excess persist or worsen with treatment. Prepare for hemodialysis or peritoneal dialysis if ordered.	Dialysis may be temporarily required to rid the body of nitrogenous waste products and excess fluid until glomeruli function is restored.

 # NURSING DIAGNOSIS: ALTERATION IN NUTRITION, LESS THAN BODY REQUIREMENTS

RELATED TO FACTORS: Anorexia and protein loss secondary to glomerular damage

DEFINING CHARACTERISTICS: Muscle wasting, weakness, sparse food intake, complains of diminished appetite, proteinuria

PATIENT OUTCOME (collaborative): Demonstrates no further nutritional deficits

EVALUATION CRITERIA: Stable weight, increased intake of food, laboratory values within normal range (BUN, serum creatinine, CBC, serum protein and albumin)

INTERVENTIONS	RATIONALE
1. Monitor: • results of serum albumin, protein, hemoglobin, hematocrit, BUN, and serum creatinine • percentage of food consumed at meal time • weight weekly	To identify indications of progress toward or deviations from expected outcome. A low hemoglobin and hematocrit cause less oxygen to be available for use by the body, resulting in fatigue. A rising BUN and serum creatinine indicate renal insufficiency and a need for dialysis.

INTERVENTIONS	RATIONALE
2. Provide a comfortable, odor-free environment at meal time.	Pain and odors cause anorexia.
3. Offer small frequent feedings. Give hard candies and ice cubes in moderation if a patient on fluid restriction becomes thirsty. Space fluid allocation so patient receives something to drink at regular intervals and with meals and medications.	Small feedings are less likely to cause gastric distention, thereby reducing nausea. Ice cubes and fluids lubricate the mouth and prevent drying of the oral mucosa. Candy also helps improve the taste in the mouth.
4. Refer the patient to a dietitian for instructions about prescribed dietary modifications, such as limited intake of sodium for acute glomerulonephritis if oliguric. Explain that sodium is restricted to help alleviate fluid retention.	A dietitian is a nutritional specialist and can assist the patient to understand the relationship between glomerular diseases and dietary restrictions and to select foods that meet nutritional needs relative to dietary restrictions. Compliance is enhanced when patients understand the relationship between their condition and prescribed therapies.
5. Provide optimal sources of protein and calories in the diet if serum albumin is significantly low.	A protein-rich diet can prevent a negative nitrogen balance, which occurs with massive proteinuria. Carbohydrates to supply calories exert a protein-sparing effect.
6. Encourage ambulation and socialization to tolerance.	Exercise promotes peristalsis that helps stimulate appetite. Socialization helps relieve depression, which often occurs in varying degrees during an acute and chronic illness.

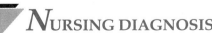

Nursing diagnosis:: activity intolerance

RELATED TO FACTORS: Altered RBC production secondary to kidney damage, inadequate nutritional intake

DEFINING CHARACTERISTICS: Tachycardia and tachypnea with minimal exertion, reports persistent fatigue

PATIENT OUTCOME: Participates in ADL without experiencing fatigue or respiratory distress

EVALUATION CRITERIA: Absence of tachycardia and tachypnea with minimal exertion, denies fatigue with activity

INTERVENTIONS | ## RATIONALE

INTERVENTIONS	RATIONALE
1. Monitor: • pulse and respiratory rate before and after activity • results of CBC reports	To identify indications of progress toward or deviations from expected outcome. Anemia, reflected by a low hemoglobin, contributes to fatigue. The amount of oxygen available to the tissue results from fewer RBCs that carry oxygen.
2. Provide periods of rest. Avoid frequent interruptions. Limit visitors if indicated.	Short periods of exertion with periods of rest conserve oxygen consumption.
3. Allow activities to tolerance. Assist with ADL as needed. Cease activity if the patient complains of fatigue, respiratory rate exceeds 24 per minute and pulse rate exceeds 100 beats per minute with minimal exertion.	These findings indicate an intolerance to the activity level.

◢ NURSING DIAGNOSIS: HIGH RISK FOR INFECTION

RELATED TO FACTORS: Immunosuppression secondary to steroid therapy, immunologic dysfunction

DEFINING CHARACTERISTICS: Elevated WBC, temperature above 99°F, malaise

PATIENT OUTCOME (collaborative): Absence of manifestations of infection

EVALUATION CRITERIA: WBC between 5,000-10,000/mm3, temperature 98.6°F

INTERVENTIONS | ## RATIONALE

INTERVENTIONS	RATIONALE
1. Monitor: • temperature q4h • CBC report, especially WBC	To identify indications of progress toward or deviations from expected outcome.

INTERVENTIONS	RATIONALE
2. Adhere to universal precautions (good handwashing technique before and after direct patient contact, wearing gloves when contact with blood or body fluid is likely to occur).	To prevent nosocomial infections. Universal precautions help protect the patient and the caregiver.
3. Consult physician if manifestations of infection are detected such as elevated temperature, WBC greater than 10,000/mm^3; cloudy, foul-smelling urine accompanied by dysuria. If urinary tract infection is suspected, obtain a clean-catch specimen for culture.	Because immunosuppressive agents weaken the patient's ability to fight infections, opportunistic infections may develop.

 # NURSING DIAGNOSIS: ANXIETY

RELATED TO FACTORS: Fear about possible progressive renal damage, knowledge deficit about diagnostic studies, treatment plan

DEFINING CHARACTERISTICS: Requests information, reports feeling nervous or anxious, verbalizes lack of understanding, tense facial expression

PATIENT OUTCOME: Demonstrates relief from anxiety

EVALUATION CRITERIA: Fewer reports of feeling anxious or nervous, relaxed facial expression, verbalizes understanding of treatment plan and diagnostic studies

INTERVENTIONS	RATIONALE
1. Encourage the patient and significant other(s) to talk about fears. Provide privacy without interruptions. Spend time with them to develop rapport.	Patients who feel comfortable talking with their nurse often can understand and incorporate needed changes in health practices with less difficulty.

INTERVENTIONS	RATIONALE

2. Provide information about:
  a. nature of the condition, especially the relationship between strepto-coccal infections of the skin or throat and glomerulonephritis.
  b. purpose of prescribed treatments.
  c. diagnostic studies, including:
    • purpose
    • brief description
    • preparation required before test
    • care after test
	Knowing expectations and the reasons why help lessen anxiety and foster patient cooperation with the therapeutic plan.

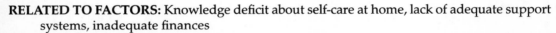

NURSING DIAGNOSIS: HIGH RISK FOR IMPAIRED HOME MAINTENANCE MANAGEMENT

RELATED TO FACTORS: Knowledge deficit about self-care at home, lack of adequate support systems, inadequate finances

DEFINING CHARACTERISTICS: Requests information, verbalizes lack of understanding about preventive measures, requests assistance in financing cost of hospitalization, may report lack of adequate transportation

PATIENT OUTCOME (collaborative): Demonstrates adequate resources for maintaining self on discharge

EVALUATION CRITERIA: Verbalizes understanding of discharge instructions, verbalizes willingness to use community resources to meet home care needs

INTERVENTIONS	RATIONALE
1. Review preventive measures for urinary tract infections (see Urinary Tract Infections, page 122).	An episode of glomerulonephritis predisposes patient to reinfection.
2. Provide information about medications prescribed for home use, including name, purpose, dose, schedule, and reportable side effects.	To ensure continued safe therapeutic benefits.

INTERVENTIONS	RATIONALE
3. Ensure the patient or significant other has a written appointment for follow-up care and written instructions for self-care at home.	Verbal instructions may be easily forgotten.
4. Instruct the patient to seek immediate medical treatment for: • sore throat or skin lesions to diagnose a streptococcal infection. • signs of excess fluid (edema), shortness of breath, daily weight gain.	Early diagnosis and treatment help preserve renal function.
5. Instruct the patient to weigh daily and keep a record of results.	To monitor fluid status.
6. Teach how to care for edematous areas and explain purpose of each. • Elevate extremities when lying down to help reduce swelling by allowing gravity to promote blood return toward to the heart. • Bathe with warm water and mild, deodorant-free soap. Dry skin thoroughly. Apply a mild emollient if skin is dry. Explain that deodorant soaps have a drying effect. Clean and lubricated skin is less likely to crack. • Avoid going barefoot to prevent accidental injury to the feet. Healing of edematous skin is prolonged because of the impaired nutritient supply. • Participate in ADL to tolerance to ensure adequate exercise. Exercise promotes circulation and a sense of well-being.	Compliance is enhanced when patients understand their condition and how to assume responsibility for promoting their recovery.
7. Initiate a referral to social services or discharge planning department if patient expresses a need for assistance with some aspect of home care management.	To ensure continuity of care on discharge.

Renal Calculi

Urolithiasis occurs when stones are present in the urinary tract. The stones themselves are called calculi. Stone formation starts with a trapped crystal somewhere along the urinary tract that grows as urine solutes precipitate. Calculi vary in size from microscopic foci to several centimeters in diameter—large enough to fill the renal pelvis.

Factors influencing stone formation include urine pH, concentration of urine solutes, urine stasis, some infections, high calcium diet, and bone demineralization. Most stones contain calcium, while the remainder contain ammoniomagnesium phosphate or struvite, uric acid, or cystine.

Hospitalization is required until the stone is removed from the urinary tract and complications resolved. The mean LOS for a DRG classification of renal calculi with extracorporeal shock-wave lithotripsy is 3.0 days (Lorenz, 1991).

The most serious complication of renal calculi is obstruction of the kidney, which can lead to permanent damage if left untreated. Bleeding and infection are other potential complications.

General Medical Management

- In most cases, no treatment because the stone may pass through the tract without medical intervention.
- Pharmacotherapy:
  a. To maintain urine pH:
    — sodium bicarbonate to make urine more alkaline, with acid-precipitating calculi
    — ascorbic acid to make urine more acid, with alkaline-precipitating calculi
  b. To reduce excretion of calculi-forming substances:
    — thiazide diuretics to lower excretion of calcium
    — allopurinol to treat uric acid stones by lowering plasma levels of uric acid
- Surgical removal of stone:
  — pyelolithotomy (stone removed from renal pelvis)
  — ureterolithotomy (stone removed from ureter)
  — cystolithotomy (stone removed from bladder)

— percutaneous ultrasonic lithotripsy (PUL) and extracorporeal shock-wave lithotripsy (ESWL) use sound waves and shock waves, respectively, to break the stone into small pieces to facilitate excretion in urine. These methods are particularly useful for patients at risk during surgical procedures.

— dissolution therapy uses a stone specific chemical solution instilled through a nephrostomy tube to irrigate the area and dissolve the stone

Integrative Care Plans

• IV therapy
• Pain
• Preoperative and postoperative care

Discharge Considerations

• Follow-up care
• Medications to continue at home
• Activity restrictions
• Measures to prevent recurrence

 # ASSESSMENT DATA BASE

1. History or presence of risk factors:
   • metabolic or dietary changes
   • prolonged immobility
   • inadequate fluid intake
   • previous history of calculi or urinary tract infections
   • family history of calculi formation

2. Physical examination based on a general survey (Appendix F) may reveal:
   • pain. A stone in the pelvis of the kidney causes dull and constant pain. A ureteral stone causes severe, intermittent colic-type pain that subsides after the stone is passed.
   • nausea and vomiting and possibly diarrhea
   • changes in urine color or voiding pattern, for example, cloudy and odorous urine if infection is present, painful urgent urination and decreased urine output if fluid intake is inadequate or if there is urinary tract obstruction, and hematuria if there is renal tissue damage

3. Diagnostic studies:
   • Urinalysis (UA) shows microscopic or gross hematuria, WBC, changes in pH, and crystals of calcium, uric acid, or cystine indicating calculi.
   • Urine culture indicates bacteria if infection is present.
   • Serum BUN and creatinine are both elevated if kidney damage has occurred.

- WBCs are elevated with infection.
- A 24-hour urine collection for creatinine clearance is decreased if kidney damage has occurred.
- Kidney, ureter, and bladder (KUB) x ray and intravenous pyelogram (IVP) detect stones and anomolies that may contribute to stone formation.
- Cystoscopy permits direct visualization of the urinary tract to detect abnormalities and, in some cases, to remove the calculi.

4. Assess the patient's feelings about condition and therapeutic plan. Patients may express concerns about recurrence and the impact on employment and other daily activities. A male patient may reveal concerns about sexual dysfunction related to pain and infection.

▌NURSING DIAGNOSIS: PAIN

RELATED TO FACTORS: Tissue injury secondary to renal calculi

DEFINING CHARACTERISTICS: Verbalizes pain that may be accompanied by tachycardia and tachypnea, frowning, moaning, crying, guarding behavior

PATIENT OUTCOME (collaborative): Demonstrates relief from pain

EVALUATION CRITERIA: Denies pain, relaxed facial expression, absence of moaning and guarding behavior, pulse rate 60-100 beats per minute, respiratory rate 12-24 per minute

INTERVENTIONS	RATIONALE
1. Monitor and document location and nature of pain. Consult physician if pain persists or worsens.	An increase in pain is indicative of obstruction, while a sudden relief of pain indicates the stone has moved. Severe pain can cause shock.
2. See Pain (page 700).	
3. Force fluids if free of nausea. Initiate and maintain prescribed IV therapy if nausea and vomiting are present.	Fluids help flush the kidney and may aid in expulsion of small stones.
4. Encourage activity as tolerated. Administer prescribed analgesic and antiemetic before moving if possible. Evaluate their effectiveness.	Movement can enhance the passage of some small calculi and deter stasis of urine. Comfort promotes rest and healing. Nausea is caused by excruciating pain.

● ●

NURSING DIAGNOSIS: HIGH RISK FOR INJURY

RELATED TO FACTORS: Presence of calculi in the renal tract

DEFINING CHARACTERISTICS: Elevated BUN and serum creatinine reflecting kidney damage, microscopic or gross hematuria, manifestations of urinary tract infection

PATIENT OUTCOME (collaborative): Demonstrates normal kidney function

EVALUATION CRITERIA: Kidney function studies within normal limits; clear amber or yellow urine; absence of painful voiding, hesitancy, frequency

● ●

INTERVENTIONS	RATIONALE
1. Monitor: • urine (color, odor) q8h • intake and output q8h • pH of urine q8h • vital signs q4h	For early detection of problems.
2. Strain **all** urine. Observe for crystals. Save crystals for physician to see, then send to laboratory for analysis of composition.	To obtain evidence of passage of calculi. Dietary changes are based on stone composition.
3. Consult physician if, • patient voids frequent, small quantities and continues to feel the urge to void after voiding • urine changes color from clear to cloudy (reddish-brownish, or bright red) with a foul-smell • oliguria (output less than 30 mL/hr) or anuria (no urine) occur • persistent pain unrelieved by analgesia Prepare the patient for prescribed surgical intervention according to facility protocol and procedures.	These findings indicate the development of an obstruction and the need for aggressive intervention (surgery or lithotripsy).

INTERVENTIONS	RATIONALE
4. Administer prescribed medication to maintain the appropriate urine pH.	By changing the urinary pH (increased acidity or alkalinity), the solubility factor for calculi can be controlled. Calcium and oxalate calculi are less likely to precipitate in an acid urine because of their alkaline chemistry. Precipitation of uric acid and cystine calculi can be controlled by maintaining an alkaline urine.

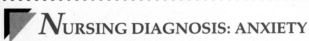

NURSING DIAGNOSIS: ANXIETY

RELATED TO FACTORS: Knowledge deficit about condition, diagnostic studies, and treatment plan

DEFINING CHARACTERISTICS: Requests information, reports feeling nervous or anxious, tense facial expression

PATIENT OUTCOME: Demonstrates less anxiety

EVALUATION CRITERIA: Verbalizes understanding of condition, diagnostic studies, and therapeutic plan; fewer reports of feeling anxious or nervous; relaxed facial expression

INTERVENTIONS	RATIONALE
1. Allow the patient and significant others to express feelings and concerns. Correct misconceptions.	The patient's problem-solving abilities are enhanced if a comfortable, supportive environment is provided.

2. Provide information about:
  a. nature of the illness
  b. purpose of prescribed treatments
  c. diagnostic studies, including
    • purpose
    • brief description of test
    • preparation required before test
    • care after test
If information must be given during a painful episode, keep instructions and explanations brief and simple. Give more detailed information when pain is under control.
	A knowledge of what to expect helps lessen anxiety. Pain interferes with learning.

◤ NURSING DIAGNOSIS: HIGH RISK FOR IMPAIRED HOME MAINTENANCE MANAGEMENT

RELATED TO FACTORS: Knowledge deficit about preventive measures on discharge

DEFINING CHARACTERISTICS: Requests information, reports routine consumption of foods that precipitate calculi formation, reports history of repeat hospitalizations for calculi

PATIENT OUTCOME (collaborative): Demonstrates ability to adhere to therapeutic home care plan

EVALUATION CRITERIA: Verbalizes understanding of instructions

INTERVENTIONS	RATIONALE
1. Arrange for a consult with dietitian for information and instructions about meal planning based on calculi composition. Have the patient identify foods high in calcium, oxalate, or purines, depending on the calculi composition and explain the reason for their restriction in the diet. Use the following list as a guide: • calcium — dairy products and green leafy vegetables • oxalate — chocolate, caffeine drinks, beets, spinach • purines (uric acid) — meats, legumes, whole grains If excess weight or compliance is a problem, consult physician about using urine-acidifying or urine-alkalizing agents instead.	A dietitian is a nutritional specialist and can assist the patient to understand prescribed dietary changes and meal planning on discharge. Patients are more likely to comply with pharmacotherapy to control urine pH rather than to make adjustments in their diets.
2. Teach the patient about prescribed medications, including, name, dosage, schedule, purpose, and reportable side effects. Teach patient how to monitor urinary pH if recommended by the physician and where to purchase supplies.	Pharmacotherapy is an important treatment adjunct. Compliance is enhanced when patients know and understand how prescribed treatments will benefit them.

INTERVENTIONS	RATIONALE
3. Teach the patient preventive measures: • Drink at least eight glasses of fluid, especially water, each day unless contraindicated. • Monitor urine pH daily. • Adhere to prescribed dietary restrictions. • Take medication as prescribed.	The risk for recurrence is high. These measures help reduce recurrence by flushing the kidneys and maintaining a urine pH inconsistent with calculi formation.
4. Instruct the patient to strain all urine through a piece of gauze and seek immediate medical attention if the following occur: • pain • urine turns reddish-brown or bright red • urine appears cloudy and is foul-smelling • painful voiding	These findings signal recurrent calculi and a need for aggressive medical intervention.

Urinary Diversion

A **urinary diversion** is any of several surgical procedures performed when it is necessary to divert urine flow away from the bladder:

1. **Ileal conduit** (also called Bricker procedure or ureteroileostomy) — the ureters are released from the bladder and anastomosed to an isolated segment of the small intestine. One end of the segment is sutured closed, and the open end is brought to the abdominal surface to form a stoma. The remaining ileum is anastomosed together. A cystectomy (complete bladder removal) is also performed.

2. **Colon loop** — same as ileal conduit, except a segment of the colon is used.

3. **Continent vesicostomy** — an internal reservoir is created from the bladder for urine. The neck of the bladder is sutured, and a nipple valve is created through which the patient catheterizes the bladder at intervals.

The physician chooses the procedure based on the individual needs of the patient and the reason for surgery. Ileal conduit is the most common urinary diversion procedure for adults. A radical cystectomy results in permanent impotence as the bladder, urethra, prostate, and seminal vesicles are removed. The mean LOS for a DRG classification of urinary diversion is 11.5 days (Lorenz, 1991).

Preoperatively, the stoma site is marked by the surgeon or the enterostomal therapist. The best location of the stoma site is determined with the patient standing and sitting. The location of skin folds and creases, clothing line, umbilicus, scars, bony prominences, and so forth are considered when selecting a stoma site. Commonly, the stoma is placed in the right lower quadrant of the abdomen.

Postoperatively, the patient often has nephrostomy tubes, a nasogastric tube, and IV fluids. The nephrostomy tubes are usually removed in about seven days. Potential postoperative complications include obstruction of the ureters, leakage at the anastomosis sites, urinary tract infections, and peritonitis.

Integrative Care Plans

- IV therapy
- Immobility
- Cancer
- Loss
- Preoperative and postoperative care

Discharge Considerations

- Follow-up care
- Medications to continue at home
- Community support groups
- Urostomy care
- Activity limitations

THE PREOPERATIVE PERIOD

 # ASSESSMENT DATA BASE

1. Review the patient's medical record to identify:
   a. Reason for the surgery:
      - cancer of the bladder (most common reason)
      - neurogenic bladder
      - congenital anomalies
      - strictures
      - trauma to the bladder
      - chronic renal infections
   b. Type of diversion being considered
   c. Presence of risk factors in the development of bladder cancer:
      - prolonged exposure to carcinogens (cigarette smoking, chemical dyes, chronic bladder infections and irritations)
      - family history of cancer
   d. Previous treatments for bladder cancer (chemotherapy using thio-THEPA or BCG Live (Thera Cys), radiation therapy, transurethral resection and fulguration, partial cystectomy)

2. Physical examination based on a general survey (Appendix F) to obtain baseline values and to identify clinical manifestations of bladder cancer:
   - painless hematuria (most frequent finding). It is usually intermittent. Severity of hematuria does not correlate with extent of the cancer.

INTERVENTIONS	RATIONALE
2. Change the stomahesive wafer weekly or when leakage is detected. Be sure the skin is clean and dry before applying the new wafer. Cut the opening in the wafer about ½ inch larger than the stoma diameter to ensure a snug fitting pouch that completely covers peristomal skin. Empty the urostomy bag when it is ¼ to ½ full.	The increased weight of urine can break the peristomal seal, allowing urine leakage. Persistent exposure of peristomal skin to the acid urine can cause skin breakdown and increase the risk of infection.

*N*URSING DIAGNOSIS: DISTURBANCE IN SELF-CONCEPT

RELATED TO FACTORS: Altered body image secondary to a urostomy

DEFINING CHARACTERISTICS: Demonstrates behaviors of body image disturbance (refuses to look at or touch the stoma, verbalizes feelings of embarrassment), withdraws from social activities (refuses visitors, verbalizes fear of rejection), verbalizes concerns about sexuality and role performance, expresses anger or denial, may refer to stoma as the "thing" or use comical terms or names instead of using term "stoma"

PATIENT OUTCOME: Demonstrates acceptance of self in current situation

EVALUATION CRITERIA: Participates in self-care, verbalizes plans for resuming social activities within recommended limitations, refers to stoma as "stoma"

INTERVENTIONS	RATIONALE
1. See Loss (page 733).	

*N*URSING DIAGNOSIS: HIGH RISK FOR IMPAIRED HOME MAINTENANCE MANAGEMENT

RELATED TO FACTORS: Knowledge deficit about self-care activities after discharge

DEFINING CHARACTERISTICS: Verbalizes lack of understanding; reports feelings of depression, lack of interest, or lack of confidence in ability to perform self-care activities; history of lack of health-seeking behavior; reports lack of personal support system or financial resources; demonstrates inability to perform psychomotor skills

PATIENT OUTCOME (collaborative): Demonstrates ability to manage health maintenance activities on discharge

EVALUATION CRITERIA: Performs ostomy self-care correctly without assistance, verbalizes understanding of discharge instructions, identifies community resources for support

• •

INTERVENTIONS	RATIONALE
1. Evaluate the patient's and significant other's ability to perform ostomy care. Have the patient and significant other demonstrate procedures for emptying the drainage bag, changing the wafer and pouch, performing peristomal skin care, attaching the nighttime bedside drainage bag. Allow them to perform these procedures two or three times without assistance before discharge. Contact social services to make arrangements for home care by a visiting nurse if the patient and significant other cannot perform ostomy care because of a physical or psychological deficit.	Psychomotor skills improve with practice. Social services is a liaison between the facility and community service agencies, making necessary arrangements for a patient's transition to home.
2. Encourage the patient to participate in ostomy self-care. Offer praise when the patient shows behaviors toward resuming a normal independent lifestyle (participating in ostomy self-care, verbalizing plans for returning to work or being involved in social activities).	Self-care fosters a sense of independence. Rewards serve to motivate an individual to learn.
3. Place written instructions for changing the urostomy appliance in the Kardex and at the patient's bedside. Encourage all caregivers to follow these steps. Do **not** interject new information or change any planned steps without first consulting the enterostomal therapist or the caregiver who planned the procedure. The caregiver who planned the procedure must introduce any new changes to resolve problems.	A consistent procedure reduces confusion and makes learning easier.

INTERVENTIONS	RATIONALE
4. Ensure the patient or significant other has: • a written appointment for follow-up care and written instructions for urostomy care • enough urostomy supplies to last at least one week • the telephone number for a contact person, preferably the enterostomal therapist • the address and telephone number for the American Cancer Society and the local ostomy association	Verbal instructions may be easily forgotten. Having sufficient supplies for physical care allows the patient and significant other(s) time to focus on readjusting to home. Contact persons can provide immediate support if problems arise. These agencies can provide continued support for the patient and significant others.
5. Provide information about medications prescribed for home use, including name, purpose, dose, schedule, and reportable side effects.	To ensure safety in self-medication administration.
6. Instruct the patient to: • empty the urostomy bag when ¼ to ½ full • connect the urostomy bag to a bedside drainage bag at night • follow the steps outlined for changing, emptying, and cleaning urostomy pouch, and performing peristomal skin care • contact enterostomal therapist at earliest signs of peristomal skin irritation (tenderness and redness) • to drink at least eight glasses of fluid daily, especially fresh water and cranberry juice	These measures help maintain kidney function and prevent peristomal skin breakdown.

Renal Failure

Renal failure occurs when the kidneys, because of damage, can no longer maintain homeostasis. For life to be sustained, a renal replacement therapy must be instituted. These therapies include hemodialysis, peritoneal dialysis, and kidney transplant. In some cases the renal failure is reversible, and the therapy is discontinued when renal function returns. However, in many cases the renal damage is permanent, and the therapy becomes the patient's lifeline.

Renal failure is acute or chronic. Acute renal failure is characterized by oliguria of rapid onset, followed by a diuretic phase lasting a few weeks to one month. If the renal failure is not reversed, chronic renal failure develops.

Chronic renal failure develops slowly over months or years, with a gradual decrease in renal function and subsequent increase in symptoms, resulting in end-stage renal disease (ESRD). The patient is asymptomatic during the initial stage of diminished renal reserve. Vague symptoms and elevated serum creatinine and BUN are noted in renal insufficiency (Zorzanello, 1989). As end-stage is reached, fluid and biochemical imbalances become more evident, and symptoms worsen.

Because of the vital role the kidney plays in many of the body's homeostatic mechanisms, complications of renal failure are varied and complex. Fluid and biochemical imbalances (hyperkalemia, hyponatremia, metabolic acidosis) occur because of the kidney's inability to excrete waste products and excess fluid and because a disruption occurs in the mechanism that maintains a normal serum pH. Excess fluid intake, without adequate removal through dialysis, leads to peripheral edema and pulmonary edema. Cardiovascular problems include hypertension and pericarditis. The excess of uremic toxins is responsible for pericarditis and irritations along the gastrointestinal tract from the mouth to the anus. Disruption in the calcium and phosphorus balance over time results in bone demineralization. Peripheral neuropathies also are common. Anemia develops because of decreased production of erythropoietin.

The mean LOS for a DRG classification of renal failure is 6.3 days (Lorenz, 1991).

General Medical Management

a. Acute Renal Failure:
- Dietary restriction of sodium and fluid
- Pharmacotherapy:
  — diuretics (mannitol)
  — antihypertensives

INTERVENTIONS	RATIONALE
• Consult physician if iron and ferritin levels are low, BP persistently elevated, or history of hypersensitivity to albumin and mammalian cell-derived products. • Administer iron supplements if prescribed. b. Stop the IV infusion and consult physician immediately if following adverse reactions occur: • headaches • worsening of hypertension • tachycardia, dyspnea • nausea and vomiting • diarrhea • hyperkalemia	These adverse reactions are more likely to occur if the patient concurrently takes aluminum hydroxide, to control serum phosphate level or if an iron or vitamin deficiency exists.
5. If the patient complains of a dry mouth, allow patient to rinse mouth with water at least hourly, or provide ice chips sparingly, or hard lemon candy.	Stomatitis can occur because of excessive uremic toxins on the oral mucosa and reduced fluid intake. In addition, anorexia is enhanced by a dry, sticky mouth. These measures promote salivation.
6. Ensure that environment is conducive for eating during meal times (free of odors, food served at appropriate temperature, foods served that patient likes).	Although anorexia results from a combination of factors such as fatigue, excess uremic toxins, and depression, adjustments can be made to enhance appetite.
7. Administer prescribed phosphate-binding agents, calcium supplements, and vitamin D supplements.	Calcium deposits account for joint discomfort. In renal failure, vitamin D metabolism is reduced, which causes decreased calcium absorption from the GI tract. When serum calcium falls parathormone production increases, resulting in increased calcium and phosphate resorption from the bone and ultimately bone demineralization.
8. Assist the patient with planning a daily activity schedule to avoid immobilization and fatigue.	Immobility promotes calcium resorption from the bone.

INTERVENTIONS	RATIONALE
9. Maintain prescribed nutritional intake, which usually includes high calorie and a specific amount of protein, sodium, potassium, and fluid. Refer the patient to the dietitian if oral intake continues to be less than 30% each meal. Consult physician about using enteral feedings or total parenteral nutrition (TPN) if dietary intake continues to be insufficient to maintain an anabolic state.	A catabolic state contributes to further fatigue, weakness, and anemia. Restricting protein and potassium helps control nitrogenous waste buildup. Restricting sodium and fluid helps control fluid retention. A dietitian is a nutritional specialist who can evaluate the patient's nutritional status and suggest appropriate foods based on the patient's preference and nutritional needs relative to the current illness.

 # Nursing Diagnosis: Anxiety

RELATED TO FACTORS: Knowledge deficit about condition, diagnostic studies, treatment plan, and prognosis

DEFINING CHARACTERISTICS: Verbalizes lack of understanding, requests information, reports feeling nervous and afraid

PATIENT OUTCOME: Demonstrates less anxiety

EVALUATION CRITERIA: Verbalizes understanding of condition, diagnostic studies, and treatment plan; fewer reports of feeling nervous or afraid

INTERVENTIONS	RATIONALE
1. If possible, arrange for a visit from an individual who is receiving the therapy being considered.	An individual who is successfully coping with ESRD can be a positive influence to help a newly diagnosed patient maintain hope and to begin adjusting to accommodate lifestyle changes.
2. Provide information about: a. nature of renal failure. Ensure the patient understands that chronic renal failure is irreversible and that lifetime treatment is required to maintain normal body function.	Patients often do not understand that dialysis will be needed forever if the renal failure is irreversible. Keeping the patient informed encourages participation in decision making and fosters compliance and maximum independence.

INTERVENTIONS	RATIONALE
b. diagnostic studies, including: • purpose • brief description • preparation required before test • care after test • results of test and significance of test results c. purpose of prescribed therapy	
3. Allow time for the patient and significant others to talk about concerns and feelings about lifestyle changes that will be needed to accommodate chosen therapy.	Expressing feelings helps lessen anxiety. Treatment for renal failure impacts the entire family.

. . . .

 # NURSING DIAGNOSIS: HIGH RISK FOR IMPAIRED ADJUSTMENT

RELATED TO FACTORS: Actual and perceived losses associated with a chronic illness

DEFINING CHARACTERISTICS: Changes in eating habits, sleep patterns, activity levels, and libido; verbalizes nonacceptance or difficulty accepting health status change; inadequate support systems

PATIENT OUTCOME: Demonstrates willingness to make lifestyle adaptations to accommodate changes imposed by a chronic illness

EVALUATION CRITERIA: Shows increasing interest in participating in self-care, verbalizes specific actions for dealing with stressful situations that impair adjustment, verbalizes strategies to incorporate health maintenance activities into daily routine, verbalizes realistic plans in view of current situation

. . . .

INTERVENTIONS	RATIONALE
1. See Loss (page 733).	

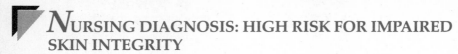

NURSING DIAGNOSIS: HIGH RISK FOR IMPAIRED SKIN INTEGRITY

RELATED TO FACTORS: Pruritus secondary to renal failure

DEFINING CHARACTERISTICS: Scratching, complains of itching, scratch marks on the skin

PATIENT OUTCOME (collaborative): Skin remains intact

EVALUATION CRITERIA: Absence of scratch marks on skin, fewer complaints of pruritus

INTERVENTIONS	RATIONALE
1. Encourage the patient: • to keep fingernails trimmed short. • keep room temperature at a comfortable setting to prevent sweating. • keep skin lubricated with an emollient lotion. • adhere to prescribed dietary restrictions. • bathe with a nondeodorant, hypoallergenic soap.	Short nails are less likely to tear the skin. Sweat, heat, and dry skin increase pruritus. Uremic toxins account for pruritus. Plain soap is less likely to dry and irritate the skin.
2. Administer phosphate-binding agents and arrange for dialysis, as prescribed. (See Dialysis, page 165).	Serum phosphate levels are too high. Because calcium and phosphorus are inversely proportional, serum calcium drops and the patient develops tremors. Dialysis removes uremic toxins and helps normalize biochemicals.

NURSING DIAGNOSIS: HIGH RISK FOR NONCOMPLIANCE

RELATED TO FACTORS: Knowledge deficit, inadequate support system

DEFINING CHARACTERISTICS: Patient or significant other verbalizes a history of failure to adhere to therapeutic recommendations, verbalizes nonacceptance of health status change, verbalizes lack of understanding of self-care management at home

PATIENT OUTCOME (collaborative): Demonstrates willingness to comply with recommended home care therapeutic regimen

EVALUATION CRITERIA: Verbalizes understanding of discharge instructions, demonstrates ability to care for vascular access site

INTERVENTIONS	RATIONALE
1. Review rationale for prescribed dietary modifications on discharge: • protein restriction to prevent tissue protein catabolism, yet avoid an excess that would elevate urea levels • sodium restriction to reduce fluid retention • potassium restriction (damaged kidney cannot clear potassium) • if oliguric, water restriction to prevent edema • high calories to ensure protein use for tissue protein synthesis and to supply energy Discuss long-term effects of noncompliance with medications and diet: • increased risk for fracture because of bone disease resulting from calcium and phosphorus imbalance • cardiac enlargement resulting from chronic fluid overload • pericarditis, dementia, GI upset, and peripheral neuropathies because of excess accumulation of nitrogenous waste products Reinforce the need to continue therapy to minimize these complications.	Compliance is enhanced when patients understand the effects of prescribed treatments on their condition.
2. Ensure that the patient or significant other has in writing: • appointment for follow-up care instructions for self-care at home • directions and telephone number of the dialysis center that provides maintenance therapy	Verbal instructions may be easily forgotten.

INTERVENTIONS	RATIONALE
3. Provide written instructions about all medications prescribed for home use, including name, dosage, schedule, purpose, and reportable side effects.	To ensure safe self-medication administration.
4. Discuss changes in daily life needed to accommodate the chosen therapy. Refer the patient to social services or discharge planning department, if concerns are expressed about financing the chosen therapy, or to arrange for visits from a home health nurse if patient and significant other cannot safely perform required home maintenance activities.	Work schedules often need changing so the patient can receive dialysis at times available in the dialysis center. Patients choosing peritoneal dialysis can schedule treatments at their convenience. End-stage renal disease patients are eligible for Medicare benefits. Medical social workers and discharge planners are specialists who help arrange for continuity of care when the patient is discharged.
5. Be sure the patient has the telephone numbers of resource persons such as the dialysis nurse or transplant coordinator, physician, renal dietitian, renal social worker, and the American Kidney Foundation.	A consistent, available support team is needed throughout the patient's life.

Dialysis

Dialysis is a process that removes solutes and fluids from the blood across a semipermeable membrane. It is based on the principles of diffusion, osmosis, and ultrafiltration. Solutes move by diffusion from an area of higher concentration to an area of lower concentration. The difference in the concentration gradient determines the amount of solute that crosses the membrane. If the size of the solute particles is larger than the openings in the membrane, the solute will not move. Fluid moves across the membrane from an area of lesser concentration of solutes to an area of greater concentration of solutes to dilute the concentrated side. A difference in the pressure across the membrane results in fluid movement called ultrafiltration. Methods of dialysis that will be discussed include hemodialysis, continuous arteriovenous hemofiltration, and peritoneal dialysis.

Dialysis is generally performed on an out-patient basis. Patients receiving dialysis have special needs when they are admitted to the facility. The mean LOS for a DRG classification of dialysis is 2.5 days (Lorenz, 1991). In addition to the reason for hospitalization, problems associated with the dialysis must be anticipated and managed. The nursing care needs are unique to each type of dialysis. Also, elderly patients requiring dialysis pose an additional challenge because of the normal physiological changes that occur with the aging process (narrowing of vessels and thickening of capillary walls, decreased number of renal nephrons).

HEMODIALYSIS

Hemodialysis is the passage of blood through tubings outside of the body to an artificial kidney where excess solute and fluid removal occurs. The blood is then returned to the patient. Specially trained nurses are required to provide hemodialysis. Patients also can be trained with a partner (usually a family member) to perform dialysis at home.

Patients who are candidates for hemodialysis must maintain access to circulation. In addition, the cardiovascular system must tolerate the large fluid volume swings that result from this treatment. Home hemodialysis candidates must have a partner who is willing to participate and who can learn the skills needed to successfully perform hemodialysis. The frequency of hemodialysis varies from two to three times a week.

There are several components to a hemodialysis system:

1. Circulatory access must be available. Two types are currently used:

   • external catheter (VasCath). This catheter is usually temporary and used when dialysis is needed immediately. It is placed via a subclavian or femoral vein.

   • internal arteriovenous (A-V) or graft fistula. An enlarged vessel is created, permitting the rapid removal of blood during dialysis. Several days or weeks must pass before the graft can be used for dialysis. Two large-bore needles are placed percutaneously so blood can be withdrawn.

2. Dialyzer and dialysate delivery system. The dialysate, with a composition similar to normal serum, flows through the dialyzer (artificial kidney) on the opposite side of the membrane from the blood. Solutes and fluid move from the blood across the membrane into the dialysate. The dialyzed blood is returned to the patient, and the spent dialysate is discarded.

3. Anticoagulant administration with heparin is necessary during hemodialysis to prevent clotting of blood when it is outside the body.

Integrative Care Plans

• Renal failure
• Loss

Discharge Considerations

• Follow-up care
• Signs and symptoms requiring medical attention
• Wound care (if A-V fistula is newly created, revised, or declotted)
• Protective measures for the extremity with the A-V fistula
• Muscle strengthening exercises for the extremity
• Care of the VasCath (if inserted)

 *A*SSESSMENT DATA BASE

Before Dialysis:

1. Review the patient's medical record to determine the reason for hospitalization:

   • noncompliance with the treatment plan

   • clotted fistula

   • fistula creation

   • new case of acute or chronic renal failure

2. Inquire about type of diet followed at home, amount of fluid allowed, medications currently taken, hemodialysis schedule, amount of urine output.

3. Assess patency of internal fistula if one is present. If patent, a thrill (pulsation) will be felt and a bruit (swishing sound) will be heard with a stethoscope over the site. Absence of a pulsation and swishing sound indicates the fistula has clotted.

4. Assess for clinical and laboratory manifestations of the need for dialysis:
   - weight gain of three or more pounds above body weight since last dialysis treatment
   - rales, rapid respirations at rest, increasing shortness of breath with minimal physical exertion
   - persistent fatigue and weakness
   - severe hypertension
   - elevated creatinine, BUN, and electrolytes, especially potassium
   - possible EKG changes in the presence of hyperkalemia

After Dialysis:

1. Assess for hypotension and bleeding. Large volumes of fluid removal during dialysis can result in orthostatic hypotension. Using anticoagulants during the treatment puts the patient at risk for bleeding from the access site and for internal bleeding.

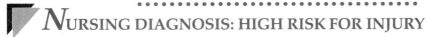

NURSING DIAGNOSIS: HIGH RISK FOR INJURY

RELATED TO FACTORS: Fluid volume deficit secondary to hemodialysis

DEFINING CHARACTERISTICS: Hypotension after dialysis, complains of light-headedness when moving from sitting to standing position accompanied by tachycardia and tachypnea

PATIENT OUTCOME: Protects self from physical injury

EVALUATION CRITERIA: Requests assistance when needed, experiences no falls

INTERVENTIONS	RATIONALE
1. On return from hemodialysis, check BP, pulse, and respiratory rate. Inquire about feelings of dizziness and light-headedness when moving from a sitting to a standing position. Explain that orthostatic hypotension may occur with hemodialysis caused by a sudden loss of large volumes of fluid. Keep call bell within patient's reach. Instruct the patient to:	To prevent falling.

INTERVENTIONS	RATIONALE
• signal for assistance before getting out of bed if feeling light-headed or dizzy when moving from a lying to a sitting position. • change from a lying to a sitting position slowly. Sit on the side of the bed until light-headedness subsides before attempting to walk.	To prevent falling.
2. After dialysis, allow the patient to rest. If hypotension is present after dialysis, allow the patient to remain in bed in a flat position. Monitor BP q15min. Raise the head of the bed gradually as the BP begins to increase.	Dialysis is fatiguing because the patient has to sit or lie still for about four hours. The sudden fluid shift from the brain to the lower extremities by the force of gravity that causes orthostatic hypotension is minimized by a gradual change of position.

• •

 # NURSING DIAGNOSIS: HIGH RISK FOR ALTERATION IN TISSUE PERFUSION.

RELATED TO FACTORS: Clotted A-V fistula, A-V fistula creation or revision

DEFINING CHARACTERISTICS: Absence of bruit and thrill, several previous admissions for declotting of A-V fistula, reports failure to follow guidelines in caring for extremity with the A-V fistula

PATIENT OUTCOME: Circulatory access remains patent

EVALUATION CRITERIA: Thrill and bruit present

• •

INTERVENTIONS	RATIONALE
1. Monitor: • patency of the A-V fistula. Palpate the fistula site for a thrill and auscultate (using the diaphragm of a stethoscope) for bruit q8h.	Access to the circulation is required for hemodialysis. The patient's blood is heparinized during dialysis, which predisposes patient to bleeding.

INTERVENTIONS	RATIONALE
• neurovascular status (Appendix D) of the extremity with the A-V fistula q8h: — color —temperature —sensation — movement of fingers —any swelling • needle insertion site every hour x 4 hours after dialysis for bleeding	
2. Protect the extremity with the A-V fistula. a. In the immediate postoperative period, elevate the extremity. b. Do **not** take blood pressure or draw blood from the extremity with the A-V fistula. c. Place a sign above the patient's bed and a Medical Alert bracelet on the unaffected arm ("Avoid Using (site) Arm for BP and Venipunctures"). d. Instruct the patient to refrain from bending the affected arm for prolonged periods and to avoid sleeping on the side of the affected arm.	Elevation helps reduce swelling. Constriction impedes blood flow, which increases the risk of clotting. Repeated venipunctures increase the risk of infection. A sign alerts all facility personnel to refrain from using the arm with the fistula.
3. Consult physician for • absence of a thrill and bruit • persistent hypotension after hemodialysis	Absence of a thrill and bruit indicates a clotted fistula. Severe hypotension causes clotting in the fistula.
4. If bleeding occurs at the needle access site, apply pressure for ten minutes. If bleeding continues, notify dialysis nurse or physician.	To prevent blood loss, protamine sulfate may be required to reverse the effects of heparin.
5. During the early postoperative period, encourage flexion and extension of the fingers on the extremity with the fistula.	To promote muscle strength and facilitate maturation of the fistula.

• •

◤ NURSING DIAGNOSIS: HIGH RISK FOR INFECTION

RELATED TO FACTORS: Central vascular access device, need for repeat venipunctures for hemodialysis, immunocompromised secondary to renal failure, peritoneal catheter placement, femoral catheter placement

DEFINING CHARACTERISTICS: A VasCath is in place, surgical incision following the creation, revision, or declotting of an A-V fistula; peritoneal catheter in place; femoral artery and vein cannulated with large-bore catheters

PATIENT OUTCOME (collaborative): Demonstrates absence of infection

EVALUATION CRITERIA: Temperature 98.6°F; WBC between 5,000-10,000/mm^3; absence of redness, drainage, and increased tenderness at surgical site

• •

INTERVENTIONS	RATIONALE
1. Monitor: • temperature q4h • appearance of skin at insertion site for the vascular access catheters, incision for the A-V fistula, peritoneal catheter	Early detection of problems facilitates early treatment.
2. Using aseptic technique, cleanse the A-V fistula incision daily with the prescribed antibacterial solution. Keep the incision covered with a sterile dressing until the sutures are removed. Avoid applying tape directly to the extremity containing the A-V fistula. Ensure that vascular access catheters (VasCath or femoral catheters) are kept securely covered with an occlusive dressing. Check facility policy and procedures to determine if the dialysis nurse provides site care for these catheters.	These measures help prevent contamination of the wound. Frequent application and removal of tape cause skin irritation that increases the risk of skin breakdown. Limiting the number of persons who manipulate the VasCath to a specialist, such as the dialysis nurse, helps reduce the risk of contamination.

INTERVENTIONS	RATIONALE
3. Consult physician if redness, swelling, and drainage at the incision or catheter insertion site, accompanied by fever, occur. Obtain a specimen of the drainage for culture. Administer prescribed antibiotic and evaluate its effectiveness.	These findings indicate infection and a need for antibiotic therapy. A culture helps identify the causative pathogen so appropriate antibiotic therapy can be prescribed. Antibiotic therapy is required to resolve an infection.
4. Use strict aseptic technique, including mask and sterile gloves, when preparing connection sites according to facility protocol and procedures. Adhere to universal precautions (good handwashing technique before and after care, wearing gloves when contact with blood or body fluid is likely to occur) when providing patient care. Protect patient from others who may have an infection.	To prevent nosocomial infection. Caregivers are the most common source of nosocomial infections.

NURSING DIAGNOSIS: HIGH RISK FOR IMPAIRED HOME MAINTENANCE MANAGEMENT

RELATED TO FACTORS: Knowledge deficit about self-care on discharge, nonacceptance of health status change, inadequate support system, inadequate finances, altered thought processes

DEFINING CHARACTERISTICS: Verbalizes lack of understanding, verbalizes difficulty in accepting illness, reports history of noncompliance, may report outstanding debts or financial crisis

PATIENT OUTCOME: Demonstrates willingness to comply with home therapeutic regimen

EVALUATION CRITERIA: Participates in self-care, asks questions, verbalizes understanding of discharge instructions

INTERVENTIONS	RATIONALE
1. Teach and have the patient practice daily self-care of the A-V fistula: a. Palpation of the thrill. Advise the patient to contact dialysis nurse or physician if unable to palpate a thrill. Explain significance of the presence of the thrill—indicates patency of the fistula. b. Inspection of the surgical site if fistula is newly created, revised, or declotted for signs of infection (redness, swelling, increased tenderness, drainage, fever). Report these findings immediately to dialysis nurse or physician.	Patency may be reestablished if clotting is detected early. Infection can ultimately lead to clotting and impair wound healing, thus delaying use of the A-V fistula.
2. Provide instructions about protecting the extremity: • Refrain from carrying purse or wearing tight restrictive clothing over the arm with the fistula. • Do **not** allow anyone to use the extremity with the fistula for assessing BP, obtaining blood samples, or giving injections. • Refrain from sleeping on the side where the fistula is located. • Keep the extremity elevated until swelling has subsided. • Wear heavy-duty gloves when gardening. • Avoid contact sports.	These measures are aimed at avoiding constriction of the extremity. The risk of clotting increases when circulation through the fistula is impaired. Maintaining skin integrity on the extremity helps reduce the risk of infection. Elevation helps reduce edema.
3. Instruct the patient to wear a Medic Alert bracelet over the unaffected arm.	To alert healthcare workers of the fistula in case of an accident.
4. Provide instructions about preventing infection: Cleanse the extremity daily with an antiseptic solution such as povidone-iodine (Betadine). Rewrap the extremity with sterile Kerlix dressing if a covering is required.	To reduce the number of transient bacteria. An antiseptic solution provides a protective barrier for the skin. Edematous skin is more susceptible to breakdown.

INTERVENTIONS	RATIONALE
5. Provide the patient and significant other with a written appointment for follow-up care and written instructions for care of the fistula site and extremity.	Verbal instructions may be easily forgotten.
6. Instruct the patient to begin resistance exercises about two weeks postoperatively: • Use the hand on the unaffected arm to tightly grasp the upper extremity that contains the A-V fistula to distend the vessel. • Then squeeze and release a rubber ball, tennis ball, or hand grips in the hand of the extremity with the fistula.	These exercises pump arterial blood against venous blood to distend the vessels.
7. Provide instructions for care of the VasCath if one is in place. • Avoid getting the dressing wet. • If tape becomes loose, reinforce the dressing with additional tape and immediately contact the dialysis nurse for further instructions. Let the patient know if the facility policy requires that only the dialysis nurse perform dressing changes. Usually site care is done each time dialysis is performed.	These measures help reduce the risk of an infection.

CONTINUOUS ARTERIOVENOUS HEMOFILTRATION

Continuous arteriovenous hemofiltration (CAVH) is a new method of removing toxic wastes from the blood of patients in acute renal failure. It is safer than conventional hemodialysis because as the patient's blood is removed for filtering it is simultaneously being replaced by a solution resembling plasma. Fluid overload is gradually alleviated, thus reducing the risk of severe hypotension from rapid fluid removal, which is common with conventional hemodialysis (Price, 1991).

CAVH is less expensive and is a simpler procedure compared with conventional hemodialysis. Two large-bore catheters are used — one inserted into the femoral artery and the other inserted into the femoral vein. The catheters are linked by a hemofilter unit. Blood is pumped out of the artery through the filter by the patient's own arterial pressure. The ultrafiltrate (water and toxic wastes) passes through the filter and collects in a special electronic collection container. To prevent sudden hypovolemia, a filter replacement fluid (FRF) is infused back to the patient through the venous circuit. The FRF is a plasma-like solution. Lactated Ringer's solution also may be used. To calculate the amount of FRF, the following parameters must be considered:

- amount of ultrafiltrate
- patient's total fluid intake and output from the previous hour
- desired net hourly fluid loss determined by the physician (Price, 1991)

 # ASSESSMENT DATA BASE

1. Before initiating CAVH, assess vital signs, pulmonary artery pressure, oxygen saturation, weight, and renal function studies (serum electrolytes, BUN, serum creatinine, coagulation factors, and CBC) to obtain baseline measurements.

NURSING DIAGNOSIS: HIGH RISK FOR ALTERED TISSUE PERFUSION

RELATED TO FACTORS: CAVH

DEFINING CHARACTERISTICS: One large-bore catheter inserted in the femoral artery and one inserted in the femoral vein

PATIENT OUTCOME: Demonstrates adequate circulation

EVALUATION CRITERIA: Pedal pulses present and equal, feet warm, color normal, wiggles toes without discomfort, denies numbness

INTERVENTIONS	RATIONALE
1. Monitor: • neurovascular status (Appendix D) of lower extremities q1h x 4 hours after catheter insertion, then q2h thereafter • BP, pulse, and respiration q1–2h • catheter insertion site q2–4h for evidence of bleeding • coagulation factors such as activated clotting time (ACT), prothrombin time (PT), and partial thromboplastin time (PTT)	For early detection of complications.

INTERVENTIONS	RATIONALE
2. Infuse prescribed amount of heparin into the infusion port on the arterial side of the hemofilter. Avoid infusing other medications or blood through the venous cannula. Consult physician immediately if the following occur: • coagulation factors above or below acceptable range • pallor, coolness, weakened or absent pedal pulse in the cannulated extremity	The extracorporeal circuit through which the blood flows, not the patient, must be anticoagulated to prevent clotting. Normally, the ACT should be maintained between 100–300 seconds, PT between 9.5–11.3 seconds, and PTT between 21–29 seconds. The risk of clotting is increased when values fall below the normal range. Bleeding may occur with values above the normal range. These abnormal physical findings signal obstruction.
3. Maintain bedrest with affected limb extended. When exercising the extremity, allow no more than a 30-degree hip flexion.	To prevent dislodgment of the femoral catheters.
4. Ensure all tubing is kept free of kinks. Adjust bed height to maintain the ultrafiltrate flow rate between 500–900 mL/hr. Raise the bed to increase the flow rate; lower the bed to decrease the flow rate.	Clotting is less likely to occur when this ultrafiltrate flow rate is maintained.

• •

◣ NURSING DIAGNOSIS: HIGH RISK FOR INFECTION

RELATED TO FACTORS: CAVH, immunocompromised state secondary to acute renal failure

DEFINING CHARACTERISTICS: Large bore-catheter inserted and kept in the femoral artery and vein for several days

PATIENT OUTCOME: Free of signs and symptoms of infection

EVALUATION CRITERIA: Temperature 98.6°F, WBC between 5,000–10,000/mm,^{3} absence of redness and drainage at insertion site

• •

INTERVENTIONS	RATIONALE
1. See **Nursing Diagnosis: High risk for infection** in the discussion on Hemodialysis.	
2. Adhere to strict aseptic technique, including gloves and mask, when preparing connection sites according to facility protocol and procedures.	Direct access to the patient's blood through these connections creates a culture medium for bacterial growth.
3. Monitor color of ultrafiltrate. If the ultrafiltrate turns pink-tinged or bloody, inspect the hemofilter for a membrane leak. If a break is detected, change the filter immediately according to facility protocol and procedures.	Normally, the ultrafiltrate should be clear yellow, with no gross blood. Blood-contaminated ultrafiltrate signals a membrane leak of the hemofilter, which leaves the compartment open for bacterial contamination.
4. Keep the connection sites always securely taped.	To prevent accidental disconnections.

PERITONEAL DIALYSIS

Peritoneal dialysis uses the highly vascular semipermeable peritoneal membrane to accomplish solute and fluid removal. Dialysate fluid is instilled into the peritoneal cavity via a silicone-rubber catheter (Tenckhoff catheter) and is left in place until solute and fluid are removed and then drained by gravity (dwell time). Fresh dialysate is then instilled, and the process repeated. The treatment can be intermittent—exchanges occur 12 hours, two or three times a week, or continuous with exchanges occurring four times daily each day. Continuous ambulatory peritoneal dialysis (CAPD) was developed and permits end-stage renal disease patients to enjoy a treatment that easily fits into their lifestyles.

Peritoneal dialysis is less efficient than hemodialysis because solute and fluid removal takes longer. But the shifts in fluid and solutes are more gradual and often better tolerated by patients. There is less incidence of hyperkalemia because potassium removal is constant. Ultrafiltration of fluid results from the osmotic effect of the glucose in the dialysate fluid instilled in the peritoneal cavity. Because protein loss occurs across the peritoneal membrane, the diet is more liberal in protein and, therefore, more tolerable for the patient.

After catheter placement, peritoneal dialysis can be instituted immediately. The procedure is not as technically involved as hemodialysis and can be performed in various settings. Patients who have had recent abdominal surgery or who have adhesions are not candidates for peritoneal dialysis. Also, patients with respiratory distress may not be able to tolerate the large volume of fluid instilled in the peritoneal cavity. Patients considering CAPD must learn the needed skills or have a significant other that can learn them.

The major complication of peritoneal dialysis is peritonitis. Hyperglycemia, hypovolemia, and hypoalbuminemia also may occur with peritoneal dialysis.

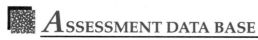

ASSESSMENT DATA BASE

1. See Hemodialysis.

• •

NURSING DIAGNOSIS: HIGH RISK FOR INFECTION

RELATED TO FACTORS: Peritoneal dialysis

DEFINING CHARACTERISTICS: Manifestations of peritonitis, including fever, persistent abdominal pain, cloudy and foul-smelling outflow, leakage of dialysate around the catheter, redness and tenderness at catheter site

PATIENT OUTCOME (collaborative): Demonstrates no manifestations of infection

EVALUATION CRITERIA: Temperature 98.6°F; WBC between 5,000–10,000/mm^3; clear outflow; no redness, drainage, or tenderness at catheter insertion site

• •

INTERVENTIONS	RATIONALE
1. Monitor: • temperature q4h • color of effluent with each exchange • results of CBC reports, especially WBC • appearance of peritoneal catheter insertion site with each dressing change	Early detection of problems minimizes complications by instituting immediate intervention.
2. Use strict aseptic technique in all aspects of care for peritoneal dialysis, including site dressing changes. Maintain a closed-sterile system. If catheter, tubing, or bag becomes contaminated, arrange for change immediately. Administer prophylactic antibiotic therapy as prescribed.	The high glucose concentration of the dialysate promotes bacterial growth.

INTERVENTIONS	RATIONALE
3. Consult physician for findings of cloudy effluent, persistent abdominal pain, redness, increased tenderness, drainage around the catheter site, and fever. Obtain a specimen of the effluent and drainage around the catheter site for culture.	These findings indicate infection. A cloudy outflow is the earliest sign of infection. Antibiotic therapy is required to resolve infection. A culture helps identify the causative organism so appropriate antibiotic therapy can be prescribed.
4. Limit the number of nurses caring for the patient, and ensure all are knowledgeable about the care required.	The chance of pathogens introduced to the patient is reduced.
5. See **Nursing Diagnosis: High risk for infection** in the discussion on Hemodialysis.	

 # NURSING DIAGNOSIS: HIGH RISK FOR FLUID VOLUME DEFICIT

RELATED TO FACTORS: Peritoneal dialysis

DEFINING CHARACTERISTICS: Hypovolemia (orthostatic hypotension, BP below normal level), hyperglycemia (blood glucose above normal range), hypoalbuminemia (serum albumin below normal level)

PATIENT OUTCOME: Demonstrates no manifestations of fluid volume deficit

EVALUATION CRITERIA: BP remains above 90/60 mm Hg, pulse rate 60–100 beats per minute, denies dizziness and light-headedness when moving from sitting or supine position to erect position

INTERVENTIONS	RATIONALE
1. Monitor: • weight before and after dialysis; compare the weight with the patient's dry body weight • BP and pulse before, during, and after dialysis • results of serum albumin and blood glucose studies	For early detection of fluid volume deficit. Body weight is the best indicator of fluid status. A weight change of 1 kg (2.2 pounds) is equivalent to 1 liter of fluid loss or gain.

INTERVENTIONS	RATIONALE
2. If body weight is increasing, arrange for consultation with the dietitian to evaluate caloric intake.	Reduction in food intake may be necessary to decrease calories.
3. Record the amount of dialysate instilled and the amount drained at the end of the dwell time. Compare the difference. Weigh the patient if the amount of effluent continually exceeds the amount instilled. Consult physician and change dialysate concentration as prescribed when the patient reaches dry weight.	To avoid dehydrating the patient by removing too much fluid.
4. Consult physician if blood glucose level is above normal range.	A change in the glucose concentration of the dialysate or adjustment in diet is required. A change in insulin dosage may be needed by diabetics.
5. Consult physician if the serum albumin value is below normal range. Arrange a consult with the dietitian to increase protein in diet.	Albumin is lost during peritoneal dialysis, especially if peritonitis occurs. Excess loss of albumin can cause hypovolemia as fluid shifts from the intravascular space to the extravascular compartments and peritoneal cavity.

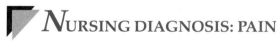

NURSING DIAGNOSIS: PAIN

RELATED TO FACTORS: Infusion of dialysate into the peritoneal cavity

DEFINING CHARACTERISTICS: Reports abdominal pain, facial frowning, moaning, distention of abdomen

PATIENT OUTCOME: Demonstrates absence of discomfort during instillation or drainage of dialysis fluid

EVALUATION CRITERIA: Denies pain, absence of moaning and facial frowning

INTERVENTIONS	RATIONALE
1. Warm dialysate to body temperature before infusing.	To prevent abdominal cramping.
2. Slow the infusion rate if the patient complains of discomfort during dialysate instillation.	Rapid infusion causes sudden abdominal distention.
3. Have the patient change position every 1–2 hours as the dialysate is drained.	To facilitate movement of the catheter tip and drainage of the solution.
4. Encourage the patient to use roughage in the diet to prevent constipation. Consult physician about using laxatives, stool softeners, or enemas if constipation is a constant problem.	Stool in the lower bowel can obstruct outflow of the dialysate.

◢ NURSING DIAGNOSIS: HIGH RISK FOR IMPAIRED HOME MAINTENANCE MANAGEMENT

RELATED TO FACTORS: Lack of knowledge about peritoneal dialysis, inability to perform peritoneal dialysis without assistance

DEFINING CHARACTERISTICS: Verbalizes lack of understanding, demonstrates inability to self-administer peritoneal dialysis, reports lack of adequate support system

PATIENT OUTCOME (collaborative): Demonstrates ability to manage peritoneal dialysis at home

EVALUATION CRITERIA: Accurately performs peritoneal dialysis without assistance or presence of a significant other who can perform the skill, verbalizes understanding of community service that assists with home peritoneal dialysis

INTERVENTIONS	RATIONALE
1. Evaluate the patient's or significant other's ability to perform peritoneal dialysis. Contact social services or discharge planning department to make arrangements for the patient to have peritoneal dialysis performed at a community dialysis	Teaching and evaluating the patient's ability to manage self-care help ensure safety in home maintenance management and improve compliance with therapy. These departments can initiate continued care activities for patient using available community resources.

INTERVENTIONS	RATIONALE
center or by a home health nurse if the patient and significant other cannot perform the procedure.	
2. Provide written instructions for steps in performing the procedure and follow-up care. Ensure the patient has the telephone number of the dialysis nurse to contact if any problems occur.	Verbal instructions may be easily forgotten.
3. Instruct the patient to keep a record of daily weights.	To monitor fluid status.
4. Emphasize the importance of adhering to aseptic technique when performing peritoneal dialysis and catheter site care. Instruct the patient to contact the dialysis nurse or physician if the following occur: • fluid excess (difficulty breathing, rales, weight gain, rising BP accompanied by tachycardia) • infection (redness, drainage, increased tenderness at the catheter insertion site accompanied by fever) • obstructed inflow or outflow of fluid • persistent pain or discomfort in abdomen, back, or shoulder • persistent constipation • leakage of dialysate around the catheter • hypotension (persistent dizziness and light-headedness especially when standing, excess weight loss)	Peritoneal dialysis predisposes a patient to these problems. Early recognition and treatment help reduce the severity of the problem.

Renal Transplantation

Renal transplantation is an alternative treatment for end-stage renal disease for those patients who meet criteria. Generally patients over the age of 65 or with metastatic diseases, advanced cardiac or pulmonary disease or infection are not candidates for a renal transplant. The donated kidney is placed in the anterior iliac fossa, and the patient's nonfunctioning kidneys are left in place unless they are infected or grossly enlarged.

The care of transplant patients is the responsibility of the transplant team—the surgeon and transplant coordinators who are clinical nurse specialists. When it is determined that renal transplant is a viable option for the patient, a donor source for the kidney must be identified. A well-matched living related donor (usually, parent, child, or sibling) ensures the best outcome. If a living related kidney transplant will be done, two family members undergo surgery. The long hospitalization and uncertain outcome place strain on the family.

If a donor is not available, the patient is put on a waiting list for a tissue-matched cadaver kidney. Cadaver kidney procurement is managed by organ procurement organizations under federal regulation. A computerized system matches cadaver donors with the best candidate for transplant.

Two major complications of renal transplant are rejection and side effects of long-term immunosuppressive drug therapy. Rejection of the graft is the most serious. There are three types of rejection. Hyperacute rejection occurs immediately after surgery and is not treatable. Acute rejection is experienced by most patients within the first few weeks after transplant. In most cases, acute rejection can be reversed with increased doses of immunosuppressive drugs. The most commonly used drugs are:

- prednisone
- azathioprine (Imuran)
- cyclosporine (Sandimmune)
- methylprednisolone (Solu-Medrol)
- antilymphocyte globulins
- muromonab-CD3 (Orthoclone OKT3)

Chronic rejection occurs over a period of months to years. It does not respond to treatment and is characterized by increasing blood chemistries and fluid retention. When the patient reaches end-stage renal disease, dialysis is resumed. Patients who are at least 12 months post-transplantation are considered long-term recipients.

Major side effects common to immunosuppressive agents are weight gain, mood changes, susceptibility to infection, ulceration and GI bleeding, and aseptic necrosis of the femoral head.

Acute tubular necrosis (ATN) is seen most often in cadaver kidneys. It is caused by prolonged ischemia and may take at least four weeks to resolve. Dialysis may be needed until ATN resolves and kidney function returns to normal.

The mean LOS for a DRG classification of renal transplantation is 13.9 days (Lorenz, 1991). The recipient is usually dialyzed 24 hours after receiving the transplant to remove uremic toxins and restore normal platelet function. Readmission for several days for treatment of rejection is common.

Integrative Care Plans

- Preoperative and postoperative care
- Dialysis
- Fluid and biochemical imbalance
- Surgery
- Loss
- Renal failure
- IV therapy

Discharge Considerations

- Medications to continue at home
- Activity limitations
- Signs and symptoms requiring medical attention
- Follow-up care

THE PREOPERATIVE PERIOD

 *A*SSESSMENT DATA BASE

1. Assess past history of compliance with treatment plan.

2. Assess patency of dialysis access device—peritoneal catheter or arteriovenous (A-V) fistula.

3. Perform a general assessment (Appendix F) to establish baseline values. Assess for clinical manifestations of infection:
   - elevated temperature
   - cold or flu
   - dysuria
   - condition of peritoneal exit site

4. See Preoperative and Postoperative Care (page 738).

THE POSTOPERATIVE PERIOD

1. See Preoperative and Postoperative Care (page 738). For assessment data base and additional nursing interventions in addition to those listed below.

● ●

◤ Nursing Diagnosis: HIGH RISK FOR ALTERED TISSUE PERFUSION

RELATED TO FACTORS: Rejection or infection secondary to kidney transplantation

DEFINING CHARACTERISTICS: Recurring manifestations of acute/chronic renal failure (rejection)

PATIENT OUTCOME (collaborative): Demonstrates adequate renal function

EVALUATION CRITERIA: Urinary output greater than 30 mL/hr; serum potassium, creatinine and BUN within normal limits; no signs of fluid retention

● ●

INTERVENTIONS	RATIONALE
1. Monitor: • intake and output qh x 48 hours, then q2h x 48 hours, then q4h if urinary output is consistently greater than 30 mL/hr • vital signs q4h • results of renal scan (evaluates excretory function of the kidney) • results of renal biopsy (helpful in diagnosing rejection) • weight daily • lung sounds q8h • results of laboratory studies (CBC, serum creatinine and BUN, urine specific gravity)	To identify indications of progress toward or deviations from expected outcomes.
2. Consult physician immediately if the following occur: • urine output less than 30 mL/hr • change in color of urine (cloudy, hematuria) • dysuria	These findings signal renal failure/rejection and a need for additional immunosuppressive agents to suppress the recipient's immune response.

INTERVENTIONS	RATIONALE
• swelling or tenderness over the kidney • elevated temperature • proteinuria • weight gain of two pounds or more per day Administer prescribed immunosuppressive agents and evaluate their effectiveness.	
3. Maintain IV therapy at prescribed rate until oral intake is adequate to maintain urine output.	Hypovolemia can lead to renal shutdown. The infusion rate is determined by the urine output rate.

• •

 # Nursing Diagnosis: High Risk for Infection

RELATED TO FACTOR: Renal transplantation, required use of immunosuppressant agents

DEFINING CHARACTERISTICS: Urinalysis reveals bacturiuria; cloudy, foul-smelling urine; reports dysuria; oral ulcerations, whitish plaques in the mouth, reports painful mouth; WBC above 10,000/ mm³; fever

PATIENT OUTCOME (collaborative): Absence of manifestations of infection

EVALUATION CRITERIA: Temperature 98.6°F; WBC between 5,000–10,000/ mm³; passage of clear, yellow urine; denies dysuria; normal urinalysis

• •

INTERVENTIONS	RATIONALE
1. See **Nursing Diagnosis: High risk for infection** in the discussion on Hemodialysis.	
2. Consult physician for early signs of infection: • WBC above 10,000/mm³ (often the first sign of rejection) • chronic cough • redness, swelling, increased tenderness, drainage of surgical incision	Immunosuppressive agents make the patient more susceptible to opportunistic infections. *Candida albicans* and herpes simplex are the most common pathogens affecting the oral cavity. Appropriate antibiotic therapy and protective care measures are required to prevent massive spread of the infection.

INTERVENTIONS	RATIONALE
• dysuria, cloudy urine, bacteriuria • elevated temperature • complaints of sore throat or mouth, accompanied by whitish plaques along the oral cavity Obtain urine, blood, and throat specimen for culture. Administer prescribed antibiotic and evaluate its effectiveness. Provide routine oral care according to facility protocol and procedures.	
3. Provide perineal care with soap and water b.i.d. Adhere to universal precautions when direct contact is required. This includes good hand-washing technique before and after patient care and wearing gloves when contact with blood or body fluid is likely to occur. Use strict aseptic technique with dressing changes — includes wearing sterile gloves and mask.	Invasive procedures and devices create a path for pathogens to enter the body. Caregivers are the most common source of nosocomial infections.
4. Initiate protective care measures: • Restrict visitors with infections from the patient. • Instruct patient and family in good handwashing techniques. • Place the patient in a private room. • Have the patient wear a mask when leaving the room; also, visitors wear masks if the patient is leukopenic.	These measures help reduce the transmission of pathogens.

●●●●●●●●●●●●●●●●●●●●●●●●●●●●●●●●

NURSING DIAGNOSIS: HIGH RISK FOR IMPAIRED HOME MAINTENANCE MANAGEMENT

RELATED TO FACTORS: Knowledge deficit about self-care, history of noncompliance.

DEFINING CHARACTERISTICS: Verbalizes lack of understanding, history of occasional noncompliance with treatment plan when on dialysis

PATIENT OUTCOME (collaborative): Demonstrates willingness to adhere to prescribed plan for home maintenance and prevention

EVALUATION CRITERIA: Verbalizes understanding of discharge instructions

●●●●●●●●●●●●●●●●●●●●●●●●●●●●●●●●

INTERVENTIONS	RATIONALE
1. Develop a teaching plan in cooperation with the transplant coordinator. Ensure the patient and family member know: • name, frequency, indications for, dosage, and reportable side effects of all prescribed medications. • signs and symptoms of infection to report. • signs and symptoms of rejection to report. • diet—usually sodium restriction; arrange for dietary consult. • how to obtain required specimens, such as 24-hour urine collection and clean-catch urine. • normal laboratory values for creatinine, and BUN. • assess weight and temperature daily. Ensure patient has a log for recording daily weights and temperature.	Patient compliance is essential for continued functioning of the transplanted kidney.
2. Review schedule for follow-up visits to the transplant office or clinic. Be sure patient knows where and how often blood needs to be drawn. Ensure all self-care instructions and follow-up appointments are written.	Frequent monitoring is required to detect and treat rejection episodes as early as possible. Verbal instructions may be easily forgotten.

INTERVENTIONS	RATIONALE
3. Encourage the patient to fully participate in self-care activities while in the hospital (self-medication, weighing, obtaining temperature, monitoring laboratory values).	These activities must become part of the patient's daily activities at home.
4. Encourage patient to increase activity level while hospitalized. If permitted, allow patient access to other areas of the facility, for example cafeteria and gift shop.	An environment conducive to self-care helps the patient incorporate changes into daily activities.
5. Remind the patient: • that immunosuppressive drugs must be taken for the life of the transplanted kidney. • to wear a Medic Alert bracelet to identify self as a kidney transplant and as a user of immunosuppressant agents. • to refrain from participating in contact sports.	Immunosuppressants help suppress rejection. Special identification quickly alerts medical personnel of health status if a medical emergency arises. Blunt trauma to the abdomen may disrupt the transplanted kidney.
6. Refer the patient to a vocational counselor for assistance in career planning when the patient feels ready.	Some patients may need assistance in redirecting their lives to accommodate the demands a kidney transplant imposes.
7. Include family members in all teaching when possible.	The patient needs continued support from the family to cope with needed changes.
8. Reinforce the need for early reporting of signs of infection and rejection and the importance of keeping all appointments for follow-up care.	Complications are often treatable if identified early.

BIBLIOGRAPHY

Blair, K. A. (1990). Aging: Physiological aspects and clinical implications. **Nurse Practitioner, 15,** 14–16, 18, 23, 26–28.

Coloski, K., Mastrianni, J., Dube, R., & Brown, L.H. (1990). Continuous arteriovenous hemofiltration patient: Nursing care plan. **Dimensions of Critical Care Nursing, 9,** 130–142.

Conway, J. (1989). Taking a look at lower UTI's—Urinary tract infections. **Journal of Urologic Nursing, 8,** 641–643.

England, G.E. (1990). Preoperative care of renal transplant patients: Physiological and psychological approach. **Journal of Urologic Nursing, 9,** 1011–1016.

Freeman, N.L. (1991). Ureteroscopic laser lithotripsy and extracorporeal shock wave lithotripsy: The advantage of both in a lithotripsy center. **Urologic Nursing, 11,** 28–29.

Feikles, R. (1991). Long-term complications of renal transplantation. **Journal of Urologic Nursing, 10,** 1086–1098.

Glassock, R. J. (1988). Pathophysiology of acute glomerulonephritis. **Hospital Medicine, 23,** 163–178.

Greig, B.J. (1990). A new option for cystectomy patients. **RN, 53,** 34–36.

Heneghan, G.M., Clark, N., Hensley, B.J., & Yang, T. (1990). The indiana pouch: A continent urinary diversion. **Journal of Enterostomal Therapy, 17,** 231–236.

Jennette, J. C., & Falk, R. J. (1990). Diagnosis and management of glomerulonephritis and vasculitis presenting as acute renal failure. **Medical Clinics of North America, 74,** 893–907.

Johnson, D.L. (1989). Nephrotic syndrome: A nursing care plan based on current pathophysiologic concepts. **Heart Lung, 18,** 85–93.

Lorenz, E.W. (1991). **1992 St. Anthony's DRG Working Guidebook.** Alexandria: St. Anthony Publishing Company.

Maidl, L. (1990). Stomal and peristomal skin complications with urostomies. **Urologic Nursing, 10,** 17–22.

Norris, M.K.G. (1989). Acute tubular necrosis: Preventing complications. **Dimensions of Critical Care Nursing, 8,** 16–26.

Price, C.A. (1991). Continuous renal replacement therapy. **Journal of American Nephrology Nurses Association, 18,** 239–244.

Rauscher, J., Farber, R.D., & Parra, R.D. (1991). Camey procedure: A continent urinary diversion technique. **Journal of American Operating Room Nurses, 54,** 34, 36–37, 39–41.

Rutherfor, C. (1991). Erythropoietin: A new frontier. **Journal of Intravenous Nursing, 14,** 163–165.

Tombasco, M.N. (1990). Postoperative nursing management following renal transplantation. **Journal of Urologic Nursing, 9,** 1034–1043.

Warren, H. (1989). Changes in peritoneal dialysis nursing. **Journal of American Nephrology Nurses Association,16,** 237–241.

Zorzanello, M.M. (1989). Preventing acute renal failure in patients with chronic renal insufficiency: Nursing implications. **Journal of American Nephrology Nurses Association, 16,** 433–438.

C

HAPTER THREE

Problems of the Gastrointestinal Tract

Gastroplasty

Gastroplasty (gastric partitioning) is a surgical procedure used for treating morbid obesity. Obesity is excess body weight. Morbid obesity refers to 100 pounds or 100% over ideal body weight for height and age. Obesity contributes to various health problems such as heart disease, diabetes, hypertension, and gallbladder disease. Also, obesity can diminish one's self-concept since obese people are often targets of ridicule and are frequently stereotyped as "comical."

Gastroplasty is done under general anesthesia via an abdominal incision. It involves placement of sutures or staples vertically or horizontally through the stomach walls to reduce the stomach size. Consequently, the intake of food and fluid is limited because of the smaller stomach.

Preoperative preparation is the same for any patient undergoing surgery. Postoperatively, the patient has a Foley catheter, nasogastric tube, IV infusion, abdominal dressing, and antiembolism stockings. Small amounts (about 10 mL) of clear liquids are given hourly on the third postoperative day, full liquids for about eight weeks, pureed food for about 12 weeks, and then a soft diet.

The mean length of stay (LOS) for a diagnostic related group (DRG) classification of gastroplasty is 6.9 days (Lorenz, 1991).

Integrative Care Plans

- Preoperative and Postoperative Care
- IV therapy

Discharge Considerations

- Follow-up care
- Dietary modifications
- Signs and symptoms indicating perforation of sutures or staples

THE PREOPERATIVE PERIOD

1. See Preoperative and Postoperative Care (page 738).

THE POSTOPERATIVE PERIOD

 ASSESSMENT DATA BASE

1. See Preoperative and Postoperative Care (page 738).
2. Assess ability to manage dietary modifications at home.

• •

NURSING DIAGNOSIS: HIGH RISK FOR ALTERATIONS IN HOME MAINTENANCE MANAGEMENT

RELATED TO FACTORS: Knowledge deficit about self-care on discharge, disturbance in self-concept

DEFINING CHARACTERISTICS: May verbalize history of noncompliance, verbalizes lack of understanding about self-care activities on discharge, requests information, may report low self-esteem, may report frustration at failed attempts to lose weight by dieting, may verbalize unrealistic expectations about surgical outcomes

PATIENT OUTCOME: Demonstrates willingness to comply with self-care maintenance and preventive measures on discharge

EVALUATION CRITERIA: Verbalizes understanding of discharge instructions, realistic weight loss goals, ways to deal with reactions of significant others to weight loss, positive statements about self, and understanding of need to adjust to new body image

• •

INTERVENTIONS	RATIONALE
1. Assist the patient with planning strategies for dealing with anticipatory reactions of friends and significant others to new body image.	Reactions from friends and family members may range from happiness to jealousy.
2. Allow the patient to express feelings about self. Assist in setting realistic weight loss goals.	Talking helps promote effective coping.

INTERVENTIONS	RATIONALE

3. Provide instructions on how to prevent perforation of the staples or sutures.
  • Consume only the prescribed volume of food.
  • Eat six small meals daily instead of three large meals.
	Gastroplasty does not alter appetite, thus, hunger is still experienced. Frequent feeding helps satisfy hunger and control overeating. Overeating is the primary cause of ruptured staples.

4. Instruct the patient to notify the physician if sudden abdominal pain that radiates to the shoulders occurs.	This finding signals perforation of the staples.

Inflammatory Bowel Disease

Inflammatory bowel disease (IBD) has an unknown etiology. The primary pathological findings are inflammation, edema, thickening, and ulceration of the intestinal mucosa. Bleeding may occur when stool passes over the inflamed areas, breaking the mucosal surface. Abscess formation occurs when the broken surfaces become infected. IBD is a chronic disorder characterized by periods of remission and exacerbation.

Crohn's disease (regional enteritis) and ulcerative colitis are the most prevalent forms of IBD. Both forms have a strong genetic predisposition. There is no single dietary cause nor cure. Some major distinguishing features for each form are (Cooke, 1991):

- **Crohn's disease**—can occur anywhere in the GI tract

  — characterized by patchy or "skip" lesions (areas of healthy tissue interspersed with areas of affected tissue)

  — high risk for fistula and stricture formation because of transmural involvement

- **Ulcerative colitis**

  — may predispose to cancer of the colon

  — extends upward from the rectum and affects only the colon

  — involves only mucosal and submucosal layers

  — characterized by a continuous lining involvement

  — a total colectomy is curative

Hospitalization is not required for patients with IBD unless IV therapy is required to correct severe fluid and biochemical imbalances or complications, such as perianal disease (anorectal fistulas and abscesses), intestinal obstruction, perforation, or hemorrhage. The mean LOS for a DRG classification of inflammatory bowel disease is 7.1 days (Lorenz, 1991).

General Medical Management

- Pharmacotherapy:

  — anticholinergic agents

  — corticosteroids such as prednisone, sulfasalazine (Azulfidine), mesalamine (Rowasa), or hydrocortisone acetate intrarectal foam (Cortenema)

  — metronidazole (Flagyl) (used to relieve perianal disease)

— sedatives or tranquilizers

— antidiarrheal agents

• Nutritional supplements of iron and vitamins

• Stress management

• Surgery if medical treatments are ineffective and complications develop:

— for Crohn's disease, a segmental resection with ileostomy if an extensive segment of the bowel must be removed

— for ulcerative colitis, a colectomy and ileostomy

Integrative Care Plans

• Bowel diversion (if ileostomy performed)

• Preoperative and Postoperative Care

• IV therapy

• Fluid and biochemical imbalance

• Loss

Discharge Considerations

• Follow-up care

• Ostomy care (if ileostomy performed)

• Measures to control exacerbations

• Medications to continue at home

• Stress management techniques

• Signs and symptoms of exacerbations

 # ASSESSMENT DATA BASE

1. History or presence of risk factors:
   • positive family history
   • inadequate intake of dietary fiber
   • food allergies
   • emotional stress

2. Inquire about the color and consistency of stools, the number of stools per day, and the presence of rectal urgency. Physical examination based on a general survey (Appendix F) may reveal:
   • reports of diarrhea accompanied by cramplike abdominal pain (most common finding). Stools may be steatorrhea, contain mucus, pus, or blood.
   • reports of painful and excoriated anus resulting from frequent stools

- malabsorption syndrome (dehydration and weight loss caused by excessive diarrhea)
- reports of rectal bleeding

3. Assess for factors that precipitate symptoms.
   - emotional upsets
   - spicy foods
   - gas-forming foods

4. Diagnostic studies:
   - Radiologic studies (barium enema, sigmoidoscopy or colonoscopy, upper GI series) identify the extent of the disease.
   - Hematest® stool for occult blood may be positive for blood.
   - Stool culture for ova and parasites rules out parasitic infections.
   - Biopsy confirms diagnosis and rules out carcinoma.
   - Complete blood count (CBC) often reveals anemia (hemoglobin, hematocrit, and RBC below normal range).
   - B_{12} level detects a vitamin B_{12} deficiency).

5. Assess the patient's understanding of condition and treatment.
6. Assess the patient's feelings about having a chronic condition and its impact on lifestyle.

▶ NURSING DIAGNOSIS: HIGH RISK FOR FLUID VOLUME

RELATED TO FACTORS: Diarrhea, inadequate fluid intake

DEFINING CHARACTERISTICS: Abnormal electrolyte values, weight loss, weakness, possibly ECG changes, dry skin, concentrated urinary output

PATIENT OUTCOME (collaborative): Fluid and biochemical status return to normal limits

EVALUATION CRITERIA: Electrolyte values within normal range, no further weight loss, denies weakness, absence of diarrhea, supple skin

INTERVENTIONS	RATIONALE
1. Monitor: • intake and output q8h • results of electrolyte reports • weight daily • stools (number, consistency, color)	To evaluate effectiveness of therapy.

INTERVENTIONS	RATIONALE
2. See Fluid and Biochemical Imbalance (page 773), especially, hypokalemia, hypernatremia, and metabolic acidosis.	Fluid, potassium, and bicarbonate ions are lost with prolonged diarrhea. An elevated serum sodium reflects dehydration.
3. Avoid rectal temperatures or anything per rectum.	Foreign objects placed in the rectum stimulate peristalsis.
4. Administer prescribed antidiarrheals and anticholinergic agents. Evaluate their effectiveness. Consult physician if diarrhea and abdominal cramps persist after 48 hours of treatment.	Antidiarrheal agents reduce the number of liquid stools and also help the stools become more formed. Often the patient has to experiment with different agents to discover the most effective one. Anticholinergic agents reduce spastic activity of the intestines; thus, the number of bowel movements.
5. Hematest stools for blood. Report positive results to physician.	Persistent bleeding can lead to anemia and possibly a need for a blood transfusion.
6. Keep nothing by mouth (NPO) and administer prescribed IV therapy with electrolyte supplements or total parenteral nutrition (TPN) (page 220) if diarrhea cannot be controlled. Initiate preventive and maintenance activities for IV therapy. (See IV Therapy, page 764).	Certain foods stimulate intestinal activity. Supplemental IV fluids with replacement of electrolytes help correct dehydration and electrolyte imbalances that occur with prolonged diarrhea.

• •

 NURSING DIAGNOSIS: HIGH RISK FOR ALTERATION IN SKIN INTEGRITY

RELATED TO FACTORS: Excessive diarrhea

DEFINING CHARACTERISTICS: Reddened and excoriated anus, reports painful anus with each bowel movement

PATIENT OUTCOME (collaborative): Perianal skin heals

EVALUATION CRITERIA: Denies painful anus with bowel movements, absence of redness and excoriation around anus

• •

INTERVENTIONS	RATIONALE
1. Instruct patient to cleanse perianal area with warm water and a mild deodorant-free soap after each stool. This may be done with the use of a sitz bath. Pat the area dry and then use Tuck's wipes. Apply a protective skin barrier (A and D ointment, Peri-care, Desitin cream) to the perianal area.	Cleansing helps to control odor and removes irritating substances. Deodorant soaps tend to dry the skin. Tuck's wipes contain a solution of witch hazel that has a soothing effect. A skin barrier reduces contact of perianal skin with acid, liquid stool.
2. Instruct the patient to wear cotton and not nylon underwear.	Cotton underwear allows for better air circulation to promote drying of the perineal area. Moisture buildup promotes bacterial growth

NURSING DIAGNOSIS: HIGH RISK FOR INFECTION

RELATED TO FACTORS: Long-term use of steroids, immunocompromised state secondary to inadequate nutritional intake

DEFINING CHARACTERISTICS: May have persistent low-grade fever, WBC above 10,000/mm^3, history of perianal abscess

PATIENT OUTCOME: Absence of manifestations of infection

EVALUATION CRITERIA: Temperature 98.6°F, WBC between 5,000–10,000/mm^3, perianal tissue intact

INTERVENTIONS	RATIONALE
1. Monitor: • CBC reports, particularly WBC • temperature q4h	To identify indications of progress toward or deviations from expected outcome.
2. Administer prescribed antibiotic and evaluate its effectiveness.	Antibiotics are required to prevent and resolve an infection.

INTERVENTIONS	RATIONALE
3. Use universal precautions (good handwashing technique before and after patient contact, wearing gloves when contact with blood or body fluid is likely to occur). When providing patient care, advise the patient about the importance of washing hands and cleansing the perianal area thoroughly after toileting.	An immunocompromised state is induced with long-term steroid therapy, thus increasing the patient's risk for infections.

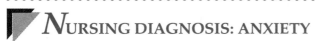

NURSING DIAGNOSIS: ANXIETY

RELATED TO FACTORS: Knowledge about diagnostic studies treatment plan, and threats to health status change

DEFINING CHARACTERISTICS: Verbalizes lack of understanding; requests information; may report feelings of nervousness, inadequacy, uncertainty, or apprehension; repetitive questioning; tense facial expression; may report insomnia

PATIENT OUTCOME: Demonstrates less anxiety

EVALUATION CRITERIA: Fewer reports of nervousness; verbalizes understanding of diagnostic studies and treatment plan; relaxed facial expression

INTERVENTIONS	RATIONALE
1. See **Nursing Diagnosis: Anxiety** (page 262).	

NURSING DIAGNOSIS: HIGH RISK FOR ALTERATIONS IN HOME MAINTENANCE MANAGEMENT

RELATED TO FACTORS: Knowledge deficit about self-care measures on discharge, inadequate support system

DEFINING CHARACTERISTICS: Verbalizes lack of understanding, reports history of noncompliance, reports difficulty accepting condition, requests information

PATIENT OUTCOME (collaborative): Demonstrates willingness to comply with self-care preventive and maintenance measures on discharge

EVALUATION CRITERIA: Verbalizes understanding of discharge instructions, verbalizes plans for normal nutritional maintenance

● ●

INTERVENTIONS	RATIONALE
1. Evaluate patient's understanding of condition. Correct any misconceptions. Emphasize there is no cure and medical treatments are aimed at controlling symptoms. If surgery is scheduled because of Crohn's disease, ensure the patient understands that surgery will not cure the disease because the lesions are scattered throughout the GI tract. If surgery is scheduled for ulcerative colitis, ensure the patient understands that surgery may provide a cure because the lesions are limited to the colon, which is removed during surgery.	A realistic understanding of the outcomes of medical intervention helps facilitate coping and patient compliance.
2. Collaborate with the patient, significant other, and dietitian in planning for a high-calorie, high-vitamin, low-residue diet. Advise use of liquid nutritional supplements, such as Ensure or Sustacal if anorexia occurs. Instruct the patient to avoid intake of alcoholic beverages and foods that cause gastric distress. Provide a list of common gas-forming foods to avoid during periods of exacerbations (for example, bananas, cabbage, raw vegetables, and milk, especially if the patient has a lactase deficiency). If a lactase deficiency exists, advise the patient to use lactose-free milk or lactase tablets. Encourage the patient to keep a diary of foods and situations that precipitate pain and diarrhea.	The dietitian is a nutritional specialist and can assist the patient in planning meals to meet caloric needs relative to the current illness. Alcohol is an irritant to an already inflamed area. Often the patient has to experiment with foods to determine which ones to avoid. Fiber tends to be poorly tolerated.

INTERVENTIONS	RATIONALE
3. Provide information about medications prescribed for home use, including name, dosage, schedule, purpose, and reportable side effects. Emphasize the importance of taking the medication as prescribed.	Medications effectively control the symptoms of inflammatory bowel disease but must be taken continuously to be effective. Side effects signal a need for a change in drug, dosage, or administration frequency .
4. Reinforce the need to drink at least eight glasses of water daily.	To combat dehydration.
5. Advise the patient to consult the physician when: • antidiarrheal medication fails to control diarrhea after 48 hours • exacerbation of IBD occurs: — diarrhea accompanied by abdominal cramping — anorexia unrelieved by prescribed medication	These findings signal worsening of the condition.
6. Assist the patient to identify ways to relieve emotional stress. • Identify common sources of stress. • Attend stress management classes. • Engage in a regular exercise program. • Plan rest periods during the day when experiencing an exacerbation of diarrhea.	Emotional stress can precipitate an attack of diarrhea.
7. Advise the patient to eat six small meals a day instead of three large meals.	Distention of an inflamed intestinal mucosa from a heavy meal can trigger nausea and vomiting.
8. See Loss (page 733).	

Abdominoperineal Resection

An **abdominoperineal resection** (APR) results in three wounds: an abdominal wound, a colostomy, and a perineal wound. The perineal wound is created by removal of the anus and rectum. A wound drainage device is placed into the perineal wound and usually removed within a few days. Wound irrigations or sitz baths are then allowed. The major complications associated with APR are impotence in males (because of dissection of sympathetic nerves), wound infection, and urinary tract infection. Sexual dysfunction may occur in females secondary to scarring and contracture of the perineum.

General preoperative preparation is the same for any patient undergoing surgery. Additional preparation may include:

1. Bowel cleansing. This usually involves:
   - low-residue diet three days before surgery
   - clear liquid diet the day before surgery
   - laxatives and enemas the day before surgery
   - antibiotics, oral and IV, the day before surgery to rid the bowel of natural bacteria flora. (Neomycin and erythromycin are commonly used).

2. Insertion of a nasogastric (N/G) tube to maintain gastric decompression postoperatively.

Postoperatively, the patient may return to the medical/surgical unit with the following:

- IV infusion
- Foley catheter
- abdominal and perineal dressings
- N/G tube for connection to intermittent suction
- antiembolism stockings
- wound drainage device

The N/G tube remains until peristalsis returns. Ice chips may be allowed while the N/G is in place, otherwise the patient is kept NPO. The Foley catheter is often removed on the second postoperative day. Prophylactic antibiotics are given IV for a few days. The wound drainage device is removed when drainage is scant. Daily dressing changes are then started. The patient is assisted out of bed (OOB) the first postoperative day, with progressive ambulation thereafter.

If no N/G is in place, the patient is kept NPO until peristalsis returns, evidenced by bowel sounds and passage of flatus. After peristalsis returns, clear liquids are allowed and advanced to a regular diet, according to the patient's tolerance.

Integrative Care Plans

- Preoperative and postoperative care
- Bowel diversion and rectal surgery
- IV therapy
- Loss
- Pain

Discharge Considerations

- Follow-up care
- Activity limitations
- Signs and symptoms of wound infection
- Wound care
- Ostomy care

THE PREOPERATIVE PERIOD

1. See Preoperative and Postoperative Care (page 738).

THE POSTOPERATIVE PERIOD

 *A*SSESSMENT DATA BASE

1. See Preoperative and Postoperative Care.

◤ *N*URSING DIAGNOSIS: HIGH RISK FOR FLUID AND BIOCHEMICAL IMBALANCES

RELATED TO FACTORS: Nasogastric suctioning, inability to intake food and fluids orally

DEFINING CHARACTERISTICS: Electrolyte values below normal range (particularly potassium and bicarbonate), weakness, possibly ECG changes

PATIENT OUTCOME (collaborative): Demonstrates fluid and biochemical equilibrium

EVALUATION CRITERIA: Stable weight, serum electrolyte values within normal range, fluid output approximates fluid intake

INTERVENTIONS	RATIONALE
1. See Fluid and Biochemical Imbalances (page 773).	
2. Administer prescribed IV therapy with prescribed amount of potassium chloride (KCL). Use an infusion pump when administering a continuous infusion of KCL. Monitor intake and output q8h while receiving KCL infusion. Notify physician if output is less than 30mL/hr.	A potassium deficit can occur with prolonged N/G suctioning. An infusion pumps allows better control of the infusion flow rate. Potassium is excreted by the kidneys. If urine output falls, hyperkalemia can develop quickly.

◤ NURSING DIAGNOSIS: HIGH RISK FOR POSTOPERATIVE COMPLICATIONS

RELATED TO FACTORS: Abdominoperineal resection

DEFINING CHARACTERISTICS: May show early signs and symptoms of atelectasis, infection, thrombophlebitis, dehiscence, paralytic ileus or peritonitis

PATIENT OUTCOME (collaborative): Demonstrates no manifestations of postoperative complications

EVALUATION CRITERIA: Absence of manifestations of infection, atelectasis, dehiscence, thrombophlebitis, peritonitis, and paralytic ileus

INTERVENTIONS	RATIONALE
1. For infection, atelectasis, dehiscence, and thrombophlebitis, see **Nursing Diagnosis: High risk for postoperative complications** in the discussion on Preoperative and Postoperative Care (page 738).	

INTERVENTIONS	RATIONALE

Paralytic Ileus:
 	
2. Monitor:
 	
  • amount of N/G tube drainage q8h
 	
  • abdominal status q8h for return of peristalsis (auscultate bowel sounds, inquire about passage of flatus, inspect abdomen size, palpate abdomen for unusual firmness)
	To identify indications of progress toward or deviations from expected outcome.

3. Irrigate N/G tube with a saline solution prn. To ensure accurate N/G tube output, measure the amount of irrigant used each time the tube is irrigated. Subtract the irrigant used during an 8-hour period from the total drainage in the collection bottle at the end of that 8-hour shift. Record the difference to reflect the exact amount of drainage.	Irrigation helps maintain patency of the N/G tube. A saline irrigant is isotonic and therefore helps prevent additional loss of electrolytes. Peristalsis is normally reduced following general anesthesia or abdominal surgery. An accurate output is needed to determine the amount of IV fluid required to prevent dehydration.
4. Initiate measures to prevent accidental dislodgment of the N/G tube. Apply wrist restraints prn, if the patient is confused, restless, or disoriented.	Safety is a priority when individuals experience altered levels of consciousness.
5. Consult physician immediately if N/G tube drainage turns bright red.	This would signal hemorrhage. A normal drainage is green or gold.
6. If no N/G tube is used, keep the patient NPO until peristalsis returns, indicated by bowel sounds and expelling flatus.	After abdominal surgery, a temporary ileus (lack of peristalsis) is expected because of interference with neuromuscular stimulation caused by manipulation of the intestines. Ileus is evidenced by lack of bowel sounds. Normally, bowel motility returns within 3–4 days.

INTERVENTIONS	RATIONALE
7. If the patient experiences nausea and vomiting accompanied by progressive abdominal distention and absence of bowel sounds, consult physician immediately. Obtain a portable abdominal x ray as prescribed. Measure and record the abdominal girth q8h if distention is suspected. Insert an N/G tube and connect to intermittent suction as prescribed.	These clinical findings may occur because of obstruction, intra-abdominal hemorrhage, or severe potassium deficit. An abdominal x ray, serum electrolytes, and CBC are needed to identify the etiology of symptoms. Gastric decompression with an N/G tube allows the bowel to rest.
Peritonitis: 1. Monitor abdominal status (Appendix B) q8h.	For early detection of peritonitis.
2. Consult physician immediately if the patient suddenly experiences severe abdominal pain, rapid shallow respirations, rigid distended abdomen, and absence of bowel sounds. Check vital signs for shock (BP less than 90/60 mm Hg, tachycardia, and tachypnea accompanied by cool clammy skin) and fever. Prepare the patient for return to surgery if ordered.	Seepage of GI contents into the peritoneal cavity (peritonitis) can cause septic shock. Inadequate suturing of the surgical site and intestinal obstruction can cause peritonitis.
3. Irrigate the N/G tube, if in place, prn to maintain patency.	Maintaining adequate gastric decompression helps prevent strain on the sutures at the anastomosis site following surgery on the GI tract.

NURSING DIAGNOSIS: ALTERATION IN ORAL MUCOSA

RELATED TO FACTORS: Nasogastric tube placement and restricted oral intake of fluids

DEFINING CHARACTERISTICS: Reports sore throat, dry mouth and lips, requests something to drink

PATIENT OUTCOME: Oral mucosa remains intact

EVALUATION CRITERIA: Fewer reports of sore throat, moist lips

INTERVENTIONS	RATIONALE
1. Provide oral care q2h while NPO or while the N/G tube is in place. Keep a moistened gauze at the bedside for the patient to moisten mouth prn. If the patient is alert and oriented, allow to rinse mouth with water prn. Apply lubricant, such as petroleum jelly to lips prn.	Moisture helps maintain integrity of the oral mucosa.
2. If an N/G tube is in place, give prn ice chips, topical anesthetic (Viscous Xylocaine), or an anesthetic throat lozenge.	An anesthetic effect is induced with cold or drug therapy.

• •

◤ NURSING DIAGNOSIS: HIGH RISK FOR IMPAIRED HOME MAINTENANCE MANAGEMENT

RELATED TO FACTORS: Knowledge deficit about self-care on discharge

DEFINING CHARACTERISTICS: Verbalizes lack of understanding, requests information, may report difficulty adjusting to altered body image

PATIENT OUTCOME (collaborative): Demonstrates willingness to comply with self-care preventive and maintenance measures on discharge

EVALUATION CRITERIA: Verbalizes understanding of discharge instructions, accurately performs required self-care procedures

• •

INTERVENTIONS	RATIONALE
1. Advise the patient to avoid heavy lifting for 6–8 weeks or as instructed by physician. Rest frequently and avoid overexertion.	To reduce strain on the suture line. Full recuperation from major surgery takes about 4–6 weeks.

INTERVENTIONS	RATIONALE
2. See Preoperative and Postoperative Care (page 738) for additional discharge instructions.	
3. See Loss (page 733) for plan of care related to altered body image.	
4. See Rectal Surgery (page 251) for plan of care related to the perineal incision.	
5. See Bowel Diversion (page 235) for plan of care related to the colostomy.	

Cancer of the Stomach

Stomach cancer has an insidious onset and an unknown etiology. It spreads rapidly and often has metastasized before the patient becomes symptomatic. The tumor may cause ulceration, perforation, obstruction, or hemorrhage. Distant metastases occurs via the lymphatics to the liver, pancreas, lungs, bone, and peritoneal cavity.

General Medical Management

- Chemotherapy
- Radiation therapy
- Surgery:
    a. Subtotal esophagogastrectomy—for operable tumors in the proximal stomach. The lower portion of the esophagus and most or all of the stomach are removed. The remaining upper portion of the esophagus is anastomosed to the duodenum or jejunum. The patient often has a chest tube following this procedure since the chest cavity is entered.
    b. Total gastrectomy—for lesions in the midportion of the stomach. The entire stomach is removed, and the esophagus is anastomosed to the jejunum.
    c. Subtotal gastrectomy—for lesions in the antrum of the stomach when the patient is elderly or debilitated. This is a Billroth I operation in which the duodenum, distal stomach, pylorus, and supporting vascular and lymphatic structures are removed, and the remaining stomach portion is sutured to the remaining duodenum.
    d. Subtotal gastrectomy—a Billroth II operation, which is a more radical procedure than the Billroth I. Operation involves removal of antrum, pylorus, upper duodenum, supporting vascular structures, and all surrounding lymphatics. The remaining stomach portion is sutured in a side-to-side fashion to the jejunum. The duodenual stump is sutured closed.

The major complications associated with these gastric surgical procedures are esophagitis (caused by reflux aspiration), anastomotic leakage, vitamin B_{12} deficiency, weight loss, and pneumonia. Additional complications associated with a subtotal gastrectomy include the dumping syndrome and steatorrhea. The mean LOS for a DRG classification of stomach cancer is 7.0 days; 14.3 days for stomach procedures with complications, and 7.7 days without complications (Lorenz, 1991).

Integrative Care Plans

- Cancer
- Chemotherapy
- Pain
- Radiation therapy
- Preoperative and postoperative care (if gastrectomy is performed)
- Loss

Discharge Considerations

- Follow-up care
- Hospice referral for end-stage disease
- Dietary modifications to continue at home
- Medications to continue at home

 # ASSESSMENT DATA BASE

1. History or presence of risk factors:
   - achlorhydria or pernicious anemia
   - history of gastric ulcers

2. Physical examination based on a general survey (Appendix F) may reveal:
   - initial complaints of a vague feeling of fullness and discomfort after meals. The patient often interprets these symptoms as "upset stomach" and uses home remedies and antacids, which provide temporary relief.

     As the tumor enlarges, the patient experiences:
   - weight loss caused by anorexia, nausea, and vomiting
   - weakness and fatigue due to nutritional deficiency anemia
   - dysphagia if the tumor is located in the proximal stomach
   - epigastric pain caused by gastric distention from the enlarging tumor
   - a palpable epigastric mass

3. Diagnostic studies:
   - Upper GI series reveals a solid mass.
   - CT scan of the abdomen reveals a solid mass.
   - Endoscopic examination provides direct visualization of the lesion and allows specimen collection for biopsy and cytology studies. (Cytology studies provide the most definitive diagnostic information).
   - CBC reveals anemia (hemoglobin, hematocrit, and red blood cell count below normal range).

4. Assess the patient's and significant other's feelings and concerns about illness.

5. Assess the patient's and significant other's understanding of illness, diagnostic studies, and treatment.

NURSING DIAGNOSIS: PAIN

RELATED TO FACTORS: Gastric distention from stomach tumor

DEFINING CHARACTERISTICS: Verbalizes pain, moaning, frowning

PATIENT OUTCOME (collaborative): Demonstrates relief from discomfort

EVALUATION CRITERIA: Reports pain less intense, absence of moaning, relaxed facial expression

INTERVENTIONS	RATIONALE
1. See Pain (page 700).	
2. Encourage rest periods at intervals.	Tissue demands for oxygen are less during rest periods because less energy is expanded. Also, gastric secretion is lessened during rest.
3. Encourage intake of six small meals a day instead of three large meals.	Excessive food intake causes gastric distention, which leads to stomach pain.

NURSING DIAGNOSIS: ALTERATIONS IN NUTRITION: LESS THAN BODY REQUIREMENT

RELATED TO FACTORS: Anorexia, nausea, and/or vomiting secondary to stomach cancer

DEFINING CHARACTERISTICS: Progressive weight loss, possibly dysphagia, weakness, anemia, persistent reports of fatigue

PATIENT OUTCOME (collaborative): Maintains optimal nutritional status

EVALUATION CRITERIA: No further weight loss, serum chemistry studies within normal limits, fewer reports of fatigue

INTERVENTIONS	RATIONALE
1. Monitor: • amount of food consumed with each meal • weight every other day or weekly • intake and output q8h • results of serum chemistry studies	To evaluate effectiveness of therapy.
2. Provide a bland diet high in calories, protein, vitamins, and minerals. Encourage use of enteral feeding supplements (Sustacal, Ensure) if dietary intake is less than 50%.	Spicy foods are gastric irritants. Cancer cells rapidly divide resulting in a rate of catabolism (tissue destruction) greater than the rate of anabolism (tissue building). A high-carbohydrate diet exerts a protein-sparing effect in the presence of a negative nitrogen (protein) balance.
3. Ensure a comfortable, odor-free environment during meal times. Provide foods that patient likes, if possible. Refer to dietitian for assistance with meal planning. If dietary intake is inadequate for more than four days and weight loss continues, confer with physician about the use of total parenteral nutrition (TPN) therapy.	Anorexia is a common finding with cancer of the GI tract. Failure to eat properly leads to malnutrition and weight loss. TPN therapy provides adequate caloric intake to spare body protein.
4. Administer prescribed antiemetic at least 30 minutes before meals if nauseated.	Nausea contributes to anorexia.
5. Provide at least 2500 mL of fluid daily.	To protect against dehydration.

NURSING DIAGNOSIS: ACTIVITY INTOLERANCE

RELATED TO FACTORS: Anemia and malnutrition secondary to cancer of the stomach

DEFINING CHARACTERISTICS: Reports fatigue and weakness when performing activities of daily living (ADL), abnormal heart rate or blood pressure response to activity, anemia (hemoglobin, RBC, and hematocrit values below normal range)

PATIENT OUTCOME (collaborative): Demonstrates increased tolerance to activities

EVALUATION CRITERIA: Fewer reports of fatigue and weakness when performing ADL

INTERVENTIONS	RATIONALE
1. Monitor: • color and consistency of stools • results of CBC reports • vital signs q4h • response to physical activities: (respiratory rate)	To identify indications of progress toward or deviations from expected outcome.
2. Provide assistance with ADL as needed. Plan rest periods during the day.	Rest reduces energy expenditure.
3. Administer prescribed treatments for anemia (iron supplements or blood transfusions).	Iron is needed for normal erythropoiesis. Whole blood may be given if massive hemorrhage occurs. Packed RBCs may be given to replace blood cell loss when fluid volume is adequate.
4. Hematest® all stools if dark. Consult physician if stools are guaiac positive.	Black, tarry stools indicate GI bleeding, reflected as positive guaiac tests.

Herniorraphy

Herniorraphy refers to surgical repair of a hernia. A hernia is a protrusion of an organ through a congenital or acquired defective opening in the wall of the cavity that normally contains the organ. Most hernias occur somewhere in the abdominal cavity and involve the intestine. A loop of intestine is forced through the defective opening as a result of increased intra-abdominal pressure (Nyhus et al, 1990).

Some hernias can be manually pushed back into the normal cavity (reducible) while others are not (irreducible). Irreducible hernias predispose persons to intestinal obstruction. Obstruction of the flow of intestinal contents occurs with strangulation of the hernia. Most hernias require surgical repair.

The hernia is named for its location:

a. indirect inguinal hernia—a loop of intestine escapes through the inguinal canal and follows the spermatic cord (males) or round ligaments (females). It results from failure of the processus vaginalis to close after the testes descend into the scrotum, or fixation of the ovaries.

b. direct inguinal hernia—the loop of intestine escapes through the posterior inguinal canal.

c. femoral hernia—a loop of intestine passes through the femoral ring down the femoral canal.

d. umbilical hernia—more common in children. A loop of intestine protrudes through the umbilical ring, which failed to close.

Preoperative preparation is the same for any patient undergoing surgery. Postoperatively, the patient returns to a medical/surgical unit with an IV infusion and a groin dressing (for inguinal or femoral hernias) or an abdominal dressing (for umbilical hernia). Because of the proximity of the surgery to urinary structures, difficulty in voiding may be encountered. Following inguinal hernia repair in males, swelling and ecchymosis of the scrotum are common. For this reason, males are often concerned about the effect of surgery on sexual functioning.

The mean LOS for a DRG classification of herniorraphy is 3.2 days (Lorenz, 1991).

Integrative Care Plans

- Preoperative and postoperative care
- IV therapy
- Pain

Discharge Considerations

- Follow-up care
- Signs and symptoms of wound infection
- Wound care
- Activity restrictions
- Pain control

THE PREOPERATIVE PERIOD

 ## ASSESSMENT DATA BASE

1. Physical assessment based on an abdominal assessment (Appendix F) may reveal:
   - a lump in the groin or umbilical area (most significant finding)
2. Inquire about activities that affect the size of the lump. The lump may be present constantly or only appear with activities that increase intra-abdominal pressure such as coughing, sneezing, lifting, or having a bowel movement.
3. Inquire about discomfort. Some discomfort may be experienced because of tension. Pain indicates strangulation and a need for urgent surgery. Additionally, manifestations of intestinal obstruction may be detected (high-pitched bowel sounds progressing to absent, nausea, vomiting).
4. See Preoperative and Postoperative Care (page 738) for additional assessments and plan of care for the preoperative period.

THE POSTOPERATIVE PERIOD

 ## ASSESSMENT DATA BASE

1. See Preoperative and Postoperative Care (page 738) for assessments and additional plans of care.

Nursing Diagnosis: HIGH RISK FOR INFECTION

RELATED TO FACTORS: Acute urinary retention, surgical incision, and inflammation of the scrotum secondary to herniorraphy

DEFINING CHARACTERISTICS: Verbalizes inability to void, suprapubic distention, swelling and ecchymosis of the scrotum, WBC greater than $10,000/mm^3$, temperature above 98.9°F, may report dysuria and frequency

PATIENT OUTCOME (collaborative): Demonstrates absence of manifestations of infection

EVALUATION CRITERIA: Clear yellow or amber urine, voiding without complaints of discomfort, scrotum of normal color and size, temperature 98.6°F, wound heals, WBC between $5,000–10,000/mm^3$

INTERVENTIONS	RATIONALE
1. Monitor: • for voiding difficulties q8h • intake and output q8h • color and size of scrotum daily • results of CBC reports • appearance of wound with dressing changes • temperature q4h	To identify indications of progress toward or deviations from expected outcome.
2. Report to physician findings of: • inability to void accompanied by suprapubic distention • frequent voiding of small amounts Catheterize as ordered.	These findings signal acute urinary retention and a need for catheterization to empty the bladder. Urinary retention increases the risk of urinary tract infection.
3. Consult physician if the patient experiences swelling and ecchymosis of the scrotum or painful voiding of a foul-smelling, cloudy urine. Apply ice packs and a scrotal support as ordered. Administer prescribed antibiotics. Increase fluid intake to at least 2–3 liters daily.	These findings signal infection. Cold and elevation help relieve swelling. Antibiotics are required to resolve an infection. Fluids help flush the kidneys and promote better distribution of antibiotics.
4. See **Nursing Diagnosis: High risk for infection** under Preoperative and Postoperative Care (page 738) for additional interventions.	

Appendicitis

Appendicitis refers to inflammation of the appendix, a nonfunctional pouchlike extension located at the inferior portion of the cecum. The most common cause of appendicitis is obstruction of the lumen by feces, which ultimately impairs blood supply and erodes the mucosa causing inflammation (Wilson & Goldman, 1989). The major complication associated with appendicitis is peritonitis, which may occur if the appendix ruptures. An appendectomy (removal of the appendix) is the only treatment.

Preoperative and postoperative care is the same for any patient undergoing surgery. The mean LOS for a DRG classification of appendicitis is 6.1 days without complications and 9.8 days with complications (Lorenz, 1991).

Integrative Care Plans

- Preoperative and postoperative care
- Pain
- IV therapy

Discharge Considerations

- Follow-up care
- Signs and symptoms of wound infection
- Wound care
- Activity limitations
- Pain control

THE PREOPERATIVE PERIOD

 ## ASSESSMENT DATA BASE

1. Physical assessment based on an abdominal assessment (Appendix F) may reveal:
   - severe and persistent, right lower quadrant abdominal pain

- rebound tenderness over the McBurney's point (midpoint between umbilicus and right iliac crest)
- increased pain when coughing
- fever
- nausea and vomiting

2. Diagnostic studies:
   - CBC reveals white blood cell count above 10,000/mm^3.
   - Ultrasound of the abdomen shows inflammatory process.

3. See Preoperative and Postoperative Care (page 738).

◤ NURSING DIAGNOSIS: HIGH RISK FOR INFECTION

RELATED TO FACTORS: Peritonitis secondary to ruptured appendix

DEFINING CHARACTERISTICS: Sudden cessation of pain accompanied by rigid boardlike abdomen, falling BP, rising pulse rate, and pale, cool, clammy, skin

PATIENT OUTCOME (collaborative): Demonstrates no manifestations of peritonitis

EVALUATION CRITERIA: Absence of manifestations of peritonitis

INTERVENTIONS	RATIONALE
1. Every hour monitor: • vital signs • bowel sounds • size of abdomen • quality of pain	To detect perforation.
2. Notify physician immediately and prepare for surgery as ordered if manifestations of perforation occur: • sudden cessation of pain. Minutes later, the pain recurs accompanied by abdominal distention, rigid abdomen, tachycardia, falling BP, tachypnea, and vomiting.	Prompt surgery is required for a ruptured appendix. Bowel contents spill into the peritoneal cavity when the appendix ruptures, precipitating peritonitis.

INTERVENTIONS	RATIONALE
3. Keep nothing by mouth (NPO). Initiate prescribed IV therapy. Prepare the patient for surgery as ordered.	Abstaining from food and liquids by mouth (NPO) before surgery reduces the risk of vomiting and aspiration when under anesthesia. Vascular access is needed if emergency drugs are needed.
4. Maintain bedrest in a semi-Fowler's position. Keep knee of bed slightly flexed.	To relieve tension on abdominal muscles.
5. Explain that pain medication cannot be given until the cause of the pain has been identified.	Pain medication masks symptoms, especially if the appendix ruptures.
6. Avoid giving an enema.	An enema can precipitate rupture of the appendix.

THE POSTOPERATIVE PERIOD

1. See Preoperative and Postoperative Care (page 738).

Total Parenteral Nutrition

Total parenteral nutrition (TPN), also called hyperalimentation, is the infusion of a concentrated nutrient solution through a catheter placed into a central vein, either the subclavian, internal jugular vein or peripherally inserted central catheter (PICC). A large vein must be used because the highly concentrated hypertonic solution causes damage to the vein wall and thrombosis if given through a peripheral vein.

TPN is used as a last resort to provide adequate nutrient intake for patients unable to tolerate oral feedings or a nasogastric tube (patients with chronic inflammatory or obstructive bowel disease, severe burns, multisystem trauma, anorexia nervosa, or carcinoma of the gastrointestinal tract).

FreAmine III is the most commonly used TPN solution. For patients with renal failure, Nephramine is used. The TPN solution is composed of proteins (essential amino acids), electrolytes, vitamins, minerals, insulin, and 20–50% glucose. Vitamin K is given weekly by intramuscular injection because it is incompatible with the TPN solution.

Essential fatty acids, called lipids or fat emulsion, are supplied as a separate infusion. Lipid solutions are available as Liposyn (composed of safflower oil) or Intralips (composed of soybean oil). Both are available in 500 mL bottles as a 10% solution providing 550 kcal, or a 20% solution providing 1000 cal. Lipids are given as supplemental calories to prevent fatty acid deficiency. The usually dose of fat emulsion is 500 mL daily.

TPN therapy is planned by a nutritional support team, a multidisciplinary team consisting of a physician, a nurse, a dietitian, and a pharmacist. The physician prescribes the composition of the TPN solution, type of solution, type and concentration of lipids, and flow rate. The solution is mixed in a special environment by the pharmacist. The nurse collects the required supplies (per facility protocol) and assists with the insertion of the central venous catheter (CVC). The nurse makes continual assessments for signs of complications and ensures the patient receives the prescribed solutions. The pharmacist prepares the TPN solution as prescribed by the physician. The dietitian monitors the nutritional status of the patient to determine when adjustments are needed in the composition of the TPN solution.

The major complications associated with TPN therapy are sepsis, fluid overload, metabolic imbalances, and catheter displacement. Pneumothorax and air embolism are complications related to initial insertion of the CVC. Allergic reaction is the major adverse reaction associated with using lipids.

This plan of care assumes the CVC has been inserted and proper placement has been confirmed by x ray.

ASSESSMENT DATA BASE

1. Ongoing assessments include:
   - weight
   - vital signs
   - level of consciousness
   - condition of the skin
   - results of serum electrolyte and glucose reports
   - intake and output
   - status of catheter insertion site
   - lung sounds

NURSING DIAGNOSIS: HIGH RISK FOR COMPLICATIONS: SEPSIS, FLUID OVERLOAD, METABOLIC IMBALANCES

RELATED TO FACTORS: TPN therapy via a central vascular access catheter, continuous infusion of a hypertonic glucose solution

DEFINING CHARACTERISTICS: May show early manifestations of sepsis, fluid overload, or metabolic imbalances

PATIENT OUTCOME (collaborative): Remains free of manifestations of sepsis, fluid overload, and metabolic imbalances

EVALUATION CRITERIA: Temperature less than 99°F; WBC between 5,000-10,000/mm^3; clear lung sounds; absence of edema; BP between 90/60–140/90 mm Hg; catheter insertion site without redness, drainage, tenderness; blood glucose within normal limits

INTERVENTIONS	RATIONALE

Sepsis:
1. Monitor:
  • For redness and drainage at insertion site on each shift; palpate site for tenderness
  • temperature q4h
  • results of CBC reports, particularly WBC
	To identify indications of progress toward or deviations from expected outcome.

INTERVENTIONS	RATIONALE
2. Consult physician of temperature above 100°F (38°C), or redness, swelling, or drainage at the insertion site. If physician orders removal of the CVC for culture, use sterile equipment and cut about four inches of the catheter tip. Place the tip in a sterile cup. Obtain blood, urine, and wound cultures as prescribed. Administer prescribed antibiotic and evaluate its effectiveness.	These findings indicated infection. If the wound shows no signs of infection in the presence of a fever, additional testing is needed to determine the source of the infection. Broad-spectrum antibiotic therapy helps resolve an infection.
3. Adhere to infection control guidelines when giving a TPN solution. • Keep the TPN solution refrigerated until ready for use. • Inspect the solution. Do not use solution if it is cloudy or contains particulate matter. • Change the TPN tubing and Leur-lok injection cap (on unused CVC ports) every 24 hours. • Wipe the Leur-lok injection cap with alcohol or povidone-iodine solution before inserting a needle to flush the unused ports or to withdraw blood. • **Always** infuse the TPN solution through IV tubing that has a 0.22 micron filter. • Change the CVC site dressing three times a week and when it becomes moist or loose. Ensure an occlusive dressing is applied. Label the dressing with the date and time changed.	A high dextrose concentration provides a good medium for bacterial growth. These measures help reduce the risk of infection.

INTERVENTIONS	RATIONALE
• Use strict aseptic technique when changing the site dressing (wear mask, sterile gloves, sterile gown, and cap). If available, use the commercially prepared "central line dressing kit." • Do **not** allow the TPN solution to hang over 24 hours.	

Fluid Overload:
 	
1. Monitor:
   • weight daily or as prescribed
   • vital signs q4h
   • general status (Appendix F) q8h
   • results of electrolyte reports, particularly the serum sodium
	To evaluate effectiveness of interventions and to detect problems early.

2. Reduce the IV flow rate and consult physician immediately if peripheral edema, neck vein distention, rales, fluid intake significantly greater than output accompanied by daily weight gain, low serum sodium, rising BP, or change in sensorium occur. Keep the patient in a semi-Fowler's position.	These findings signal fluid overload and a need to restrict fluid intake, or administer diuretic therapy, or both. An erect position reduces venous return to the heart.
3. **Always** use an infusion pump to administer the TPN solution, fat emulsion, and other solutions that are infused through the CVC.	An infusion pump provides the best control of the flow rate.

Metabolic Imbalances (hyperglycemia and hypoglycemia):
 	
1. Monitor:
   • blood glucose levels q6h using a capillary blood glucose monitoring device, and record results on facility's flow sheet
   • CVC insertion site q8h for signs of infiltration
	To detect potential problems early.

INTERVENTIONS	RATIONALE
2. Report blood glucose values above normal range. Administer regular insulin as prescribed for persistent blood glucose values above normal range.	Hyperglycemia reflects inability of the pancreas to handle the increased amount of glucose. Insulin helps maintain adequate glycemic control.
3. Adhere to guidelines to prevent hypoglycemia. • Keep the TPN line open with a 10% dextrose solution at the same rate as the TPN solution if the next bottle of TPN solution is not available. • Ensure a bottle of TPN solution is always available. • If the patient has been NPO during TPN therapy and no peripheral IV infusion is in place that contains dextrose, reduce the flow rate of the TPN solution to 50 mL/hr while increasing oral intake or tube feeding intake before discontinuing the TPN infusion. Allow four hours for this change over.	Normally, the pancreas secretes insulin to maintain the serum glucose between 80–120 mg/dL. When TPN is given, insulin secretion is sustained at a high level. Discontinuing a TPN solution abruptly while insulin secretion is high results in a rapid depletion of serum glucose, evidenced by symptoms of hypoglycemia.
4. Do **not** try to "catch up" if the TPN infusion falls behind schedule.	A rapid infusion of the solution can cause a rapid rise in serum glucose or hyperglycemia.
5. After the TPN solution is discontinued, obtain a blood glucose sample immediately and consult physician if nausea, blurred vision, light-headedness, diaphoresis, weakness, or tachycardia occur. Administer orange juice or initiate an IV of 5% dextrose in water (D-5-W) at 100 mL/hr if the patient is NPO. Retest blood glucose level within 15 minutes.	These findings indicate hypoglycemia and a need for rapid glucose replacement.

INTERVENTIONS

6. Ensure catheter patency:

   a. Notify physician if the following occur:

      • leaking of solution at site

      • swelling or pain around site during infusion

   b. Never infuse any other solution or blood except lipids through the TPN line. Consult pharmacy about compatibility of medications with TPN solutions.

   c. Do not draw blood through the TPN line if a single lumen CVC is used.

   d. Flush unused ports of the multilumen CVC with the appropriate solution according to facility protocol and procedures, depending on the type of central vascular device:

      • heparinized solution for the Hickman central venous catheter CVC, the standard triple lumen CVC, and the implanted port.

      • saline only for the Groshong catheter.

   e. After withdrawing blood or injecting medication through a port, **always** flush the port with at least 10 mL of bacteriostatic saline, followed by a heparin flush solution.

   f. If a multilumen CVC is used, use the port according to its indicated use specified by the manufacturer. Label each port to indicate how it is to be used.

RATIONALE

These findings indicate catheter displacement and a need to remove the catheter. Other solutions may be incompatible with the TPN solution. Frequent use of the CVC for blood sampling increases the risk of clotting. Heparin prevents blood clots from occluding the lumen of the catheter. Each port has a different size lumen.

INTERVENTIONS	RATIONALE
7. If a lumen of the CVC becomes occluded, follow facility protocol and procedures for declotting the lumen with streptokinase or urokinase. Notify physician if unable to reestablish patency. Label the port as "Clotted—Do Not Use." If streptokinase is to be used, ask patients if they have had a streptococcal infection recently.	These fibrinolytic agents may be used to dissolve clots to reestablish patency of a CVC. Ports on a mutilumen CVC that are not clotted may continue to be used. Antibodies produced with a streptococcal infection make streptokinase less effective in declotting.

NURSING DIAGNOSIS: HIGH RISK FOR IMPAIRED GAS EXCHANGE

RELATED TO FACTORS: Possible air embolism, pneumothorax secondary to insertion of a CVC, possible allergic reactions and fat emboli secondary to lipid infusions

DEFINING CHARACTERISTICS: Dyspnea, chest pain, cyanosis, diminished lung sounds, hives, itching, pain in the lower back or chest, petechiae

PATIENT OUTCOME (collaborative): Respiratory function remains intact

EVALUATION CRITERIA: Respiratory rate 12–24 per minute, clear breath sounds bilaterally, absence of chest pain, normal skin color, absence of subcutaneous emphysema, denies dyspnea, absence of hives, petechiae

INTERVENTIONS	RATIONALE
Pneumothorax: 1. Monitor lung sounds, BP, pulse, and respiration q2h for the first eight hours after insertion of the CVC. Notify physician immediately of dyspnea, decreased breath sounds, or asymmetrical chest expansion. Keep the patient in a Fowler's position. Start supplemental oxygen at 2 L/min via nasal cannula. Obtain a portable chest x ray immediately as prescribed.	These findings signal pneumothorax that can occur immediately during catheter insertion or hours later. It is the result of accidental puncture of the lung during catheter insertion. Chest x ray confirms a pneumothorax.

INTERVENTIONS	RATIONALE

Air Embolism:
 	
1. Adhere to guidelines to prevent air embolism:
  • Prime all IV tubing.
  • Tape all IV tubing connections to ensure tubing does not become accidentally disconnected.
  • Clamp the CVC **before** disconnecting the IV tubing.
  • Keep a Leur-lok injection cap on each unused port of the CVC.
  • When removing the CVC:
    — Place the patient in a supine position if tolerated.
    — Remove the sutures.
    — Instruct patient to perform the Valsalva maneuver (take a deep breath and hold while bearing down as if having a bowel movement) while pulling the catheter out.
    — Immediately apply pressure for five minutes to the site followed by a small pressure dressing.
    — Inspect the entire length of the catheter to ensure all of the catheter has been removed.
	Large amounts of air may block the outflow or inflow of blood to the heart or lungs and cause ischemia or even death. Small amounts of air usually produce no symptoms because it passes into the pulmonary circulation where it is eventually reabsorbed. The Valsalva maneuver causes normal negative intrathoracic pressure to increase above that of positive atmospheric pressure, thus guarding against the entry of air into the bloodstream.

2. Notify physician immediately if the patient suddenly experiences chest pain, dyspnea, cyanosis, and confusion. If air embolism is suspected, place the patient in a Trendelenburg position on the left side. Start oxygen via nasal cannula at 4–6 L/min. Obtain a portable chest x ray immediately as prescribed.	Air embolism may occur when air enters the vascular system either during catheter insertion or before initiating the infusion if failure to prime the TPN tubing occurs. A Trendelenburg position increases intrathoracic pressure preventing the embolus from entering cardiopulmonary circulation. A left lateral position allows air to rise, thus reducing the risk of air entering the pulmonary artery. A chest x ray establishes the diagnosis of air embolism. Cardiac catheterization may be required to aspirate large air emboli from the heart.

INTERVENTIONS	RATIONALE
Fat Emboli: 1. Inspect each bottle of lipid solution for appearance and expiration date before infusing. Discard solution if it is outdated, appears oily or to have separated, because fat emulsion is normally opaque and milky white.	To avoid infusing a solution that can increase the risk of infection if outdated, or fat emboli if oily separation is present.
2. Administer the fat emulsion through a separate line or piggyback through the TPN line **below the filter. Never infuse fat emulsion through a filter.**	The isotonic lipid emulsion is compatible with TPN solution. Because it is isotonic, it will not irritate veins when given peripherally. The fat globules will clog the filter.
3. Do **not** allow the fat emulsion to hang over 24 hours.	Normally, fat emulsion is infused over 4–8 hours, depending on the concentration. Allowing it to run longer does not allow adequate time for the liver to metabolize the product and affects the results of serum lipid studies.
4. Do **not** refrigerate Liposyn.	Refrigeration causes separation and hardening of the fat globules.
5. **Always** use an infusion pump to infuse the fat emulsion.	To ensure control of the flow rate and reduce risk of inadvertent fluid overload.
6. Start the initial lipid infusion at 1 mL/min for the first 15 minutes. Observe the patient for adverse reactions: dyspnea, cyanosis, nausea, vomiting, fever, sweating, pain in the chest or back, pressure over the eyes, flushing, skin rash, or hives. If these findings occur, **stop the infusion** and notify physician. If no reaction occurs after 15 minutes, increase the infusion to the prescribed flow rate.	Slow administration allows time for early detection of allergic reactions. Symptoms representing an allergic reaction are due to fat globules blocking microcapillaries.

Enteral Feeding

Enteral feeding, commonly termed tube feeding, is indicated for patients with a function gastrointestinal tract but who:

- are unable to swallow
- have had aerodigestive tract surgery
- have an endotracheal tube
- are comatose
- are mentally disturbed and do not eat
- have severe facial fractures

Enteral feeding may be done through a feeding tube surgically inserted into the stomach through the abdominal wall (gastrostomy) or through a nasogastric (N/G) tube. A gastrostomy may be performed through a laporotomy or by a less expensive procedure that involves less risk called percutaneous endoscopic gastrostomy (PEG).

PEG Tube

A PEG tube is inserted under local anesthesia with minimal sedation in the GI lab. Two physicians perform the procedure—an endoscopist and an assistant. An IV infusion is usually started for administration of an anesthetic or sedative, usually diazepam (Valium). A 16-F mushroom catheter is passed into the stomach through a small abdominal incision. The catheter is held in place by two rubber bumpers—one placed around the catheter inside the stomach and the other placed around the catheter on the outside of the abdomen. A topical anesthetic is sprayed on the patient's throat to reduce discomfort and to prevent gagging as the endoscopic tube is passed into the stomach. The light source at the tip of the endoscopic tube shines through the abdominal wall. A small stab incision is made over the light source, and the catheter is inserted into the stomach.

Preoperative preparation is the same for any patient undergoing surgery. Postoperatively, feeding is initiated early if no abdominal discomfort occurs.

Feeding Tubes

Small-bore feeding tubes such as the Dubbhoff, Entriflex, Duo-tube, or Kuofeed are safer than traditional feeding tubes. These long tubes rest in the duodenum instead of the stomach, thus reducing the risk of regurgitation into the esophagus and aspiration into the trachea. Traditional feeding tubes rested in the stomach.

The small-bore tubes have a mercury-weighted tip to enhance passage into the duodenum. These tubes are inserted in the same manner as other N/G tubes. Tube placement must be confirmed by an abdominal x ray before beginning the feeding. The tube should be securely taped to the nose once duodenal placement is confirmed.

This plan of care reflects care after insertion of the feeding tube.

ASSESSMENT DATA BASE

1. Before insertion of a feeding tube, perform an abdominal assessment to establish baseline values: auscultate bowel sounds, inspect the abdomen size, palpate for tenderness. Note date of last bowel movement.

NURSING DIAGNOSIS: HIGH RISK FOR INFECTION

RELATED TO FACTORS: Insertion of PEG tube or gastrostomy tube

DEFINING CHARACTERISTICS: Purulent drainage at insertion site, redness, increased tenderness, leakage of tube feeding at site, fever, WBC above 10,000/mm^3

PATIENT OUTCOME (collaborative): Absence of infection

EVALUATION CRITERIA: Temperature 98.6°F, absence of redness and drainage at insertion site, WBC between 5,000–10,000/mm^3

INTERVENTIONS	RATIONALE
1. Monitor: • temperature q4h • appearance of insertion site during dressing changes • results of CBC studies	To detect beginning of problems.
2. Cleanse the incision of the PEG site daily with an antiseptic solution using sterile technique. Apply a fenestrated dressing, such as a tracheostomy dressing, to absorb any drainage.	A fresh incision is an ideal culture medium for microbes. Adhering to aseptic technique reduces the risk of contamination.

INTERVENTIONS	RATIONALE
3. Consult physician for leakage of feeding around the tube, fever, or redness and increased tenderness at the PEG site. Administer antibiotics as prescribed.	These findings signal infection and a need for antibiotic therapy. Persistent leakage can cause skin irritation.
4. If a PEG tube is in place, do **not** place the dressing between the rubber bumper and the skin surface. Place the dressing **over** the tip of the rubber bumper.	This prevents free play of the PEG tube and reduces the risk of constant irritation to the incision.
5. Adhere to universal precautions (good handwashing technique before and after patient contact, wearing gloves when contact with blood or body fluid is likely to occur) when providing patient care.	Patients requiring feeding by alternative routes are considered immunocompromised because they are often experiencing a chronic illness. Caregivers are the most common source of nosocomial infections.
6. Provide oral care q2–4h. Apply a moisturizing lubricant to lips prn.	To minimize proliferation of normal bacteria flora in the mouth. Moist, supple tissue is less likely to break down.
7. Do **not** allow the formula for a continuous feeding to hang more than four hours. Keep ½ strength tube feeding formulas refrigerated until ready for use. Change the tube feeding administration set every 48 hours or per facility protocol.	Tube feeding formula is a good culture medium for microbes.

*N*URSING DIAGNOSIS: HIGH RISK FOR COMPLICATIONS

RELATED TO FACTORS: Continuous tube feedings

DEFINING CHARACTERISTICS: Abdominal cramping, diarrhea, aspiration, occlusion of the tube, hyperglycemia

PATIENT OUTCOME: Demonstrates absence of complications

EVALUATION CRITERIA: Denies abdominal cramping, passage of soft-formed stool, patent tube

INTERVENTIONS	RATIONALE
Abdominal Cramping: 1. Always give the formula at room temperature. If abdominal cramping occurs, reduce the flow rate of the feeding.	A cold formula or too rapid a volume causes abdominal cramping.
2. Following insertion of a PEG, administer small amounts of water as the first feeding. If no abdominal distention or vomiting occurs, increase volume to deliver prescribed amount of feeding.	Rapid distention of the stomach can cause cramping and vomiting.
3. Always check for residual q8h with a continuous feeding and before each intermittent feeding. If the residual for the continuous feeding is more than twice the hourly infusion rate, stop the infusion for two hours. Recheck the residual. If it is still large, inform physician. If the residual for an intermittent feeding is greater than 100 mL, hold the feeding for 2–3 hours, then recheck. If it is still large, notify physician.	The amount of feeding given or the interval of the feeding will need to be adjusted to prevent gastric distention.
Aspiration: 1. Keep head of bed elevated about 35–45 degrees when giving a continuous feeding. When giving intermittent feedings, maintain an elevated position during the feeding and for 30 minutes afterwards.	An elevated position aids movement of the formula by gravity.
2. **Always** obtain an abdominal x ray following initial insertion of a small-bore feeding tube and when tube displacement is suspected.	Small-bore feeding tubes rest in the duodenum, which are confirmed only by x ray.

INTERVENTIONS	RATIONALE

Diarrhea:
 	
1. Monitor:
  • skin turgor
  • weight weekly
  • serum electrolyte reports, especially serum sodium
  • intake and output q8h
	To detect fluid and electrolyte disturbances if diarrhea occurs.

2. Give extra water between each bottle of formula. If diarrhea occurs, give prescribed antidiarrheal agent after each loose stool. Confer with physician about changing the formula if diarrhea persists despite antidiarrheal agent.	The hyperosmolar tube feeding pulls water into the intestine, precipitating diarrhea. Providing extra water dilutes the formula, thus reducing its osmotic action.

3. Increase amount of water given, if signs of dehydration occur:
  • elevated serum sodium
  • poor skin turgor
  • diminished urinary output
  • concentrated urine
  • dry skin
  • constipation
	Extra fluid is needed to resolve dehydration.

4. **Always** use an infusion pump when giving a continuous feeding.	The small-bore feeding tube can easily become obstructed because of its small diameter. Continuous tube feedings help keep these small tubes patent. An infusion pump ensures better control of the flow rate.

Occlusion:
 	
1. Never heat the formula. If refrigerated, allow to warm to room temperature before administering. Always flush the tube with water:
  • before and after administering medication.
  • after administering an intermittent feeding.
	Heat and medications can cause the formula to coagulate and can also destroy nutrients. Cold formula can cause stomach cramping.

INTERVENTIONS	RATIONALE
2. Use liquid medication when available. Crush pills (unless contraindicated) finely and mix with water. Administer medication by bolus. Check with pharmacy to determine if pills can be crushed.	Liquids pass through the tube with ease. Solid substances block the tube.
3. If the tube becomes clogged, administer a carbonated beverage such as ginger ale by bolus method through the tube. Use diet carbonated beverage if patient is diabetic. If unable to reestablish patency, remove the tube and insert a new one.	The fizzing action of the beverage often helps loosen coagulated substances. The tube will have to be changed if unable to unclog it.

Hyperglycemia:
 	
1. Monitor:
  • intake and output q8h
  • blood glucose level, especially if diabetic
	To identify indications of progress toward or deviation from expected outcome.

2. If hyperglycemia is suspected, assess blood glucose using a blood glucose monitor and report results to physician: • urinary output significantly higher than fluid intake, accompanied by complaints of thirst, dry mucous membranes, change in level of conciousness, reports of weakness, rapid pulse, rapid breathing	Hyperglycemia indicates the patient cannot produce sufficient insulin to handle the increased carbohydrate load from the tube feeding. Insulin must be given to lower the blood glucose by facilitating glucose metabolism.

B owel Diversion

Bowel diversion, commonly called ostomy surgery, may be permanent or temporary. It is done primarily for mechanical obstructions of the intestine, most commonly cancer of the colon, ulcerative colitis, diverticular disease, and trauma to the intestine. For a DRG classification of major small and large bowel procedures without complications, the mean LOS is 8.9 days; with complications, the mean LOS is 13.5 days (Lorenz, 1991).

Ostomy is the surgical creation of an opening (stoma) through the abdominal wall using the proximal segment of the intestine. Feces is then expelled through the stoma. The prefix indicates the segment of the intestine brought out through the abdominal wall:

- **Ileostomy** — permanent opening created from the ileum
- **Cecostomy** — temporary opening created from the cecum
- **Colostomy** — opening created from a segment of the colon (ascending, transverse, or sigmoid); usually, ascending and transverse colostomies are temporary, whereas sigmoid colostomy is permanent

There are three types of colostomies:

1. Single-barreled — the stoma is created from the proximal portion of the bowel. The distal segment may be removed or closed.

2. Double-barreled — usually involves the transverse colon. Both ends of the resected colon are brought out through the abdominal wall resulting in two stomas. The distal stoma drains only mucus and is termed a mucous fistula. A small dressing can be placed over the mucous fistula and an ostomy bag over the proximal stoma (which drains feces).

3. Loop colostomy — a loop of transverse colon is brought out through the abdominal wall and held in place by a glass rod. About 5–10 days later after the bowel forms an adhesion to the abdominal wall, an opening is created in the exposed surface of the bowel with use of a cautery. This type of colostomy is usually temporary.

Because of the normal physiological differences between the large and small intestines, some variations between an ileostomy and a colostomy are expected:

- Ileostomy:
    - semiliquid stool expelled
    - no irrigation required to regulate bowel movements

235

— no bowel cleansing needed before or after test, even for barium contrast studies of the GI tract

— incontinence of stool unless a Koch pouch or ileoanal reservoir pouch was created. With the ileoanal reservoir, a colectomy is performed and an internal pouch is created from the loops of the distal ileum and sutured to the anus, forming an ileoanal ananstomsis. A temporary loop ileostomy is created to divert fecal material until the pouch and ileoanal suture lines heal. With perianal muscle exercises to strengthen the rectal sphincter, fecal continency may again be achieved.

Colostomy:
— formed stool expelled

— irrigation required to regulate bowel movements

— bowel cleansing required before barium contrast studies of the GI tract

— incontinence of stool, however, reasonable continence often is achieved with regular irrigations

Ascending or transverse:

— semiformed stool expelled

— incontinence of stool

Integrative Care Plans

• Loss

• Cancer

• Preoperative and postoperative care

• Fluid and biochemical imbalance

• IV therapy

• Immobility

• Pain

THE PREOPERATIVE PERIOD

1. See Preoperative and Postoperative Care (page 738) and Loss (page 733).

2. Perform specific preoperative preparation as prescribed that may include:

   • low-residue diet several days before surgery

   • clear liquids the day before surgery

   • antibiotics to sterilize intestinal tract

   • laxatives and enemas to remove intestinal contents and reduce the risk of infection from spillage of intestinal contents into the peritonial cavity

THE POSTOPERATIVE PERIOD

 # ASSESSMENT DATA BASE

1. Inspect the stoma for color, size, and drainage.

2. See Preoperative and Postoperative Care (page 738).

NURSING DIAGNOSIS: HIGH RISK FOR COMPLICATIONS

RELATED TO FACTORS: Bowel diversion procedure

DEFINING CHARACTERISTICS: Peristomal skin irritation, strangulation of the stoma, paralytic ileus

PATIENT OUTCOME: Demonstrates absence of complications

EVALUATION CRITERIA: Peristomal skin intact, pink and moist stoma, passage of stool

INTERVENTIONS	RATIONALE
Peristomal Skin Breakdown: 1. Use the stoma measuring card to measure the stoma. Then cut hole in the stomahesive wafer the size of the stoma so it fits snugly around the stoma and covers the peristomal skin surface. Cleanse the skin around the stoma with warm water and mild soap when changing the ostomy bag. Change the stomahesive wafer weekly and when leakage occurs. If peristomal skin appears reddened, tender, and with denuded areas, contact the enterstomal therapist for suggested skin care.	Peristomal skin breakdown is due to continuous exposure of peristomal skin to proteolytic enzymes from the intestine. Early detection and prompt intervention when redness occurs prevent further loss of skin integrity.
2. Empty the ostomy bag at regular intervals or when ¼ to ½ full. Use a two-way ostomy pouch system.	Excessive weight can break the peristomal seal. With a two-way pouch system, removal of the pouch is not necessary when emptying is required. The pouch can be emptied from the bottom prn by removing and reapplying the special clamp that comes with the pouch.

INTERVENTIONS	RATIONALE
Strangulation of the Stoma: 1. Inspect and record the color of the stoma on each shift. Notify physician if the stoma shows signs of inadequate blood supply (pale, dusky gray, light pink, purplish, or black).	The stoma is the everted mucosal layer of the intestine. This tissue has no sensation but is fragile and bleeds when rubbed too hard. Normally, the stoma is brick red, protrudes, and is swollen because of surgical trauma. Within 6–8 weeks, the swelling subsides.

Paralytic Ileus:
 	
1. Monitor:
  • color, consistency, and number of stools
  • bowel sounds and abdomen size on each shift
	To detect problems early and avoid irreparable damage.

2. Notify physician of absence of bowel sounds, absence of stool for more than three days, or abdominal distention accompanied by abdominal pain. Measure circumference of the abdomen on each shift if distention is suspected.	These findings signal paralytic ileus. Peristalsis is normally diminished after bowel surgery due to interference with nerve supply with manipulation of the bowel. The ostomy should begin to function within 3–4 days when peristalsis normally returns.
3. Keep NPO until bowel sounds return and the ostomy begins to function. Provide prescribed IV fluids until the patient can take oral feedings.	Giving oral feedings when peristalsis is absent causes distention, nausea, and vomiting.

• •

▶ NURSING DIAGNOSIS: DISTURBANCE IN SELF-CONCEPT

RELATED TO FACTORS: Altered body image secondary to an ostomy

DEFINING CHARACTERISTICS: Refusal to look at or touch stoma, verbal statements of shame, reports low self-esteem, may verbalize concerns about impact of ostomy on social and sexual functioning

PATIENT OUTCOME: Demonstrates effective coping with altered body image

EVALUATION CRITERIA: Participates in ostomy self-care, requests information, verbalizes plans for resuming presurgical lifestyle within context of limitations

• •

INTERVENTIONS	RATIONALE
1. If the patient desires, plan a visit from an ostomate through the local ostomy association if available.	A support system helps reinforce coping mechanisms. Individuals who have experienced the surgery and successfully adapted are often the best source of support.
2. Assist the patient in reexamining own sexuality. Initiate a discussion about concerns patients commonly want to know but often may be too embarrassed to discuss: When can sexual activity be resumed? Will it be possible to have sexual intercourse again? How can they make others see them as still being attactive or desirable? Is pregnancy still possible? Emphasize that there are a wide range of sexual expressions. Encourage the patient and significant other to be open and to explore different alternatives for expressing intimacy. Emphasize that intimacy is the key to enjoying a sexual relationship and that intimacy entails embracing, kissing, talking, and touching. Acts of intimacy do not have to end in intercourse. Emphasize good personal hygiene and wearing clothing that conceals the pouch while complimenting one's physical appearance. Suggest using decorative belts made of cloth to cover the ostomy bag or using an opaque pouch. Refer the patient and significant other to a local ostomy support group through the United Ostomy Association of the American Cancer Society.	Sexuality refers to who a person is in all aspects of life. A sense of well-being is enhanced by learning how to make adjustments to compliment one's current lifestyle rather than giving up the activity.

INTERVENTIONS

RATIONALE

INTERVENTIONS	RATIONALE
3. See Loss (page 733).	
4. Encourage the patient to refer to the stoma as a stoma.	Some patients show difficulty in adjustment to a stoma by calling the stoma "the thing" or "Joey" instead of using the appropriate term. Using the appropriate term helps facilitate acceptance.

NURSING DIAGNOSIS: HIGH RISK FOR IMPAIRED HOME MAINTENANCE MANAGEMENT

RELATED TO FACTORS: Difficulty coping with altered body image secondary to ostomy, inadequate support system, lack of adequate finances, knowledge deficit about self-care activities

DEFINING CHARACTERISTICS: May verbalize fears and doubts of ability to manage the ostomy, may report feeling anxious, verbalizes lack of understanding about ostomy self-care

PATIENT OUTCOME (collaborative): Demonstrates willingness to manage ostomy self-care

EVALUATION CRITERIA: Performs ostomy care without assistance, verbalizes awareness of community resources that can provide assistance, verbalizes understanding discharge instructions

INTERVENTIONS

RATIONALE

INTERVENTIONS	RATIONALE
1. Refer the patient to an enterostomal therapist (ET) nurse, if available, for instructions on ostomy care. If unavailable, provide ostomy care instructions per facility protocol.	An ET is a registered nurse who has received special training in the physical and psychosocial care of the ostomy patient.
2. When the procedure for ostomy care has been developed by the ET nurse or primary nurse, follow the procedure step-by-step. Do **not** interject new information or change any of the planned steps without first consulting with the ET nurse or the nurse who devised the	

INTERVENTIONS	RATIONALE
teaching plan. Let the nurse initiating the teaching plan introduce new changes to resolve problems. Ask the nurse to leave written step-by-step instructions at the bedside for changing the ostomy bag, peristomal skin care, and irrigations (if required).	A consistent procedure reduces confusion and makes learning easier.
3. Offer praise when the patient shows behaviors toward resuming a normal independent lifestyle (participating in ostomy self-care, verbalizing plans for returning to work or being involved in social activities).	Reward serves to motivate an individual to learn.
4. Ensure the patient has been instructed in methods to control odor and prevent accidental spillage: • Empty the ostomy bag when ¼ to ½ full. • Irrigate the colostomy, as prescribed, using the same technique as a regular enema, except sit on the toilet and use the specially designed irrigation set for ostomies. • Use deodorizers in the ostomy bag, such as charcoal, or use bags containing a deodorizer. • Consume a bland, low-residue diet. Avoid foods that cause gas, diarrhea, and constipation. For constipation, use prune juice or a stool softener. Refer the patient to a dietitian for assistance in planning meals to support passage of normal stools.	Odor and accidental spillage are major concerns of all ostomy patients. Learning how to effectively control these two problems can facilitate acceptance of the ostomy.

INTERVENTIONS

5. On discharge, ensure the patient or significant other:

- has the address of businesses that sell ostomy supplies.

- has the telephone number for a contact person, preferably the ET nurse, if problems arise with the ostomy at home.

- can perform ostomy care independently, or arrangements have been made for home care by a visiting nurse or significant other. Contact social services to make arrangements for home care by a visiting nurse if needed.

- has the address and telephone number of the local American Cancer Society and the local ostomy association.

- has enough ostomy supplies to last at least one week.

- has a written appointment for follow-up care and written instructions for ostomy care.

- knows characteristics of a normal stoma.

- knows how to manage diarrhea and constipation.

- knows how to control odor and flatulence.

- knows the type of ostomy, its purpose, and characteristics of a normal stool from the ostomy.

RATIONALE

Discharge teaching is essential for promoting safety during recovery and rehabilitation. Written information is required as verbal instructions may be easily forgotten.

Cancer of the Colon

Adenocarcinomas of the colon form hard, nodular bulky masses that grow irregularly and often ulcerate and lead to bleeding. The cancer is relatively slow growing. It may be confined to the intestinal mucosa and submucosa, or invade the entire bowel wall and metastasize to distant sites via the lymphatics. Common sites of metastases are the lungs, bone, liver, and peritoneum (Fry, 1989). As the mass grows, it obstructs the lumen of the bowel.

The mean LOS for a DRG classification of cancer of the colon is 3.6 days without complications and 7.0 days with complications (Lorenz, 1991).

General Medical Management

- Bowel resection (only curative treatment):
  — right or left hemicolectomy for lesions located in the right or left colon
  — abdominal-perineal resection with permanent colostomy often for lesions located in the rectosigmoid less than 6 cm from the anus
  — radiation treatments (for inoperable adenocarcinomas) used for palliation and shrinkage of the tumor

Integrative Care Plans

- Cancer
- Bowel diversion
- Rectal surgery
- Preoperative and postoperative care
- Loss
- Radiation therapy

THE PREOPERATIVE PERIOD

 # ASSESSMENT DATA BASE

1. History or presence of risk factors:
   - positive first line family history of colorectal cancer
   - diet deficient in plant fiber and high in fat
   - ulcerative colitis
   - familial polyposis (inherited disorder characterized by hundreds of adenomatous polyps in the colon)

2. Physical examination based on an abdominal assessment (Appendix B) may reveal various manifestations of colon cancer, depending on the segment of the colon involved:

   a. ascending colon
   - vague dull pain in the right lower quadrant of the abdomen
   - a palpable tender abdominal mass (late finding)
   - a history of bloody stools

   b. transverse or descending colon
   - constipation alternating with diarrhea
   - blood or mucus in the stools
   - symptoms of partial obstruction (increasing constipation and passage of narrow, pencil-like stools)

3. Diagnostic studies:
   - Barium enema reveals abnormal growths in the colon.
   - Sigmoidoscopy with biopsy and cytology provides the most conclusive evidence of cancer cells.
   - Serum iron level is low, reflecting anemia caused by the bleeding.
   - CBC shows low RBC, hemoglobin, and hematocrit caused by the bleeding.
   - Stool guaiac is positive for blood.
   - Alkaline phosphatase may be elevated, suggesting metastases to the liver or bone.

4. See Integrative Care Plans (Cancer, Bowel diversion, Rectal surgery, Abdominoperineal resection) to complete this plan of care.

*I*ntestinal Obstruction

An **intestinal obstruction** may be complete or partial. It occurs when intestinal contents are prohibited from passing through the intestinal tract as a result of a mechanical, neurogenic, or vascular pathology. The pathology interferes with peristalsis, causing an accumulation of intestinal contents, fluid, and gas proximal to the obstruction. This leads to distention. As intestinal pressure increases, capillary permeability increases, allowing fluid and electrolytes to shift into the peritoneal cavity. If the obstruction is not relieved, blood supply to the intestine can be impaired and lead to necrosis and possibly rupture of the bowel. Fluid and biochemical deficits may occur, especially with an obstruction of the proximal small bowel caused by vomiting and see page of fluid and electrolytes into the bowel lumen.

The mean LOS for a DRG classification of intestinal obstruction without complications is 3.8 days and 5.8 days with complications (Lorenz, 1991).

General Medical Management

- Nasogastric intubation with suction using a Salem sump tube or a long intestinal tube (Cantor tube, Harris tube, Miller-Abbott tube)
- IV therapy with electrolyte replacement
- Bedrest
- Analgesics
- Surgery, such as bowel resection (removal of affected segment and anastomosis to remaining bowel segment) or temporary colostomy or cecostomy, for obstructions caused by mechanical and vascular factors

Integrative Care Plans

- Bowel surgery
- Preoperative and postoperative care
- IV therapy
- Fluid and biochemical imbalances
- Immobility
- Pain

Discharge Considerations

• See respective integrative care plan listed above

ASSESSMENT DATA BASE

1. Physical examination based on an abdominal assessment (Appendix B) may reveal:
   • copious vomiting of fecal-smelling material (characteristic finding with small bowel obstruction)
   • change in bowel pattern (prominent feature with colon obstruction): pencil-shaped or ribbon-shaped stools, later bowel movements cease
   • abdominal distention
   • colicky, intermittent abdominal pain
   • initially, high-pitched rapid bowel sounds above site of obstruction; later, bowel sounds cease

2. Diagnostic studies:
   • Abdominal x rays reveal the presence and pattern of gas and fluid in the intestines.
   • CT scan, magnetic resonance imaging (MRI), or ultrasound helps confirm the diagnosis.
   • Proctosigmoidoscopy helps determine the cause of the obstruction if in the colon.
   • Barium enema helps determine if the obstruction is in the colon. It is usually done after the proctosigmoidoscopy if results are inconclusive.
   • Upper GI series reveals obstructions located in the small intestines, stomach, or esophagus.

NURSING DIAGNOSIS: PAIN

RELATED TO FACTORS: Abdominal distention secondary to intestinal obstruction

DEFINING CHARACTERISTICS: Taunt and distended abdomen, diminished or absent bowel sounds, verbalizes pain, frowning, guarding behavior, moaning

PATIENT OUTCOME (collaborative): Demonstrates relief from pain

EVALUATION CRITERIA: Denies pain, absence of abdominal distention, presence of bowel sounds, passing flatus, denies nausea

Rectal Surgery

Rectal surgery is performed for a variety of conditions: to remove painful hemorrhoids (hemorrhoidectomy), to repair an anal fissure, to correct an anal fistula, or to remove the rectum and anus when an abdominoperineal resection is performed for treatment of colorectal cancer.

Preoperative preparation is the same for any patient undergoing surgery. In addition, bowel cleansing procedures (laxative and enema) are included in preoperative preparation.

Postoperatively, the patient returns to a medical/surgical unit with an IV solution, and possibly rectal packing. The packing usually is removed within a few hours. Sitz baths are then started. Diet progresses from clear liquids to regular if no nausea or vomiting occur. Stool softeners are given as soon as oral feedings are tolerated.

The mean LOS varies depending on the type of procedure. For rectal resection without complications LOS is 9.0 days and 12.4 days with complications. For anal procedures without complications LOS is 2.5 days and 4.6 days with complications (Lorenz, 1991).

Integrative Care Plans

- Preoperative and postoperative care
- Immobility
- Pain
- IV therapy

Discharge Considerations

- Follow-up care
- Activity limitations
- Medications to continue at home
- Reportable signs and symptoms
- Measures to prevent constipation
- Wound care

THE PREOPERATIVE PERIOD

 ASSESSMENT DATA BASE

1. See Preoperative and Postoperative Care (page 738).

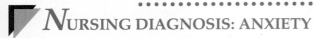

NURSING DIAGNOSIS: ANXIETY

RELATED TO FACTORS: Knowledge deficit about preoperative and postoperative events

DEFINING CHARACTERISTICS: Verbalizes lack of understanding, reports feeling anxious or nervous, expresses concern about effect of surgery on sexual functioning, tense facial expression

PATIENT OUTCOME: Demonstrates less anxiety

EVALUATION CRITERIA: Verbalizes understanding of preoperative and postoperative events, reports feeling less anxious, relaxed facial expression

INTERVENTIONS	RATIONALE
1. Reassure the patient that sexual functioning is not affected by rectal surgery and bowel continence remains intact, unless the patient is having an abdominoperineal resection in which case impotence is an outcome of surgery.	Men are commonly concerned about the effect of the surgery on sexual functioning: Is impotence or sterility an outcome? Will bowel control be lost permanently?
2. See Preoperative and Postoperative Care (page 738).	

THE POSTOPERATIVE PERIOD

 ASSESSMENT DATA BASE

1. Perform a routine postoperative assessment (Appendix L).

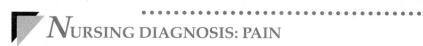

NURSING DIAGNOSIS: PAIN

RELATED TO FACTORS: Hemorroidectomy, repair of anal fissure or fistula, abdominoperineal resection

DEFINING CHARACTERISTICS: Frowning, moaning, verbalizes pain, tense body posture

PATIENT OUTCOME (collaborative): Demonstrates relief from pain

EVALUATION CRITERIA: Denies pain, absence of moaning, relaxed facial expression, relaxed body posture

INTERVENTIONS	RATIONALE
1. Administer prescribed analgesic prn and especially before the first bowel movement. Evaluate its effectiveness.	Fear of discomfort is common with the first bowel movement. The patient often tenses and tightens the anal sphincter, which increases discomfort with defecation. Effective analgesia promotes relaxation and less discomfort with defecation.
2. Administer prescribed stool softener and laxative. Ensure daily oral intake of at least 2–3 liters of fluid.	These measure are aimed at ensuring passage of a soft stool early.
3. Provide a sitz bath as ordered. Teach the patient how to prepare the sitz bath.	Warmth promotes circulation and helps relieve discomfort. Teaching self-care promotes independence.
4. Ensure the patient voids.	A full bladder can cause pain.
5. **Avoid** taking a rectal temperature.	Inserting a thermometer can traumatize already compromised tissue.

NURSING DIAGNOSIS: HIGH RISK FOR ALTERATION IN HOME MAINTENANCE MANAGEMENT

RELATED TO FACTORS: Knowledge deficit about self-care measures on discharge, inability to perform self-care activities

DEFINING CHARACTERISTICS: Verbalizes lack of understanding about self-care activities on discharge, requests information

PATIENT OUTCOME: Demonstrates willingness to comply with self-care preventive and maintenance measures on discharge

EVALUATION CRITERIA: Verbalizes understanding of discharge instructions, performs required self-care activities correctly

• •

INTERVENTIONS	RATIONALE
1. Instruct the patient to: • continue with a high-fiber diet • drink at least eight glasses of fluid daily • take stool softeners as ordered	These measures help ensure passage of a soft stool.
2. Advise the patient to contact the physician if fever, rectal bleeding, or pain unrelieved by prescribed analgesia occur.	These findings signal a need for further examination.
3. Ensure the patient has: • a written appointment for follow-up care. • supplies for a sitz bath (if continued at home). • prescription for a mild analgesic if needed. • prescription for a stool softener.	Verbal instructions may be easily forgotten. Thorough preparation can help minimize anxiety associated with self-care after surgery. Mild discomfort may be experienced for a few weeks after discharge. Passage of a soft stool helps minimize discomfort.

Peptic Ulcer Disease

Peptic ulcer is an erosion of the mucosa of the GI tract caused by too much hydrochloric acid and pepsin. Although ulcers may occur in the esophagus, the most common locations are the duodenum and stomach (Wardell, 1990).

Chronic ulcers may penetrate the muscular wall. Healing results in the formation of fibrous tissue and eventually a permanent scar. The ulcer may recur and heal several times throughout the person's life.

The major complications associated with peptic ulcer disease, in the order of prevalence, are:

1. **Hemorrhag**e — evidenced by hematemesis and a guaiac positive stool

2. **Perforation** — evidenced by sudden onset of excruciating pain accompanied by a rigid boardlike abdomen and symptoms of shock

3. **Obstruction** — (See Intestinal Obstruction, page 245). This complication is more common with duodenal ulcers located near the pylorus. It is caused by constriction of the gastric outlet as a result of edema and scarring from recurring ulcers.

Patients are generally treated on an outpatient basis. Hospitalization is required for treatment of complications. The mean LOS for a DRG classification of uncomplicated peptic ulcer disease is 5.1 days; with complications, the mean LOS is 5.9 days (Lorenz, 1991).

General Medical Management

- Pharmacotherapy:
  - histamine receptor antagonists such as cimetidine (Tagamet), ranitidine (Zantac), famotidine (Pepcid), nizatidine (Axid)
  - antacids such as magnesium hydroxide antacids (Maalox or Mylanta), or aluminum hydroxide antacids (Amphojel or Alternagel)
  - sucralfate (Carafate)
  - anticholinergics such as propantheline bromide (Pro-Banthine)
- Reduction or elimination of ulcerogenic factors, such as smoking, discontinuing ulcerogenic medication while the ulcer is still active
- Dietary modifications

- Stress management
- Surgery if complications occur:
  - — subtotal gastrectomy (removal of a portion of the stomach)
  - — vagotomy (severing of the vagus nerve to reduce secretion of hydrochloric acid) with pyloroplasty (surgical enlargement of the pyloric sphincter to allow increased gastric emptying in the presence of decreased gastric motility, which occurs following a vagotomy)

Integrative Care Plans

- Loss
- Preoperative and postoperative care, if surgery is planned

Discharge Considerations

- Follow-up care
- Reportable signs and symptoms
- Medications to continue at home
- Stress management

ASSESSMENT DATA BASE

1. History or presence of risk factors:
   - first line family history of peptic ulcers
   - chronic use of drugs that irritate the stomach mucosa (for example, aspirin, steroids, or indomethacin)
   - heavy cigarette smoking
   - exposure to chronic emotional stress

2. Physical assessment based on a general survey (Appendix F) may reveal:
   - epigastric pain. This is the most prominent symptom during periods of exacerbations. With duodenal ulcer, pain occurs 2–3 hours after eating and is often accompanied by nausea and vomiting. With gastric ulcer, pain occurs immediately after eating. The pain may be described as nagging, dull, aching, or burning. It is often relieved by food and aggravated by smoking and emotional stress. During remission, the patient is asymptomatic.
   - weight loss
   - bleeding as hematemesis or melena (if the ulcer is active)

3. Diagnostic studies:
   - Upper GI series shows an ulcer crater but does not indicate if it is benign or malignant. Malignant and benign ulcers produce the same symptoms. Often a benign ulcer heals with medical therapy in a few weeks, whereas a malignant ulcer does not heal with therapy.

- Endoscopy with brush cytology is done to accurately differentiate between a benign and malignant ulcer when symptoms persist.
- Stool guaiac may be positive for occult blood if the ulcer is active.

4. Assess typical diet and eating patterns for 72 hours prehospitalization.

5. Assess the patient's emotional response and understanding of the condition, treatment plan, diagnostic studies, and preventive self-care measures.

6. Assess the patient's methods of dealing with stressful events and perceptions about the impact of illness on lifestyle.

NURSING DIAGNOSIS: PAIN

RELATED TO FACTORS: Active peptic ulcer disease

DEFINING CHARACTERISTICS: Verbalizes discomfort, moaning, guarding behavior, frowning

PATIENT OUTCOME (collaborative): Demonstrates relief from discomfort

EVALUATION CRITERIA: Denies pain, relaxed facial expression, absence of moaning

INTERVENTIONS	RATIONALE
1. Administer prescribed medication (histamine receptor antagonists, Carafate, antacids, or anticholinergics) and evaluate its effectiveness.	Antacids and Carafate coat the ulcer crater. Histamine receptor antagonists reduce gastric acidity by blocking the secretion of histamine, a gastric acid stimulant. Anticholinergics reduce secretion of hydrochloric acid and slow motility of the GI tract.
2. Notify physician if gastric pain persists or worsens. Guaiac all stools if pain persists. Report positive guaiac stools.	These findings indicate a need for prompt medical attention.
3. Keep NPO as prescribed when active bleeding is present. Encourage oral care: • brushing teeth b.i.d. and rinsing mouth with cool water • lubricating lips with petrolatum ointment prn • keeping a moistened gauze at the bedside for the patient to moisten mouth prn	Brushing removes plaque. Restricting oral feedings causes the mouth and lips to dry. Frequent replenishing of moisture helps relieve dryness.

INTERVENTIONS	RATIONALE
4. If bloody diarrhea occurs, provide perineal care after each loose stool—cleanse with warm water and mild soap. With physician permission, apply anesthetic ointment, such as dibucaine HCl (Nupercainal), to the anus if the patient complains of soreness. Use a room deodorizer to control odor.	Frequent diarrhea causes irritation to the anus. Bloody stools can produce a foul odor.

◤NURSING DIAGNOSIS: HIGH RISK FOR FLUID VOLUME DEFICIT

RELATED TO FACTORS: Excess blood loss secondary to peptic ulcer disease

DEFINING CHARACTERISTICS: Guaiac positive stools, passage of black tarry stools, coffee-ground color emesis, falling BP accompanied by tachycardia, tachypnea, and cool clammy skin, verbalizes thirst, diminished urinary output

PATIENT OUTCOME (collaborative): Demonstrates no further signs of bleeding

EVALUATION CRITERIA: Passage of soft brown stools, hemoglobin and hematocrit within normal limits

INTERVENTIONS	RATIONALE
1. Monitor: • vital signs q4h, if stools guaiac positive • intake and output q8h • color and consistency of stools (guaiac all stools if bleeding is not visible) • color of emesis; Hematest® coffee-ground color emesis. • results of CBC reports	To evaluate effectiveness of therapy.

INTERVENTIONS	RATIONALE
2. Notify physician of coffee-ground emesis, black tarry stools, bright red emesis or stools, falling BP accompanied by tachycardia and tachypnea, cool clammy skin, or hemoglobin and hematocrit values below normal range. Administer blood transfusions as prescribed and monitor for adverse reactions.	Coffee-ground colored emesis reflects blood mixed with gastric juice. Black tarry stools (melena) indicate bleeding in the GI tract. Bright red emesis or stools indicate active bleeding. Excessive blood loss can lead to anemia, evidenced by low hemoglobin and hematocrit and symptoms of shock.
3. To control bleeding, administer prescribed medication that may include: • vitamin K (AquaMEPHYTON) if the prothrombin time is prolonged • histamine receptor antagonist such as cimetidine (Tagamet), ranitidine (Zantac), famotidine (Pepcid) • vasopressin (Pitressin Synthetic/Pitressin Tannate) Evaluate effectiveness of prescribed medication. Use an infusion pump when giving these drugs by continuous drip.	Vitamin K helps restore clotting factors. Histamine receptor antagonist reduces gastric acid production. Vasopressin causes constriction of blood vessels thereby helps control bleeding.
4. Insert an N/G tube and connect to intermittent suction as prescribed if bright red emesis occurs. Maintain tube patency by irrigating with cold, normal saline prn. Provide gastric lavage as prescribed: • Instill about 60–100 mL of the prescribed agent (iced saline, antacid, or vasopressin). • Clamp the tube for 10–15 minutes, then connect to suction. • Repeat lavage at prescribed intervals. • Inspect color of gastric output when suctioning is resumed.	N/G intubation provides a route for gastric lavage. Cold solutions and vasopressin cause vasoconstriction. Antacids coat the stomach lining to prevent further erosion by exposure to hydrochloric acid.

INTERVENTIONS	RATIONALE
5. Keep NPO as ordered if vomiting occurs. Initiate prescribed IV therapy. Use an 18-gauge needle to start the IV infusion if a blood transfusion is required.	Rapid blood loss leads to hypovolemia. IV fluids help restore intravascular volume until bleeding can be controlled. Blood transfusions should be given through a large-bore needle because of its high viscosity.
6. If the patient experiences weakness and dizziness, place a bedside commode at the bedside and assist with toileting as needed. Instruct the patient to signal for help when getting out of bed.	Excessive blood loss causes weakness and dizziness, which places the patient at risk for falling.
7. Maintain bedrest when active bleeding is present.	Bedrest reduces energy expenditure and activity of the GI tract.
8. Prepare the patient for gastric surgery or endoscopic sclerosing as ordered.	Surgery is required if drug therapy is ineffective in controlling severe bleeding after 24 hours.

◣NURSING DIAGNOSIS: HIGH RISK FOR ALTERATION IN HOME MAINTENANCE MANAGEMENT

RELATED TO FACTORS: Knowledge deficit about condition, treatment plan, and preventive self-care measures

DEFINING CHARACTERISTICS: May report difficulty in coping with a chronic illness, history of noncompliance, verbalizes lack of understanding, requests information, may verbalize fear of bleeding to death

PATIENT OUTCOME: Demonstrates willingness to comply with self-care preventive and maintenance measure on discharge

EVALUATION CRITERIA: Verbalizes understanding of condition and prescribed treatment plan, verbalizes plans for lifestyle changes to reduce risk of exacerbations

INTERVENTIONS	RATIONALE
1. Evaluate patient's understanding of condition and therapeutic plan. Correct any misconceptions. Emphasize that drug therapy does not cure the ulcer but does help heal. Let the patient know that peptic ulcer can recur if the treatment plan is not followed. Review purpose of prescribed treatments.	An understanding of one's condition and prescribed therapies promotes compliance.
2. Provide instructions about dietary modifications to prevent recurrences. Instructions should include avoiding foods that cause discomfort. Some common foods causing discomfort are chocolate, caffeine, spices, alcohol, fried foods, aspirin, and products containing aspirin. Eat three well-balanced meals daily, with snacks at regular, frequent intervals. Refer the patient to a dietitian for assistance in planning a well-balanced diet if diet history reveals inadequacy. Discourage intake of large quantities of dairy products.	There is no scientific proof that a specific diet promotes healing. Certain foods stimulate gastric secretion and precipitate gastric discomfort. Aspirin prevents platelet adhesion and can precipitate bleeding. Excessive calcium and protein from a large intake of milk and dairy products stimulate stomach acid secretion. A dietitian is a nutritional specialist and can assist the patient in planning meals to meet daily nutritional needs relative to financial status and illness.
3. Encourage the patient who smokes to take steps to stop smoking.	Nicotine stimulates gastric acid secretion that interferes with ulcer healing.
4. Emphasize the importance of taking medication as prescribed. Advise to take antacid or histamine receptor antagonist with meals.	Food delays gastric emptying, thus increasing the effectiveness of the medication.
5. Assist the patient with identifying undue stressful situations and developing a plan to modify lifestyle to reduce stress. Emphasize the importance of expressing feelings with someone. Refer the patient to stress management classes. Encourage the patient to engage in a regular exercise program and to take time for leisure activities.	Emotional stress activates adrenergic responses. Secretion of hydrochloric acid is increased, which further aggravates an already inflamed gastric mucosa.

INTERVENTIONS	RATIONALE
6. Provide instructions for relieving constipation. If taking an aluminum hydroxide antacid, drink at least eight glasses of fluid daily and eat high-fiber foods.	Constipation is a major side effect of aluminum hydroxide antacids.
7. Advise the patient to seek medical attention if the following occur: • sudden onset of gastric pain unrelieved by prescribed medication • coffee-ground or bloody emesis • black tarry stools	These findings indicate ulcer recurrence and GI bleeding. Prompt medical attention is required.

• •

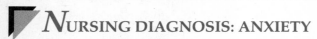

NURSING DIAGNOSIS: ANXIETY

RELATED TO FACTORS: Fear of bleeding to death, perceived loss of some aspect of independence due to chronic illness

DEFINING CHARACTERISTICS: May report difficulty in accepting condition, may report feeling nervous or anxious, tense facial expression

PATIENT OUTCOME (collaborative): Demonstrates relief from anxiety

EVALUATION CRITERIA: Relaxed facial expression, fewer reports of feeling anxious or nervous, verbalizes understanding of therapeutic plan

• •

INTERVENTIONS	RATIONALE
1. See Loss (page 733).	
2. Use a calm, reassuring approach when providing information. Encourage questions.	Problem solving is difficult for anxious people because anxiety impairs learning and perception. Clear, simple explanations are best understood. Medical and nursing jargon may confuse the patient and increase anxiety.
3. Explain purpose of all prescribed treatments and diagnostic studies, including: • brief description of test • purpose of test • preparation required before test • care after test	A knowledge of what to expect helps reduce anxiety.

Diverticular Disease

Diverticula are saclike herniations of the mucosa and submucosa of the GI tract. They may occur along any portion of the GI tract but occur most commonly in the sigmoid colon. They produce no symptoms unless a complication develops. The major complications are (Wilson & Goldman, 1989):

* diverticulitis —infection of the diverticuli due to blockage by hard feces, which causes walled-off abscesses to develop
* peritonitis — results from rupture of pericolon abscesses
* fistula formation —an opening created between the affected colon and a proximal structure, which may be the bladder, anus, or abdominal wall
* obstruction—due to stricture formation from recurrent episodes of diverticulitis

The mean LOS for a DRG classification of diverticular disease is 4.9 days (Lorenz, 1991).

General Medical Management

* For mild symptoms:
  — clear liquid diet
  — oral antibiotics
* For severe symptoms:
  — hospitalization
  — bedrest
  — NPO
  — IV therapy
  — antibiotics
* Surgery:
  — right or left hemicolectomy for recurrent attacks characterized by severe hemorrhage or fistula formation

Integrative Care Plans

- Preoperative and postoperative care, if surgery is planned
- IV therapy
- Rectal surgery (for repair of anal fistula)

Discharge Considerations

- Follow-up care
- Measures to prevent constipation

ASSESSMENT DATA BASE

1. Physical examination based on a general survey (Appendix F) may reveal:
   - mild, left lower quadrant tenderness with palpation of the abdomen
   - fever (this signals diverticulitis)
   - crampy, left lower quadrant abdominal pain
   - sudden onset of painless bleeding from the rectum if the diverticula rupture
   - history of constipation

2. Obtain a diet history. Inquire about the type of foods normally consumed. The disease is less common in vegetarians and persons who consume a high-fiber diet.

3. Assess the patient's understanding of the disease.

4. Diagnostic studies:
   - CBC reveals leukocytosis.
   - Abdominal x rays are taken to rule out appendicitis.
   - Barium enema provides the most diagnostic information by pinpointing the site and extent of the disease.
   - Proctosigmoidoscopy is done if the barium enema is inconclusive. It allows direct visualization of the colon.
   - CT scan helps to reveal abscess formation.

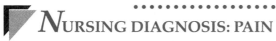

NURSING DIAGNOSIS: PAIN

RELATED TO FACTORS: Diverticulitis

DEFINING CHARACTERISTICS: Verbalizes discomfort, facial frowning, moaning, tense body posture

PATIENT OUTCOME (collaborative): Demonstrates relief from discomfort

EVALUATION CRITERIA: Denies pain, relaxed facial expression

INTERVENTIONS	RATIONALE
1. Monitor: • abdominal status (Appendix B) q8h	To evaluate effectiveness of therapy.
2. Notify physician of diminished or absent bowel sounds accompanied by abdominal distention, nausea, vomiting, and increasing discomfort. Insert a N/G tube and connect to intermittent suction as prescribed.	These findings suggest intestinal obstruction. N/G suctioning promotes gastric decompression.
3. Administer prescribed analgesic and evaluate its effectiveness.	Analgesics help block the pain pathway.

4. Keep NPO as prescribed if nausea or vomiting occur. Provide oral care while NPO:
  • allow patient to moisten mouth with a wet gauze prn
  • apply petroleum ointment to lips prn
  • allow patient to brush teeth and rinse mouth with cool water b.i.d.
  • Initiate prescribed IV therapy while NPO.
	Restricting oral feedings allows the bowel time to rest. Oral care helps relieve dryness of the mouth and reduces chance of gum disease. Supplemental fluid therapy helps maintain adequate fluid volume.

5. Provide a clear liquid diet as prescribed. Advance to solid foods as tolerated. Withhold foods if nausea or increased abdominal cramping recur.	Clear liquids require less GI activity for digestion and absorption.

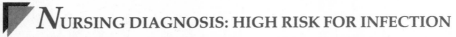

▶ NURSING DIAGNOSIS: HIGH RISK FOR INFECTION

RELATED TO FACTORS: Complication secondary to diverticular disease (diverticulitis, peritonitis, obstruction, fistula formation)

DEFINING CHARACTERISTICS: Low-grade fever, WBC above 10,000/mm^3

PATIENT OUTCOME: Infection resolves

EVALUATION CRITERIA: Temperature below 99°F, WBC within normal range

• •

INTERVENTIONS	RATIONALE
1. Monitor: • results of CBC reports • temperature q4h	To identify indications of progress toward or deviations from expected outcome.
2. Administer prescribed antibiotics and evaluate effectiveness. Notify physician if fever persists.	Diverticulitis is an infectious process thus requires antibiotics. Persistent fever indicates a need for further evaluation.
3. Implement measures to prevent constipation: • increase fluid intake to at least 2-3 liters daily • increase intake of fiber in the diet (fresh fruit, vegetables, whole wheat bread, high-fiber cereals) • use stool softeners if history of chronic constipation	Hard stool increases the possibility of rupture of the diverticuli, thus predisposing patient to diverticulitis.

• •

NURSING DIAGNOSIS: HIGH RISK FOR ALTERATION IN HOME MAINTENANCE MANAGEMENT

RELATED TO FACTORS: Knowledge deficit about condition, treatment plan, and preventive self-care measures on discharge

DEFINING CHARACTERISTICS: May report a history of noncompliance, verbalizes lack of understanding, may express a negative reaction to dietary changes

PATIENT OUTCOME: Demonstrates willingness to comply with treatment plan

EVALUATION CRITERIA: Verbalizes understanding of condition, treatment plan, and self-care measures for prevention

• •

INTERVENTIONS	RATIONALE
1. Provide information about: 　a. nature of condition 　b. purpose of prescribed treatments 　c. diagnostic studies, including: 　　• brief description of test 　　• purpose of test 　　• preparation required before test 　　• care after test	A knowledge of what to expect helps lessen anxiety and enhances patient cooperation.
2. Allow patient to express feelings about condition.	Expressing concerns helps relieve anxiety.
3. Teach the patient how to prevent recurrent attacks: 　• Avoid constipation by adhering to a high-fiber diet (fruits, vegetables, and whole grain breads and cereals), drink at least eight glasses of water daily, and use a stool softener or bulk-forming laxative (Metamucil) if needed.	Avoiding constipation is the most important measure to prevent diverticular disease.

BIBLIOGRAPHY

Blair, K.A. (1990). Aging: Physiological aspects and clinical implications. **Nurse Practitioner, 15,** 14–16, 18, 23, 26–28.

Bockus, S. (1991). Troubleshooting your tube feedings. **American Journal of Nursing, 91,** 24–29.

Cooke, D.M. (1991). Inflammatory bowel disease: Primary health care management of ulcerative colitis and Crohn's disease. **Nurse Practitioner, 16,** 27–30, 35–39.

Fry, R. D. (1989). Cancer of the colon and rectum. **Clinical Symposium, 41,** 2–32.

Johns, J.L. (1991). When the patient has an ulcer. **RN, 54,** 44–50.

Long, L. (1991). Ileostomy care: Overcoming the obstacles. **Nursing, 21,** 73–79.

Lorenz, E.W. (1991). **1992 St. Anthony's DRG Working Guidebook.** Alexandria: St. Anthony Publishing Company.

Massoni, M. (1990). Nurses' GI Handbook: Gastrointestinal. **Nursing, 20,** 65–80.

Nyhus, L.M., Klein, M.S., Rogers, F.B., & Kowalczyk, S. (1990). Inguinal hernia repairs: Types, patient care. **Journal of the Association of Operating Room Nurses, 52,** 292–3, 295–302, 304.

Wardell, T.L. (1990). Assessing and managing a gastric ulcer. **Nursing, 21,** 34–41.

Wilson, J.E., & Goldman, G.E. (1989). Appendicitis/diverticulitis. **Emergency Care Quarterly, 5,** 49–56.

Worthington, P.H., & Wagner, B.A. (1989). Total parenteral nutrition. **Nursing Clinics of North America, 24,** 355–371.

C

HAPTER FOUR
Problems of the Musculoskeletal System

Fractures

A **fracture** is a break in the continuity of bone. Most fractures are the result of traumatic injuries; some fractures are secondary to disease processes such as osteoporosis, which causes pathological fractures (Barrett and Bryant, 1990).

Hospitalization is required for reduction of a fracture since general anesthesia is required, except for a hairline fracture that can be managed on an outpatient basis.

The healing time for a fracture varies from 6–24 weeks, depending on the severity of the fracture. The major complications associated with a fracture, especially of long bones, are fat emboli, compartment syndrome, and venous thromboembolism (Slye, 1991).

Compartment syndrome is a serious neurovascular complication that occurs more commonly with severe trauma or long bone fractures. It refers to a condition in which pressure in a given anatomical space (or compartment) increases. It develops when tissue within the compartment becomes compressed within the fascia, compromising nerves and blood supply. Anatomically, bone is surrounded by muscle, nerves, and blood vessels, encased by inelastic connective tissue (fascia). Neurovascular defects are experienced distal to the pressure source, which can be external (cast or circumference bandage too tight, excessive traction) or internal (swelling or bleeding). If not relieved, permanent paralysis occurs (Slye, 1991).

Permanent loss of motor function is a common fear expressed by most patients. When the bone has healed, the patient can resume unrestricted activities.

The mean LOS varies according to the type of fracture (Lorenz, 1991). For fractures of the lower extremity and humerus (except hip, foot, femur), LOS is 4.6 days without complications and 7.2 days with complications. For knee procedures, the mean LOS without complications is 3.9 days and 7.7 days with complications. For shoulder, elbow, and other upper extremity procedures, the mean LOS without complications is 2.5 days and 3.3 days with complications. For foot procedures, the mean LOS is 3.3 days. For fracture of femur, LOS is 7.4 days. For removal of an internal fixation device, the mean LOS is 4.0 days.

General Medical Management

- Traction
- Closed reduction with application of a cast or external fixator (metal device attached to the bone by pins)
- Open reduction with insertion of a pin, screw, rod, wires, or nail

Integrative Care Plans

* Fat embolism syndrome
* Immobility
* Traction
* Cast care

Discharge Considerations

* Follow-up care
* Activity limitations
* Crutch walking (for lower extremity fractures)
* Wound care (for open reduction or application of external fixator)
* Cast care

 # ASSESSMENT DATA BASE

1. Physical examination based on a neurovascular assessment (Appendix D) of the fractured limb may reveal:
   * pain at fracture site, especially with movement
   * swelling
   * shortening of affected extremity
   * paralysis (loss of limb motion)
   * angulation of affected extremity
   * crepitations (crunching sensation produced when palpating bony fragments)
   * muscle spasms
   * paresthesia (diminished sensation)
   * pallor and pulselessness distal to fracture site if arterial blood flow is disrupted by fracture

2. Assess history of tetanus immunization if an open fracture (bone protruding through skin) exists.

3. Diagnostic studies:
   * X rays of the affected extremity reveal the type and location of the fracture.

4. Assess ability to perform activities of daily living (ADL), for example, bathing, toileting, eating, and dressing.

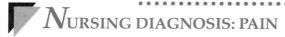

NURSING DIAGNOSIS: PAIN

RELATED TO FACTORS: Muscle spasms and tissue damage secondary to fracture

DEFINING CHARACTERISTICS: Verbalizes pain, facial frowning, moaning, guarding behavior

PATIENT OUTCOME (collaborative): Demonstrates relief from pain

EVALUATION CRITERIA: Denies pain, relaxed facial expression, absence of moaning

INTERVENTIONS	RATIONALE
1. Maintain bedrest until the fracture is reduced.	Pain and muscle spasms are controlled by immobilization.
2. Maintain prescribed traction and support devices, for example, splint, external fixator, or cast.	To immobilize the fractured extremity and decrease pain.
3. See Pain (page 700).	

NURSING DIAGNOSIS: IMPAIRED PHYSICAL MOBILITY

RELATED TO FACTORS: Traction or casting

DEFINING CHARACTERISTICS: Restricted to bed due to traction, cast on lower extremity or extremities, requests assistance with mobility

PATIENT OUTCOME: Demonstrates no complications associated with immobility.

EVALUATION CRITERIA: Intact skin, clear lung sounds, denies muscle fatigue and joint stiffness, passage of soft stools

INTERVENTIONS	RATIONALE
1. See Immobility (page 725).	
2. When ambulation is allowed, place the patient on "Falls Protocol" according to facility protocol.	One main function of the skeletal system is mobility. The risk of falling is increased when there is disruption of the skeletal system.

Nursing Diagnosis: Self-Care Deficit

RELATED TO FACTORS (collaborative): Traction or cast on an extremity

DEFINING CHARACTERISTICS: May request assistance with bathing, eating, toileting, dressing, or mobility

PATIENT OUTCOME: Demonstrates absence of self-care deficits

EVALUATION CRITERIA: Reports that ADL are being met, absence of body odor, moist oral mucosa, skin intact

INTERVENTIONS	RATIONALE
1. Provide assistance with ADL as needed. Allow the patient to do self-care within limits.	ADL are those functions that people normally perform each day to meet basic needs. Caring for one's own basic needs helps maintain self-esteem.
2. After reduction, place a plastic bag over the affected extremity to keep the cast/splint/external fixator dry when the patient takes a shower. Refer to physical therapy department as ordered for instructions in crutchwalking and exercises. Ensure the patient has crutches for ambulation and can use them properly.	A plastic bag protects the device from excess moisture that can precipitate an infection or cause softening of a plaster cast. Also, it prepares the patient for self-care on discharge. Physical therapists are exercise specialists who assist patients in mobility rehabilitation.

Nursing Diagnosis: High Risk for Impaired Tissue Integrity

RELATED TO FACTORS: Altered circulation secondary to fracture, fat embolism syndrome, or infection

DEFINING CHARACTERISTICS: May demonstrate manifestations of fat emboli, compartment syndrome, or infection

PATIENT OUTCOME (collaborative): Demonstrates adequate tissue perfusion

EVALUATION CRITERIA: Absence of manifestations of fat emboli, compartment syndrome, and infection

INTERVENTIONS	RATIONALE
Fat Emboli: 1. See Fat Embolism Syndrome (page 311).	
Compartment Syndrome: 1. Monitor neurovascular status (Appendix D) of the affected extremity q2h for first 24 hours, then q4h thereafter.	To detect early manifestations of compartment syndrome.
2. Consult physician for: • persistent pain unrelieved by narcotic analgesics (most significant finding) accompanied by swelling, numbness and tingling • cyanotic nailbeds • cool skin with poor capillary refill • loss of sensation • diminished pulse • diminished ability to wiggle toes, fingers, or both • increased pain with passive extension of the fingers/toes of the affected extremity (confirms compartment syndrome)	These findings signal inadequate circulation. If not relieved, permanent functional impairment can occur.
3. Keep fractured extremity elevated and apply ice pack	To relieve swelling.
4. If manifestations of compartment syndrome occur, take appropriate action to relieve the cause: • Elevate the limb above the level of the heart and apply ice. • Reduce weight of the traction as prescribed. • Loosen a tight bandage. • Contact orthopedic technician to split the cast as prescribed. • Assist physician with a fasciotomy (splitting the fascia to relieve compression edema).	Compartment syndrome can lead to severe tissue and nerve damage.

INTERVENTIONS	RATIONALE

Infection:
 	
1. Monitor:
  • CBC reports
  • temperature q4h
  • appearance of wound during each dressing change
	To detect early signs of infection.

2. Consult physician for signs of infection (redness, drainage, fever, increased pain). Obtain wound specimen for culture and sensitivity test. Administer antibiotics as prescribed.	Antibiotic therapy is required to resolve infections. A wound culture helps identify the causative organism so effective antibiotic therapy can be initiated.
3. If an open fracture exists (bone protruding through the skin), administer tetanus toxoid if no booster dose within past ten years, or tetanus immune globulin human (TIGH) if wound is severe or over 24 hours old.	Open wounds occurring from trauma are tetanus-prone.
4. Adhere to universal precautions (good handwashing technique before and after patient care and wearing gloves when contact with blood or body fluid is likely to occur) with direct patient contact procedures. Maintain strict aseptic technique with wound care.	Caregivers are the most common source of nosocomial infections. Open wounds are a good culture medium for bacterial growth.

· ·

NURSING DIAGNOSIS: HIGH RISK FOR ALTERATIONS IN HOME MAINTENANCE MANAGEMENT

RELATED TO FACTORS: Knowledge deficit about self-care measures on discharge, lack of adequate support system

DEFINING CHARACTERISTICS: Verbalizes lack of understanding, requests information, may verbalize need for assistance with some aspect of physical care

PATIENT OUTCOME (collaborative): Demonstrates willingness to comply with treatment plan

EVALUATION CRITERIA: Participates in self-care activities, verbalizes understanding of treatment plan, seeks additional information

● ●

INTERVENTIONS	RATIONALE
1. Explain all procedures and purpose of all treatments. Encourage patient involvement as much as possible. Evaluate patient's ability to perform self-care activities. Initiate a consult with social services or discharge planning department to make arrangements for home care assistance if unable to perform ADL independently and no reliable support system is available.	To promote cooperation, independence, and compliance.
2. On discharge, ensure the patient knows: • how to do pin care if an external fixator is in place. • signs and symptoms of neurovascular compromise that should be reported: — pain unrelieved by analgesia — persistent numbness and tingling — increased swelling — cool skin — diminished sensation — cyanosis of nailbeds • who to contact if a problem occurs: — physician — orthopedic clinic	Compliance with home care activities that are essential for maximizing a full recovery are likely to be improved when patients have a thorough understanding of what they are to do and know how to do it.

INTERVENTIONS	RATIONALE
• signs and symptoms of infection if open reduction was performed or an external fixator is in place: — increased tenderness — redness — drainage — fever • how to ambulate with assistive device (crutches, cane) on a flat surface and stairs. • how to care for a cast if applied.	
3. Provide written instructions for follow-up care and appointments.	Verbal instructions may be easily forgotten.
4. Ensure the patient has: • one week's supply of wound care supplies on discharge. • a prescription for analgesia.	To minimize anxiety commonly associated with self-care activities at home. Mild pain is expected to continue for several weeks after open reduction.
5. For a lower extremity with an external fixator or cast, ensure the patient is discharged with crutches.	To prevent placing excess weight on the weakened bone until complete healing has occurred.

*T*raction

Traction refers to using a pulling force on a part of the body. It is achieved by applying sufficient weights to overcome muscle pull. Traction is applied to minimize muscle spasms, to reduce and maintain body alignment, to immobilize a fracture, and to lessen deformity.

Two categories of traction are skin and skeletal. The maximum allowable weight for skin traction is 5–7 pounds. Skeletal traction is needed when greater amounts of weight are needed to achieve and maintain bone alignment over a long time. Skeletal traction involves inserting a Steinmann pin or Kirschner wire through the bone, with attachment to its respective holder and then attachment to weights.

To maintain effective traction, countertraction (force acting in the opposite direction) must also be established. This is accomplished by the weight of the patient's body or repositioning the bed.

In most facilities, after the physician determines the type of traction and the amount of weight, an orthopedic technician sets up the traction.

Integrative Care Plans

• Immobility
• Fractures

*A*SSESSMENT DATA BASE

1. After the traction has been applied, ongoing assessments include:

   a. Assessing the patient:

      • neurovascular status (Appendix D) of the tractioned extremity q2h for the first 24 hours, then q4h
      • mental and emotional status q8h for loneliness, boredom, and depression
      • skin for irritation q8h if skin traction is used
      • pin sites q8h for infection if skeletal traction is used

b. Assessing the traction setup:
- Weights hang freely.
- Ropes are in the pulleys, footplates, and spreader blocks.
- Knots are free from the pulleys.
- Bed linens do not interfere with the traction force.
- Countertraction is maintained.

NURSING DIAGNOSIS: HIGH RISK FOR ALTERATION IN TISSUE INTEGRITY

RELATED TO FACTORS: Traction

DEFINING CHARACTERISTICS: Red abraded skin beneath traction, reports tenderness or persistent pain

PATIENT OUTCOME (collaborative): Circulation remains intact

EVALUATION CRITERIA: Absence of signs of skin irritation, warm extremity with normal color, no further swelling, palpable pulses

INTERVENTIONS	RATIONALE
1. Monitor neurovascular status (Appendix D) q2h during first 24 hours after traction applied, then q4h thereafter. Inspect pressure points for redness q8h.	Early detect of possible complications can avert serious tissue damage.
2. Notify physician if manifestations of compartment syndrome (page 275) are detected. Reduce the amount of traction weight as ordered.	Inadequate circulation can cause permanent functional impairment.
3. **Never** interrupt traction when used to immobilize a fracture. Transport the patient to the operating room in the bed when surgery is planned.	Disrupting traction can cause misalignment of the fracture.
4. Maintain countertraction by: • keeping patient pulled up in bed so the feet are not resting against the foot of bed. • placing shock blocks beneath the foot of bed.	Countertraction helps ensure maintenance of tension on the limb thereby promoting bone alignment.

INTERVENTIONS	RATIONALE
5. Keep ropes free of obstructions. If the patient complains of being cold, use a sheet to cover the body part in traction. Do **not** drape the sheet over the traction ropes.	Excess weight on the traction ropes can reduce the pull.
6. Keep toes pointed toward the ceiling. Encourage flexion and extension exercises of digits on the affected extremity.	To ensure correct body alignment, prevent foot-drop and promote circulation.
7. Ensure that a trapeze bar is applied to the bed.	To allow the patient to assist in moving self in bed and lifting hips off the mattress for placement of the bedpan, back care, and linen change.
8. Place a special decubitus prevention mattress (egg crate, air mattress) on the bed.	To prevent skin breakdown.
9. Contact orthopedic technician to provide extra padding if signs of skin irritation occur. Loosen elastic bandage for skin traction and resecure if the patient reports persistent numbness and tingling.	Persistent skin irritation causes skin breakdown. An elastic bandage that is too tight can cause peroneal nerve damage, which can cause foot-drop.
10. Follow special considerations for the specific type of traction: • Use a footboard to prevent foot-drop. • Have the patient flex the knee of the unaffected limb and use the overbed trapeze bar to lift hips off the bed for placement of the bedpan, linen change, and back care. • Use a fracture bedpan for elimination. • With balanced suspension traction, the head of bed may be elevated 30–40 degrees for meals. • With Buck's traction, keep the bed flat with patient supine.	The line of pull must be maintained when moving the patient in bed and differs with each type of traction setup. Suspension of the limb allows the patient to move in bed without disturbing the direction of pull.

INTERVENTIONS   RATIONALE

- With a pelvic sling, apply a waterproof drape between the patient's buttocks and the sling to prevent soiling. Change a soiled pelvic sling by first anchoring the clean sling in place. Then, have someone hold the patient and the clean sling steady as the soiled sling is removed.

- With Dunlop's traction, ensure the patient's elbow does not touch the bed to ensure counter-traction is maintained.

- With cervical traction (skeletal), monitor neurological status qh for first 24 hours, then q2–4h if stable. If patient is not on a special turning bed, turn the patient with the assistance of two other persons. One person supports the head while two persons turn patient using a log-roll technique. Avoid neck flexion. Maintain alignment throughout the turn (nose in line with sternum).

- With halo traction (skeletal), always keep head of bed at 30–40 degree angle. Administer prescribed analgesic to control headache or pressure sensation that is expected for several days following application of the device. Reassure the patient that a "caged in" feeling passes with adaptation to the device. Keep a torque screwdriver at the bed-side so the physician may tighten the frame as needed.

INTERVENTIONS	RATIONALE
Monitor neurological status qh following initial application of the device, then q2–4h if stable. Notify physician if abducens nerve palsy occurs (nystagmus and asymmetrical extraocular eye movements). Instruct patient to move to the edge of the bed and then roll on side to a sitting position to get out of bed.	

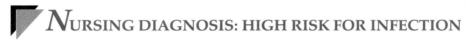

NURSING DIAGNOSIS: HIGH RISK FOR INFECTION

RELATED TO FACTORS; Insertion of pins in bone through skin surface for skeletal traction.

DEFINING CHARACTERISTICS: Pain unrelieved by analgesia, redness and drainage at pin sites, temperature above 99°F, WBC above 10,000/mm^3

PATIENT OUTCOME (collaborative): Demonstrates absence of infection

EVALUATION CRITERIA: Temperature below 99°F, WBC between 5,000–10,000/mm^3 formation of granulation tissue at pin site

INTERVENTIONS	RATIONALE
1. Monitor: • temperature q4h • CBC reports, especially WBC count • appearance of skin around pin sites on each shift	To detect early signs of infection.
2. For external fixators and skeletal traction, provide pin care at least b.i.d. Teach the patient how to do pin self-care, if possible and if pin site care is prescribed by physician.	Cleansing pin sites with an antibacterial solution helps reduce chance of infection. Self-care helps maintain self-esteem and promotes active exercise.

INTERVENTIONS

RATIONALE

3. Notify physician if signs of infection or osteomyelitis occur: redness, drainage, fever, increased pain unrelieved by narcotic analgesia, and WBC count above 10,000/mm.^{3} Obtain a wound specimen for culture and sensitivity (C&S) test and an x ray as ordered. Notify infection control nurse if the wound culture is positive. Place the patient on "Drainage and Secretion Precautions." Administer prescribed antibiotic and evaluate its effectiveness.

A wound culture helps identify the causative pathogen. The sensitivity report indicates which antibiotic is most effective against the causative pathogen. An x ray confirms the presence of osteomyelitis. The infection control nurse maintains surveillance of nosocomial infections for quality control purposes.

Cast Care

A **cast** is a stiff dressing used to immobilize a body part. The orthopedic physician determines the type (plaster or fiberglass) of casting material. The cast is applied by an orthopedic technician or the physician, depending on the problem. Periodic x rays are taken of the casted part to evaluate healing. The physical therapist instructs the patient in crutchwalking (when the lower extremity is casted) and independent transfer from bed to wheelchair if a cast is applied to both lower extremities.

After obtaining a physician order, the orthopedic technician removes the cast. A special cast saw cuts through the cast down to the first layer of padding. The blade of the saw does not revolve but merely shakes the rigid plaster apart. Thus, there is no danger of the patient's skin being cut by the blade. The patient will feel increased warmth beneath the cast during the "cutting."

The major complication associated with a cast is compartment syndrome.

Integrative Care Plans

- Fracture
- Immobility

Discharge Considerations

- Follow-up care
- Cast care
- Skin care after cast removal

 # ASSESSMENT DATA BASE

1. Presence of factors contributing to the need for casting (for example, fracture, to correct skeletal deformity, severe sprain, or dislocation).

2. Perform a neurovascular assessment (Appendix D) after the cast has been applied. Assessment of distal pulses may not be possible if the hand or foot is enclosed in the cast.

3. Assess cast edges to ensure that padded stockinette extends over edges and that raw edges do not rub against the patient's skin.

4. Assess patient's knowledge of cast care and skin care after cast removal.

5. Assess need for assistance with ADL (eating, bathing, turning, walking, toileting, writing, dressing).

▶ NURSING DIAGNOSIS: HIGH RISK FOR ALTERATIONS IN HOME MAINTENANCE MANAGEMENT

RELATED TO FACTORS: Knowledge deficit about cast care and skin care after cast removal

DEFINING CHARACTERISTICS: Verbalizes lack of understanding, requests information, observation of improper cast care

PATIENT OUTCOME: Demonstrates understanding of cast care and skin care after cast removal

EVALUATION CRITERIA: Verbalizes understanding of instructions, performs recommended exercises, follows instructions for skin care

INTERVENTIONS	RATIONALE
1. Provide written instructions for cast care at home: a. Report the following occurrences to physician: • object dropped inside or stuck inside the cast • foul smell coming from inside the cast • weakened, cracked, loose, or very tight cast • excess swelling not relieved by elevating the casted extremity and applying an ice bag • increasing pain not relieved by medication • numbness, tingling, or burning not relieved after taking pain medication and elevating the extremity for about 20 minutes • decreased movement or loss of movement in fingers or toes or both	Verbal instructions may be easily forgotten. Health teaching is essential for ensuring safety in self-care of the cast.

INTERVENTIONS	RATIONALE
b. Never get the cast wet even if the water-resistant fiberglass cast is used. The stockinette and cotton padding beneath the cast are not water-resistant and may not dry thoroughly, thus predisposing patient to skin breakdown.	
c. Never trim or remove any part of the cast.	
d. In several days, skin beneath the cast may begin to itch and have a slight odor because of the secretion of body oils and perspiration beneath the cast. Never put anything into the cast to relieve itching. Itching may be relieved by: • applying an ice pack over the cast • using a fan or blow dryer on the cool setting to vent cool air down the cast.	
e. Do not put powder down the cast. It may clump and lead to skin irritation.	
f. Keep the casted extremity elevated above chest level when possible to minimize swelling. Some swelling is expected.	
g. Flex and extend fingers and toes several times during the day to maintain joint flexibility.	
h. Avoid weight bearing on a new cast for 48 hours.	
i. Keep appointments to have cast and fracture checked.	

INTERVENTIONS	RATIONALE
2. After cast removal, provide written instructions about skin care: • Exercise the extremity gradually to help relieve the painful stiffness resulting from prolonged immobility of the limb in one position and muscle atrophy from disuse. • Cleanse the skin daily. Gently use warm water and mild soap followed by an emollient lotion to help the skin return to its normal appearance. Explain that the skin will initially be foul smelling, tender, and appear grayish, dirty, and hairless due to the buildup of body oils, perspiration, and desquamated epithelium beneath the cast. Within a few days, normal skin color and texture will return. • Avoid rubbing the skin to dry it. Blot the skin to dry. • Avoid scratching the skin. • Elevate the extremity above chest level if swelling occurs. Explain that some swelling may occur because of fluids redistribution to a previously compressed area.	Skin beneath the cast is fragile and must be treated gently to prevent skin breakdown. Verbal instructions may be easily forgotten.

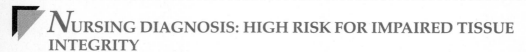

NURSING DIAGNOSIS: HIGH RISK FOR IMPAIRED TISSUE INTEGRITY

RELATED TO FACTORS: Compartment syndrome secondary to tight fitting cast

DEFINING CHARACTERISTICS: Presence of neurovascular deficits

PATIENT OUTCOME (collaborative): Demonstrates adequate tissue perfusion

EVALUATION CRITERIA: Absence of manifestations of compartment syndrome

INTERVENTIONS	RATIONALE
1. Monitor neurovascular status (Appendix D) qh for the first 24 hours after application of the cast, then q4h.	To detect early findings of compartment syndrome.
2. Keep the extremity elevated above chest level. Apply ice packs.	Elevation promotes venous and lymphatic drainage by gravity.
3. If symptoms of compartment syndrome (page 275) occur, notify physician. Contact orthopedic technician to slit the cast if ordered.	Normally, some swelling occurs after application of a cast. Excessive swelling can cause compartment syndrome. Permanent nerve and tissue damage can occur if the pressure is not relieved.
4. Avoid use of heat to hasten drying of a wet cast.	This may cause burns under the cast. It also may cause uneven drying, causing the cast to be weak in some places.
5. When handling a wet cast, use palms rather than fingers.	Using of fingers can create indentations in the cast that can become potential pressure areas when the cast dries.
6. Avoid getting the cast wet during and after the drying period. Use plastic material (such as a plastic garbage liner bag) to cover the cast when bathing or to cover that part of the cast that may become soiled by urine or feces.	The shape of the cast can be altered when wet.
7. Reposition the casted part q2h during the first 24 hours.	To promote even drying of the cast and reduce continuous pressure on the dependent area.
8. Cover the patient, not the cast. Keep the cast exposed to air to hasten the drying time.	Drying time varies from 24–48 hours.
9. Contact orthopedic technician to trim and pad cast edges if the rim is not covered and skin irritation occurs.	Persistent irritation from rough cast edges causes skin breakdown.

INTERVENTIONS	RATIONALE
10. If the patient complains of increased warmth beneath the cast after initial application, explain that this exothermic discomfort is normal because of the reaction of chemicals that hardens the cast. As the cast dries, the discomfort gradually dissipates. Keep ice applied to the cast to lessen exothermic discomfort.	A knowledge of what to expect helps lessen anxiety.
11. When applying ice bags to a wet cast, place them along the sides of the cast, not the top. After the cast dries, ice bags may be placed on the top.	Applying weight to a wet cast causes potential pressure areas when the cast dries.
12. If itching occurs, apply ice bags or use a blow dryer on the cool setting to direct cool air down into the cast.	Itching occurs because of heat buildup beneath the cast.

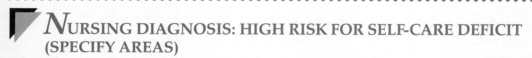

NURSING DIAGNOSIS: HIGH RISK FOR SELF-CARE DEFICIT (SPECIFY AREAS)

RELATED TO FACTORS: Casted extremity

DEFINING CHARACTERISTICS: Requests assistance with some aspect of activities of daily living (ADL)

PATIENT OUTCOME: Demonstrates absence of deficits in ADL

EVALUATION CRITERIA: Reports that ADL are met, performs self-care activities within level of ability

INTERVENTIONS	RATIONALE
1. Assist patient with ADL as needed. Teach the patient how to perform self-care activities within limitations imposed by the cast.	Encouraging active participation with ADL helps maintain joint flexibility and self-esteem.
2. Arrange a consult with occupational therapy to assist patient in learning how to be independent with ADL if needed.	An occupational therapist is a specialist who can assist the patient with necessary adaptations to accomplish ADL.
3. Allow time for the patient to accomplish tasks to fullest extent of ability.	To reduce frustration that often accompanies the difficulty encountered when learning to adapt to limitations.

Total Hip Arthroplasty

Total hip arthroplasty is the surgical replacement of the hip joint (ball and socket) with a prosthetic hip joint. The ball and stem are often made of metal and the cup of plastic. The cup and stem may be secured with a fast drying cement.

Total hip replacement (THR) is indicated when disease of the hip results in severe, chronic pain, restricted motion, loss of stability, and deformity. The leading indication for most THR is severe, chronic pain at rest and on ambulation, which has been unresponsive to analgesics and anti-inflammatory drugs.

THR may be done on both hips at the same time. Or surgery may be performed on one hip and then the other hip after the initial hip has healed. THR is performed through a lateral incision over the affected hip.

Generally, on the day of hospital admission, the patient visits the physical therapy department where instructions are given about the following postoperative activities:

- use of the continuous passive motion (CPM) device if used
- use of a walker and crutches at prescribed weight bearing
- isometric and isotonic bed exercises
- do's and don'ts following THR (Table 4–1).

Preoperative preparation is the same for any patient undergoing surgery. Postoperatively, the patient returns to a medical/surgical unit with:

- IV infusion
- antiembolism stockings to prevent thrombophlebitis
- dressing over operative site
- abduction pillow between legs
- Foley catheter (if female)
- wound drainage device

The patient may be placed on a standard orthopedic bed (bed with a trapeze setup) or a special bed such as a Cir O lectric® bed. On the first postoperative day, the physical therapist assists the patient to dangle or stand with weight-bearing to tolerance. However, if an Austin-Moore hip prosthesis is inserted, the patient remains on bedrest for usually three days to prevent dislodgment of the device.

Gait training with a walker is initiated on the second postoperative day. As weight bearing progresses to full status, the assistive devices are changed from walker to crutches or a cane. Occupational therapy assists the patient with learning how to make adjustments to be independent with ADL. The mean LOS for a DRG classification of THR is 10.1 days (Lorenz, 1991).

The major complications associated with THR are infection, fat emboli, hemorrhage, thrombophlebitis, and prosthesis dislocation.

Integrative Care Plans

- Immobility
- Pain
- Preoperative and postoperative care
- IV therapy

Discharge Considerations

- Follow-up care
- Use of assistive devices
- Signs and symptoms of wound infection and prosthesis dislocation
- Actions if infection or dislocation occur
- Activity limitations
- Measures to prevent prosthesis dislocation
- Muscle strengthening exercises

THE PREOPERATIVE PERIOD

 *A*SSESSMENT DATA BASE

1. History of conditions for which THR is performed:
   - rheumatoid arthritis
   - osteoarthritis
   - congenital hip dysplasia
   - avascular necrosis of the hip

2. Physical examination based upon a neurovascular assessment (Appendix D) and a general survey (Appendix F) to establish baseline values.

3. Assess the patient's feelings and expectations about the surgery.

4. See Preoperative and Postoperative Care (page 738).

NURSING DIAGNOSIS: ANXIETY

RELATED TO FACTORS: Knowledge deficit about preoperative and postoperative events

DEFINING CHARACTERISTICS: Verbalizes lack of understanding, requests information, reports feeling nervous about some aspect of surgery

PATIENT OUTCOME: Demonstrates relief from anxiety

EVALUATION CRITERIA: Verbalizes understanding of preoperative and postoperative events, denies feelings of nervousness, cooperates with preoperative instructions

INTERVENTIONS	RATIONALE
1. See Preoperative and Postoperative Care (page 738).	
2. Teach and have the patient practice postoperative exercises that are not taught by physical therapy: • turning with abduction pillow between legs • using the incentive spirometer for deep breathing. • using the trapeze to lift hips off the bed for placement of the bed-pan. Instruct the patient to flex the unaffected knee and hip to lift hips off the bed for bedpan placement. If the patient is too weak to lift hips, tilt the patient to the **unaffected** side for bedpan placement. Explain that the abduction pillow is kept between the legs when turning.	Practicing these activities facilitates postoperative recovery.

THE POSTOPERATIVE PERIOD

ASSESSMENT DATA BASE

1. On receiving the patient, perform a:
   • routine postoperative assessment (Appendix L)
   • neurovascular assessment (Appendix D) of both lower extremities
2. Assess ability to meet ADL

NURSING DIAGNOSIS: PAIN

RELATED TO FACTORS: THR

DEFINING CHARACTERISTICS: Verbalizes pain, frowning, moaning, guarding painful site, unwilling to turn or participate in exercise regimen

PATIENT OUTCOME (collaborative): Demonstrates relief from pain

EVALUATION CRITERIA: Denies pain, relaxed facial expression, absence of moaning and guarding behavior with movement, able to participate in exercise program and turning

INTERVENTIONS	RATIONALE
1. See Pain (page 700).	

NURSING DIAGNOSIS: HIGH RISK FOR IMPAIRED TISSUE INTEGRITY

RELATED TO FACTORS: THR complications: infection, fat embolism syndrome, thrombophlebitis, hemorrhage, prosthesis dislocation

DEFINING CHARACTERISTICS: Signs and symptoms of infection, fat embolism, thrombophlebitis, hemorrhage, or prosthesis dislocation

PATIENT OUTCOME (collaborative): Intact tissue integrity

EVALUATION CRITERIA: Absence of infection, fat embolism syndrome, thrombophlebitis, hemorrhage, prosthesis dislocation

INTERVENTIONS	RATIONALE
Infection and Hemorrhage: 1. See Preoperative and Postoperative Care (page 738).	
Fat Embolism Syndrome: 1. See (page 311).	
Thrombophlebitis: 1. See (page 381).	

INTERVENTIONS	RATIONALE
Hip Dislocation: 1. Adhere to safety measures to prevent hip dislocation: • Keep the operative leg in a position of **abduction**. When repositioning, keep the abduction pillow always between the legs when in bed. Use a regular pillow when sitting in a chair to maintain abduction. • Avoid flexing the hip beyond 90 degrees. • Avoid crossing legs. • Place a raised toilet seat cover on the commode. • Ensure that physical therapy provides the patient with a reacher. Have the patient demonstrate how to use the reacher and explain its use. • Support the operative leg in abduction as the patient exits and enters the bed. • Use a wheelchair with a hard seat when transporting the patient. • Avoid turning the patient to the operative side. When repositioning the patient, use a back-lying or side-lying position on the nonoperative side.	To ensure the hip prosthesis remains in a natural position.
2. Consult physician if signs of prosthesis dislocation are suspected: • sudden, sharp, persistent pain unrelieved by narcotic analgesia accompanied by a clicking or popping sound (most prominent finding) • shortening of affected extremity with foot in external rotation	Surgical replacement of the prosthesis is the only treatment for prosthesis dislocation.

INTERVENTIONS	RATIONALE
• loss of leg motion • a palpable lump over affected hip • swelling of affected hip If hip dislocation is suspected, refrain from moving the patient. Keep the abduction pillow between the legs. Obtain an x ray of the hip as ordered. Prepare the patient for return to surgery if x ray confirms dislocation.	

NURSING DIAGNOSIS: HIGH-RISK FOR COMPLICATIONS ASSOCIATED WITH IMPAIRED PHYSICAL MOBILITY

RELATED TO FACTORS: Limited physical activity secondary to THR

DEFINING CHARACTERISTICS: Inability to perform some ADLs independently, requires assistance with turning and ambulation, restricted weight bearing on one limb, constipation, orthostatic hypotension, flank pain, skin breakdown

PATIENT OUTCOME (collaborative): Demonstrates no complications associated with immobility

EVALUATION CRITERIA: Absence of flank pain, intact skin, passage of soft formed stool, absence of orthostatic hypotension and thrombophlebitis, denies muscle weakness and joint stiffness

INTERVENTIONS	RATIONALE
1. See Immobility (page 733).	
2. Provide assistance with ADL as needed. Encourage the patient to do as much as possible for self. Refer patient to occupational therapy for further instructions on rehabilitation training to resume ADL within current limitation.	Self-care and active exercise promote independence. An occupational therapist is a specialist who can assist the patient in learning how to resume independence within current limitations.

INTERVENTIONS	RATIONALE
3. Elevate head of the bed 45 degrees while patient is on the bedpan and for meals.	To promote comfort.
4. If a standard orthopedic bed is used, keep a draw sheet on the bed. Apply a special mattress (egg crate, air mattress) to minimize skin pressure.	A draw sheet can make turning easier. These special mattress help minimize skin breakdown.

· ·

◤NURSING DIAGNOSIS: HIGH RISK FOR ALTERATION IN HOME MAINTENANCE MANAGEMENT

RELATED TO FACTORS: Knowledge deficit about self-care on discharge, inadequate support system

DEFINING CHARACTERISTICS: Verbalizes lack of understanding, requests information

PATIENT OUTCOME (collaborative): Demonstrates understanding of self-care preventive and maintenance measures upon discharge

EVALUATION CRITERIA: Verbalizes understanding of discharge instructions, demonstrates appropriate and safe use of assistive devices

· ·

INTERVENTIONS	RATIONALE
1. Before discharge, ensure the patient: a. has the following for home use: • raised toilet seat • reacher to pick items off the floor • plump bed pillow that is used between legs to maintain the hip in abduction • an assistive device (walker or crutches) for ambulation b. knows to contact physician if a problem arises	Discharge teaching is essential for safe rehabilitation. Verbal instructions may be easily forgotten.

INTERVENTIONS	RATIONALE
c. knows signs and symptoms of prosthesis dislocation and who to contact if this problem occurs d. has written instructions about do's and don'ts for a THR e. has a written appointment for initial follow-up visit f. knows to contact physician if wound infection occurs (fever, redness, increased tenderness, purulent drainage)	Discharge teaching is essential for safe rehabilitation. Verbal instructions may be easily forgotten.
2. Evaluate patient's ability to care for self independently and availability of support system to provide necessary assistance. Contact social services or discharge planning department to arrange for assistive devices or home care assistance if the patient cannot perform ADL independently and support system is inadequate.	These departments ensure continuity of care on discharge to support the patient during the recovery period by arranging for needed care through a local home health agency or temporary placement in an extended care facility.

Total Knee Arthroplasty

Total knee arthroplasty is the surgical replacement of the knee joint with a prosthetic joint. It is performed through a straight midline incision over the affected knee. Preoperative preparation is the same for any patient undergoing surgery. Postoperatively, the patient returns to a medical/surgical unit with:

- IV infusion
- antiembolism stocking on the nonoperative extremity
- Ace bandage on the operative leg wrapped from foot to midthigh. A gauze dressing is beneath the Ace bandage
- wound drainage device
- continuous passive motion (CPM) machine

The CPM machine is applied in the recovery room by the physical therapist at the prescribed flexion and extension setting. The degree of flexion and extension on the machine is increased daily until full knee flexion is achieved. Usually, the CPM machine is used intermittently (on four hours, off two hours) per physician orders. When the device is not in use, a canvas knee splint (CKS), also called a knee immobilizer, is applied to the leg to keep the knee straight and to prevent twisting.

Usually, ambulation with minimal weight bearing is initiated by the physical therapist on the second postoperative day. The mean LOS for a DRG classification of total knee arthroplasty is 10.1 days (Lorenz, 1991).

Integrative Care Plans

- Immobility
- Preoperative and postoperative care
- Pain
- IV therapy

Discharge Considerations

* Follow-up care
* Signs and symptoms of wound infection
* Activity limitations
* Muscle-strengthening exercises
* Use of assistive devices for ambulation

THE PREOPERATIVE PERIOD

 # ASSESSMENT DATA BASE

1. History of conditions for which the surgery is performed:
   * osteoarthritis
   * rheumatoid arthritis
2. Physical examination based on a neurovascular assessment (Appendix D) and a general survey (Appendix F) to establish baseline values.
3. See Preoperative and Postoperative Care (page 738).

 # NURSING DIAGNOSIS: ANXIETY

RELATED TO FACTORS: Knowledge deficit about preoperative and postoperative events

DEFINING CHARACTERISTICS: Verbalizes lack of understanding, requests information, may report feelings of nervousness or fear about some aspect of surgery, tense posture and facial expression

PATIENT OUTCOME: Demonstrates less anxiety

EVALUATION CRITERIA: Verbalizes understanding of preoperative and postoperative events, fewer reports of feeling nervous or anxious, relaxed posture and facial expression

INTERVENTIONS	RATIONALE
1. See Preoperative and Postoperative Care (page 738).	
2. Teach and have the patient practice: • turning with leg straight. • using trapeze bar to lift hips off mattress (for bedpan placement or linen change).	Preoperative teaching helps promote postoperative recovery.

THE POSTOPERATIVE PERIOD

 ASSESSMENT DATA BASE

1. See Preoperative and Postoperative Care (page 738).
2. After receiving the patient, perform a neurovascular assessment (Appendix D) of the legs. Check and record setting on the CPM machine to ensure setting is at the prescribed degree of flexion and extension.

 NURSING DIAGNOSIS: PAIN

RELATED TO FACTORS: Total knee arthroplasty

DEFINING CHARACTERISTICS: Verbalizes discomfort, facial frowning, moaning, guarding of painful site, unwillingly to perform prescribed exercises

PATIENT OUTCOME (collaborative): Demonstrates relief from pain

EVALUATION CRITERIA: Denies discomfort, relaxed facial expression, no moaning, able to perform prescribed exercises

INTERVENTIONS	RATIONALE
1. When the patient is not on the CPM machine: • apply the CKS. • assist patient to assume a position of comfort. • place a pillow between legs when turning patient to a lateral position.	A CKS and pillow supports when turning protect the knee from twisting and help maintain full extension.
2. See Pain (page 700).	

NURSING DIAGNOSIS: HIGH RISK FOR ALTERATIONS IN TISSUE INTEGRITY

RELATED TO FACTORS: Complications associated with total knee arthroplasty: infection, fat emboli, hemorrhage, thrombophlebitis

DEFINING CHARACTERISTICS: Signs and symptoms of infection, fat emboli, hemorrhage, thrombophlebitis

PATIENT OUTCOME (collaborative): Intact tissue integrity

EVALUATION CRITERIA: Absence of infection, thrombophlebitis, fat emboli, hemorrhage

• •

INTERVENTIONS	RATIONALE
1. Monitor neurovascular status (Appendix D) q2h x 24 hours, then q4h thereafter. If manifestations of neurovascular deficits occur (pain unrelieved by analgesia, cool extremity accompanied by swelling, diminished pulse, diminished sensation, persistent numbness and tingling, cyanosis), loosen the elastic bandage. If no relief of symptoms occurs in 5–10 minutes, notify physician.	Prompt medical intervention is required to avoid permanent tissue damage.
2. Ensure that settings for flexion and extension on the CPM machine are posted at the bedside.	So all persons involved in the patient's care are informed.
3. Place the patient on facility protocol for "Falls Precautions."	Procedures that impair motor function of the lower extremities increase the risk of falling.
Infection and Hemorrhage: 1. See Preoperative and Postoperative Care (page 738).	
Thrombophlebitis: 1. See page 381.	
Fat Embolism Syndrome: 1. See page 311.	

• •

NURSING DIAGNOSIS: HIGH RISK FOR ALTERATION IN HOME MAINTENANCE MANAGEMENT

RELATED TO FACTORS: Knowledge deficit about self-care activities on discharge, lack of adequate support system

DEFINING CHARACTERISTICS: Verbalizes lack of understanding, requests information, unsafe behaviors observed

PATIENT OUTCOME (collaborative): Verbalizes understanding of home care instructions, demonstrates compliance with activity limitations.

EVALUATION CRITERIA: Verbalizes understanding of discharge instructions, demonstrates appropriate and safe use of assistive devices

INTERVENTIONS	RATIONALE
1. Instruct the patient to: • continue leg exercises at home as taught by physical therapy. • avoid running, jumping, and heavy lifting. • report signs and symptoms of wound infection to the physician: — fever — redness — increased tenderness — purulent drainage	To prevent undue stress on the artificial knee joint. Infections require treatment with an antibiotic to reduce the risk of osteomyelitis.
2. Provide a written appointment for initial follow-up visit and written self-care instructions.	Verbal instructions may be easily forgotten.
3. Teach and have the patient practice wound care. Clean, dry dressing changes daily are sufficient until the sutures or staples are removed. Emphasize the importance of handwashing before and after wound care.	To reduce risk of infection.
4. Provide the patient with sufficient supplies for dressing changes.	Searching for medical supplies can be stressful for the patient just discharged from the hospital.
5. Ensure the patient has an assistive device for ambulation (cane, walker, or crutches). Evaluate the patient's use of the device. Contact physical therapy to assist patient in safe use of the devices if improper technique is observed.	Use of an assistive device increases the risk for injury.
6. Allow the patient to apply and remove the CKS.	To evaluate proper application of the device.

Arthritis

Arthritis is inflammation of a joint. Rheumatoid arthritis (RA), osteoarthritis (OA), and gout are the more prevalent forms. There are many other connective tissue diseases characterized by arthritis, such as systemic lupus erythematosus, dermatomyositis, scleroderma, rheumatic fever, and ankylosing spondylitis.

The course of the disease is slow and progressive. There is no cure for arthritis. Medical treatments control discomfort and maintain joint function. Hospitalization is not required for treatment unless complications occur or surgery is planned.

Rheumatoid arthritis is a chronic, systemic connective tissue disease characterized by inflammation of the synovial membrane of diarthrodial joints. RA is characterized by periods of remission and exacerbation. With repeated exacerbations, the articular cartilage is eventually destroyed and replaced by fibrous tissue. Muscle spasms and the replacement of normal tissue with scar tissue (pannus) leads to flexion contracture deformities, which predisposes to subluxation and dislocation. The etiology of RA is unclear but is believed to be an immune response to some unknown antigen or some infectious agent. It is also believed to be linked to heredity owing to the finding of specific histocompatibility antigens (HLA) in family members.

The disease occurs bilaterally with symmetrical joint involvement. Small joints of the hands, wrist, knees, shoulders, and feet are most commonly affected.

Osteoarthritis (also called degenerative joint disease) is a noninflammatory disorder characterized by degenerative changes in the articular cartilage and bony overgrowths (osteophytes) at the joint margins. It affects any joint in the body, especially weight-bearing joints such as the spine, hips, and knees. Unlike RA, there is no systemic involvement with OA.

General Medical Management

- Rest
- Exercise
- Heat
- Well-balanced diet
- Pharmacotherapy:

a. nonsteroidal anti-inflammatory drugs (NSAIDs):

— aspirin (drug of choice)

— ibuprofen (Motrin)

— indomethacin (Indocin)

— naproxen (Naprosyn)

b. corticosteroids:

— prednisone

• For RA only, the following may be prescribed:

a. gold salts

— auranofin (Ridaura)

b. antimalarials:

— hydroxychloroquine sulfate (Plaquenil)

c. Immunosuppressive agents:

— azathioprine (Imuran)

— cyclophosphamide (Cytoxan)

Integrative Care Plans

• Loss

ASSESSMENT DATA BASE

1. Physical examination based on a general survey (Appendix F) and an assessment of the musculoskeletal system (Appendix C) may reveal:

   a. early nonspecific symptoms, such as malaise, fatigue, and diffuse musculoskeletal pain, or

   b. more defined symptoms that indicate progressive disease:

   • joint pain and tenderness accompanied by redness and swelling of soft tissue around joints

   • joint stiffness after periods of inactivity and on arising that may last 30 minutes or longer

   • low-grade fever (during periods of exacerbations)

   • bony enlargements of distal interphalangeal joints (Heberden's nodes) and proximal interphalangeal joints (Bouchard's nodes), both specific for OA.

   c. manifestations indicating advanced systemic involvement with RA:

   • eyes — scleritis, keratoconjunctivitis

   • lymph nodes — lymphadenopathies

   • spleen — splenomegaly

- bone marrow — anemia, thrombocytopenia
- blood vessels — vasculitis (ulcers around the nailbeds), Raynaud's phenomenon
- pulmonary — pleural effusion, pulmonary fibrosis
- heart — pericardial effusion, pericarditis
- renal — amyloidosis
- muscles — muscle wasting, myositis
- skin — subcutaneous nodules of bony prominences

2. Assess for factors or situations that precipitate exacerbation of joint pain, such as emotional stress, cold weather, overexercising, and extreme fatigue.

3. Assess the patient's understanding of condition and its impact on lifestyle and ability to perform ADL (bathing, dressing, walking, toileting, feeding, sleeping) and social ADL (writing, working, sexual activities, cooking, recreation).

4. Diagnostic studies:

    a. There is no single diagnostic test for OA. X rays often show bone spurs (osteophytes), degeneration of cartilage and denuded bone.

    b. There is no single test for RA. In conjunction with the patient's history and physical findings, several tests provide positive indicators:

       - Erythrocyte sedimentation rate is increased, indicating inflammation.
       - Latex agglutination test reveals high levels of immunoglobulin IgG or IgM (major rheumatoid factors). The higher the titer, the more severe the disease.
       - CBC reveals normocytic hypochromic anemia.
       - Synovial fluid analysis reveals increased amount of synovial fluid that is thin and opaque (it is normally viscous and clear), excess polymorphonuclear leukocytes, and decreased complement.
       - X rays of involved joints reveal soft tissue swelling, erosion of the articular cartilage and osteoporosis in acute disease. In chronic disease, x rays reveal narrowing of joint spaces, subluxation, and ankylosis.

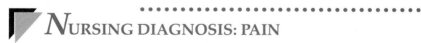

NURSING DIAGNOSIS: PAIN

RELATED TO FACTORS: Chronic arthritis

DEFINING CHARACTERISTICS: Redness and swelling of joints, verbalizes discomfort and stiffness, slow movement, limited range-of-motion exercises, moaning with movement

PATIENT OUTCOME (collaborative): Demonstrates relief from discomfort

EVALUATION CRITERIA: Denies pain, absence of moaning, relaxed facial expression, able to perform ADL

INTERVENTIONS	RATIONALE
1. Administer prescribed arthritis medication and evaluate its effectiveness. Apply prescribed method of moist heat.	To reduce inflammation thereby relieving pain. Heat helps stimulate circulation and promotes muscle relaxation.
2. Refer the patient to the physical therapy department as prescribed.	The physical therapist can evaluate the patient's degree of mobility and plan an exercise program that fits the patient's specific needs within the framework of the limitations. Regular exercise helps maintain joint flexibility.
3. Provide rest during painful episodes. Assist with ADL as needed.	Rest reduces energy expenditure.

◥ NURSING DIAGNOSIS: HIGH RISK FOR ALTERATION IN HOME MAINTENANCE MANAGEMENT

RELATED TO FACTORS: Knowledge deficit about condition and treatment plan, ineffective coping

DEFINING CHARACTERISTICS: Verbalizes lack of understanding, reports using fad diets and treatments, requests information, may verbalize feelings of depression

PATIENT OUTCOME (collaborative): Demonstrates an understanding of self-care maintenance and preventive measures

EVALUATION CRITERIA: Verbalizes understanding of self-care instructions, performs recommended exercises correctly, verbalizes willingness to comply with prescribed therapeutic plan

INTERVENTIONS	RATIONALE
1. Provide instructions on how to care for arthritic joints: a. Use heat or cold treatments to relieve joint stiffness and pain (warm shower or bath, whirlpool, paraffin bath, moist hot packs, cold packs).	To avoid further damage to compromised joints. Exercise tolerance is improved when pain is absent.

INTERVENTIONS	RATIONALE
b. Do exercises prescribed by the physical therapist **after** heat treatments. c. Avoid exercising painful joints. Begin activity slowly in the mornings. d. Avoid activities that involve: • impact or jolting of joints (running, contact sports). • use of heavy appliances/equipment (heavy pans for cooking).	To reduce inflammation thereby relieving pain. Heat helps stimulate circulation and promotes muscle relaxation.
2. Encourage the patient to plan rest periods during the day, especially during episodes of exacerbations.	To prevent excess fatigue and improve endurance for engaging in activities.
3. Emphasize the importance of engaging in a daily exercise program, for example, walking, swimming, bicycling, golfing, or gardening.	To maintain joint flexibility and muscle tone.
4. Advise the patient to take arthritis medication as ordered and to notify physician if adverse reactions occur. Provide written information about prescribed medications including name, dosage, purpose, frequency, and reportable side effects.	Medications help reduce inflammation and control pain and stiffness.
5. Refer the patient to the local chapter of the Arthritis Foundation.	This organization provides information about arthritis and its self-management.
6. Encourage the patient to seek medical attention if arthritic pain is unrelieved by medication or persistent fever develops.	These findings may signal advancement of the disease and a need for medication adjustment.

INTERVENTIONS	RATIONALE
7. Evaluate dietary history. Refer the patient to a dietitian for assistance with meal planning if patient's dietary intake does not follow the criteria for being well-balanced (foods from the five recognized food groups), or the patient is obese. Suggest a weight reduction diet for obese individuals.	There is no special diet for arthritis. A well-balanced diet is essential to effect control of the disease. Meals should include foods high in vitamins, protein, and iron for tissue building and repair. Obesity contributes to OA by placing undue stress on joints.
8. If joint contractures are present, arrange consult with an occupational therapist for assistance in devising orthotic devices as needed. Provide suggestions for more independent functioning such as using Velcro fasteners on clothing instead of buttons or ties, wearing slip-on shoes with a flat or very low (one-inch) heel instead of shoes that tie, and wearing clothing that zips or buttons down the front instead of the back.	The occupational therapist can evaluate the patient's need for orthotic devices, such as hand splints, and design one to meet the patient's needs. Orthotic devices help maintain normal alignment of contracted body parts. The therapist also can help the patient make adjustments in ADL to function more independently.
9. Evaluate understanding of condition. Provide information about the nature of the disease and purpose of prescribed treatments. Emphasize there is no cure for arthritis. Stress the importance of following the treatment plan to maintain joint function.	An understanding of the relationship between the disease process and treatment program helps promote patient cooperation and compliance.

*F*at Embolism Syndrome

Fat embolism syndrome is an important cause of acute respiratory syndrome in postskeletal trauma. It is most likely to occur within 24–72 hours postskeletal trauma.

Although the exact pathogenesis of fat emboli remains unclear, fat globules are believed to be released from the bone marrow directly into the bloodstream through severed veins at the fractured site. Another theory maintains that stress induced by trauma triggers the release of high levels of catecholamines that, in turn, trigger the release of free fatty acids and neutral fats. These fatty substances form fat globules that are then coated by platelets as they enter the circulation through severed veins at the fractured site (Slye, 1991).

As prevention, some physicians give steroids to multiple skeletal trauma patients beginning in the emergency room. The major complications associated with fat embolism syndrome are pulmonary edema, disseminated intravascular coagulation, and adult respiratory distress syndrome (ARDS). For this reason, patients are commonly placed in an ICU.

General Medical Management

- Supplemental oxygen
- IV therapy
- Bedrest
- Pharmacotherapy:
  - corticosteroids (drugs of choice)
  - low molecular weight dextran (improves microcapillary blood flow)
  - heparin (breaks down fat globules)

Integrative Care Plans

- IV therapy
- Immobility

Discharge Considerations

• Follow-up care

 # ASSESSMENT DATA BASE

1. Physical examination based on a respiratory status assessment (Appendix A) may reveal:
   • tachypnea and dyspnea accompanied by cyanosis
   • temperature above 100°F
   • BP significantly higher than the patient's baseline value
   • alterations in mental status (drowsiness, restlessness, confusion caused by cerebral hypoxia)
   • bilateral basilar rales
   • petechiae— one of the most characteristic findings that helps differentiate fat embolism from embolism caused by a blood clot in the lungs. It may occur on the second or third day post-trauma. Common sites for petechiae are neck, axillae, and lower conjunctiva (assessed by retracting the lower eyelids).

2. Presence of risk factors:
   • long bone fractures, orthopedic surgery, or multiple fractures

3. Diagnostic studies:
   • Arterial blood gases (ABG) reveal hypoxemia.
   • Brain and lung scans detect sites of vessel occlusion.
   • Chest x ray shows infiltrates in the lungs.
   • CBC reveals low hemoglobin, hematocrit, and platelet count.

4. Assess emotional response to condition.

NURSING DIAGNOSIS: IMPAIRED GAS EXCHANGE

RELATED TO FACTORS: Altered pulmonary blood flow secondary to fat emboli

DEFINING CHARACTERISTICS: Dyspnea, tachypnea, cyanosis, rales, restlessness, diminished sensorium, abnormal ABG (below normal PaO_2, above normal range $PaCO_2$)

PATIENT OUTCOME (collaborative): Demonstrates adequate gas exchange

EVALUATION CRITERIA: ABG within normal range, respiratory rate 12–24 per minute, absence of cyanosis, mentally alert and oriented

INTERVENTIONS	RATIONALE
1. Monitor: • results of ABG reports • respiratory status (Appendix A) and vital signs q2h	To evaluate effectiveness of therapy.
2. Place in a Fowler's position and administer oxygen via nasal cannula at 6 L/min immediately when respiratory distress first occurs.	To facilitate breathing.
3. If no IV site is in place, initiate an IV infusion at slow rate until a specific IV fluid order is obtained.	To provide vascular access for administration of emergency medication.
4. Maintain bedrest until symptoms of respiratory distress resolve and ABG return to within normal limits.	Bedrest reduces oxygen tissue demands.
5. Administer prescribed medication such as heparin or corticosteroids and evaluate its effectiveness.	These drugs enhance the breakdown of fatty acids and fat globules.
6. Notify physician if symptoms persist or worsen.	This indicates a need for additional testing to rule out development of complications.

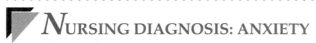

NURSING DIAGNOSIS: ANXIETY

RELATED TO FACTORS: Fear of uncertainty of outcome, feelings of suffocation

DEFINING CHARACTERISTICS: Tense facial expression; may report feeling afraid, may become demanding or show increasing irritability

PATIENT OUTCOME: Demonstrates relief from anxiety

EVALUATION CRITERIA: Reports feeling less nervous, relaxed facial expression, verbalizes understanding of condition and treatment plan

INTERVENTIONS	RATIONALE
1. Provide simple explanations about treatment plan and nature of condition during episode of acute respiratory distress. When respiratory distress is resolved, provide more indepth information based on the patient's level of comprehension.	Anxiety interferes with learning.
2. Allow the patient to express feelings about condition and perceptions of outcomes. Correct any misconceptions. Explain that transfer to ICU is to closely monitor the condition.	A knowledge of what to expect helps lessen anxiety.
3. See Nursing Diagnosis: Anxiety (page 262) for additional interventions.	

Integrative Care Plans

- Fracture
- Total hip arthroplasty
- Pain
- Traction (Buck's or Russell)
- Preoperative and postoperative care
- Immobility

Discharge Considerations

- Activity limitations
- Use of assistive device for ambulation
- Follow-up care
- Signs and symptoms of wound infection
- Muscle-strengthening exercises

THE PREOPERATIVE PERIOD

 ASSESSMENT DATA BASE

1. Physical examination based on a neurovascular assessment (Appendix D) of the affected limb and a general survey (Appendix F) may reveal:
   - shortening of the extremity on affected side
   - loss of limb motion
   - pain at the site, especially with passive movement
   - external rotation of the leg

2. See Preoperative and Postoperative Care (page 738).

3. Diagnostic studies:
   - X ray of the hip confirms the type of hip fracture.

4. See integrative care plans for the remainder of this preoperative and postoperative plan of care.

Facial Fractures Requiring Jaw Wiring

Facial fractures are seldom fatal. They may affect any bone in the face but more commonly affect the nose, zygomatic arch, maxillary bone, and mandible.

If the patient has sustained a mandibular fracture, a Barton's bandage may be applied in the emergency department to stabilize the fracture until surgery is performed. The mean LOS for a DRG classification of fractured mandible is 3.8 days (Lorenz, 1991).

Preoperative preparation of the patient requiring surgical repair is the same for any patient undergoing surgery. Postoperatively, the patient returns to a medical/surgical unit with the teeth wired together. After nausea has subsided, clear liquids are allowed, using a straw. The diet then progresses to full liquids and then pureed foods until the wires are removed. Special oral care is required until the wires are removed, usually in 4–8 weeks, depending on the extent of the fracture.

General Medical Management

a. Facial fractures:
- analgesia
- antibiotics
- ice pack
- bedrest in semi-Fowler's position

b. Nasal fractures:
- nostril packed with cotton pledget soaked in lidocaine
- closed reduction under local anesthesia with application of a plaster splint for 2–3 weeks

c. Zygomatic arch fracture:
- open reduction with internal fixation using wires or pins

d. Maxillary or mandible fracture:
- wiring of the jaws

Integrative Care Plans

- Fractures
- Preoperative and postoperative care
- Pain
- IV therapy

Discharge Considerations

- Follow-up care
- Preparation of diet following jaw wiring
- Activity limitations
- Signs and symptoms of infection
- Oral care

THE PREOPERATIVE PERIOD

(NOTE: This care plan is specific to jaw wiring.)

 *A*SSESSMENT DATA BASE

Regardless of the facial fracture, the patient assessments are the same when brought to the facility.

1. Assess airway patency and breathing. Noisy breathing indicates obstruction. Patient may complain of difficulty breathing through the nostril.

2. Assess level of consciousness (LOC) and if the patient is alert, oriented, disoriented, confused, lethargic, stuporous, semiconscious, or comatose.

3. Inquire about discomfort. Expect the patient to verbalize pain.

4. Assess vision:
   - Check field of gaze. Instruct patient to move eyes up, down, side-to-side, and in a circular motion.
   - Inquire about the presence of diplopia — double vision and limited eye movement in the upward gaze are common findings with zygomatic arch fracture.

5. Inspect the face for any obvious abnormalities:
   - malocclusion of the teeth (common with mandible and LeFort I maxillary fracture)
   - asymmetry
   - deviation of nasal ridge (with nasal fracture)
   - swelling
   - epistaxis

- drainage from nose or ears. If drainage is noted, determine if it is cerebrospinal fluid (CSF) using Tes-Tape. Drainage is positive for CSF if Tes-Tape is positive for glucose.
- movement of nose with dental arch as patient attempts to talk (common finding with LeFort II maxillary fracture)
- movement of the nose and dental arch (a common finding with LeFort III maxillary fracture)

6. Palpate for crepitations, paresthesia, and displacement.

7. Diagnostic studies:
- X rays determine if cervical spine injury is present and the extent of facial fractures.

• •

NURSING DIAGNOSIS: HIGH RISK FOR INEFFECTIVE AIRWAY CLEARANCE

RELATED TO FACTORS: Facial swelling secondary to fractured mandible, aspiration due to inability to open mouth

DEFINING CHARACTERISTICS: Inability to open mouth to expectorate secretions coughed up or vomited, may demonstrate noisy breathing, may communicate difficulty breathing

PATIENT OUTCOME: Airway remains patent

EVALUATION CRITERIA: Clear breath sounds, normal skin color, respiratory rate 12 –24 per minute, denies difficulty breathing

• •

INTERVENTIONS	RATIONALE
1. Avoid hyperextension of the neck until cervical spine injury has been ruled out. Immobilize the neck with trochanter rolls, cervical collar, or sandbags.	A neck injury is always suspected with facial or head injuries.
2. Keep suction equipment at the bedside. Suction gently if the patient coughs up mucus but is unable to expectorate it.	Suctioning removes secretions.
3. Keep NPO. Maintain a semi-Fowler's position.	Restricting oral feedings helps reduce the possibility of vomiting. An erect position enhances lung expansion.

NURSING DIAGNOSIS: PAIN

RELATED TO FACTORS: Fractured jaw

DEFINING CHARACTERISTICS: Verbalizes pain (that which is aggravated by talking), moaning, guarding painful site, facial frowning

PATIENT OUTCOME (collaborative): Demonstrates relief from discomfort

EVALUATION CRITERIA: Positive nod when asked if pain relieved, relaxed facial expression, absence of moaning

INTERVENTIONS	RATIONALE
1. Administer prescribed narcotic analgesic prn and evaluate its effectiveness.	Narcotic analgesics are required for severe pain. Analgesics block the pain pathway.
2. Keep head of bed elevated 45 degrees and apply ice packs.	To reduce swelling.
3. Instruct the patient to avoid talking.	Movement of the lower jaw while talking causes further tissue damage.

NURSING DIAGNOSIS: ANXIETY

RELATED TO FACTORS: Knowledge deficit about preoperative and postoperative events and inability to verbally communicate

DEFINING CHARACTERISTICS: Tense facial expression, may communicate fear of some aspect of surgery

PATIENT OUTCOME: Demonstrates less anxiety

EVALUATION CRITERIA: Relaxed facial expression, positive nod when understanding of preoperative and postoperative events evaluated, acknowledges feeling less anxious

INTERVENTIONS	RATIONALE
1. Provide a pad and pencil for writing. Keep call bell at bedside and go to patient's bedside when signaled instead of using the intercom system. Place a note on the intercom system such as "Fractured Jaw" or "Cannot Talk" to let all persons responsible for the patient's care know that they need to go to the patient's room instead of using the intercom system.	Communicating needs through alternative methods helps lessen anxiety and reduces feelings of helplessness.
2. Teach and have the patient practice deep breathing through the mouth by keeping the teeth together, opening the lips, and then inhaling deeply.	Practice facilitates postoperative performance of activities.
3. See Preoperative and Postoperative Care (page 738).	

THE POSTOPERATIVE PERIOD

 ## ASSESSMENT DATA BASE

1. After receiving the patient, perform a routine postoperative assessment (Appendix L).
2. Check postoperative orders to ensure an antiemetic has been prescribed.

• •

NURSING DIAGNOSIS: HIGH RISK FOR INEFFECTIVE AIRWAY INTERFERENCE

RELATED TO FACTORS: Aspiration secondary to jaw wiring

DEFINING CHARACTERISTICS: Dyspnea and possible cyanosis if vomiting occurs

PATIENT OUTCOME (collaborative): Airway remains patent

EVALUATION CRITERIA: Clear breath sounds, normal skin color, respiratory rate 12–24 per minute

• •

INTERVENTIONS	RATIONALE
1. Keep a pair of wire cutters and suction equipment at the bedside. If the patient begins to vomit, suction immediately with a tonsilar suction catheter. If airway problems develop, use the wire cutters to cut the vertical wire loops. Notify surgeon as soon as possible so the loops can be replaced.	To prevent aspiration, the vertical loops are cut to allow the patient to open the mouth.
2. If the patient complains of nausea, administer the prescribed antiemetic and withhold oral feedings until nausea subsides.	To prevent vomiting that increases the risk for aspiration.
3. When oral feedings are allowed, place in a Fowler's position and instruct the patient to sip liquids slowly through a straw.	To prevent vomiting.
4. Maintain a semi-Fowler's position.	To facilitate breathing and to prevent choking and aspiration.

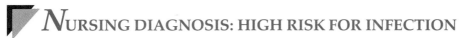

NURSING DIAGNOSIS: HIGH RISK FOR INFECTION

RELATED TO FACTORS: Surgery for fractured mandible

DEFINING CHARACTERISTICS: Fever, WBC above 10,000/mm,[3] increased discomfort, foul-breath odor

PATIENT OUTCOME (collaborative): Demonstrates absence of infection

EVALUATION CRITERIA: Temperature 98.6°F, WBC between 5,000-10,000/mm,[3] absence of foul-breath odor

INTERVENTIONS	RATIONALE
1. Monitor: • temperature q4h • results of CBC reports, especially WBC	To identify indications of progress toward or deviations from expected outcome.
2. Provide oral care after each meal and at bedtime. Irrigate the mouth with prescribed solution; • one part povidine-iodine mouthwash and two parts warm water, or • one part hydrogen peroxide and two parts water Using a bulb syringe, squirt about 15 mL of the solution into each quadrant of the mouth and suction, if necessary, with a tonsilar suction catheter. Provide the patient with a soft bristle toothbrush to brush the outer surface of the teeth after swelling has subsided. Inform the patient that the gums will be tender at first.	Oral care reduces bacteria and plaque formation.
3. Allow the patient to apply a lubricant to the lips prn. Avoid use of lemon glycerin swabs to clean the teeth.	A lubricant helps combat dryness. Lemon glycerin swabs do not clean sufficiently and get snagged on the wires.

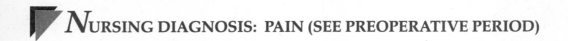

NURSING DIAGNOSIS: PAIN (SEE PREOPERATIVE PERIOD)

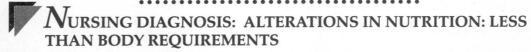

NURSING DIAGNOSIS: ALTERATIONS IN NUTRITION: LESS THAN BODY REQUIREMENTS

RELATED TO FACTORS: Inability to chew solid foods secondary to jaw wiring
DEFINING CHARACTERISTICS: Weight loss

PATIENT OUTCOME (collaborative): Demonstrates adequate nutritional status
EVALUATION CRITERIA: Stable weight

INTERVENTIONS	RATIONALE
1. Monitor weight weekly and the amount of food consumed with each meal.	To evaluate effectiveness of interventions.
2. Refer the patient to a dietitian for assistance with planning liquid or pureed meals that meet the patient's energy needs. Provide several small feedings throughout the day.	Some weight loss is expected with a liquid diet. Significant weight loss can be prevented by ensuring adequate caloric intake with commercially prepared liquid meals (Ensure, Isocal). A dietitian is a nutritional specialist who can plan a liquid and pureed diet to meet the patient's energy needs in view of current health situation. Small feedings reduce the risk of gastric distention, which causes nausea and vomiting.

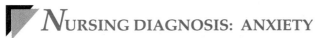

NURSING DIAGNOSIS: ANXIETY

RELATED TO FACTORS: Impaired verbal communication secondary to jaw wiring
DEFINING CHARACTERISTICS: Inability to speak clearly, facial tension and restlessness when attempting to communicate
PATIENT OUTCOME: Demonstrates less anxiety when attempting to communicate needs
EVALUATION CRITERIA: Relaxed facial expression, absence of restlessness, denies feelings of nervousness and frustration

INTERVENTIONS	RATIONALE
1. See preoperative interventions.	To evaluate effectiveness of interventions.
2. Instruct the patient to verbalize by pronouncing words slowly moving lips and tongue. Remind the patient that opening the mouth will not be possible.	After swelling has subsided, most patients are able to pronounce words through their teeth by moving their lips and tongue.

▶ NURSING DIAGNOSIS: HIGH RISK FOR IMPAIRED HOME MAINTENANCE MANAGEMENT

RELATED TO FACTORS: Knowledge deficit about self-care on discharge, lack of adequate support system or finances

DEFINING CHARACTERISTICS: Acknowledges lack of understanding, requests information, acknowledges lack of adequate support system, expresses financial difficulties

PATIENT OUTCOME (collaborative): Demonstrates willingness to comply with recommended home care plan

EVALUATION CRITERIA: Acknowledges understanding of self-care instructions, correctly performs required self-care skills

INTERVENTIONS	RATIONALE
1. Evaluate patient's ability to perform oral self-care. Teach and have patient practice oral care. Suggest use of a water pik to rinse teeth after brushing with a soft bristle toothbrush. Advise to do oral care after each meal and at bedtime.	Good oral hygiene helps control infection.
2. Suggest use of a blender to puree foods.	Commercially prepared nutritional beverages can be costly.
3. Advise the patient to avoid swimming and water sports.	Clearing the airway of water is difficult with the teeth wired.
4. Advise the patient not to drink alcoholic beverages.	These may cause nausea and impair judgment. Patients are more likely to engage in unsafe practices when judgment is impaired.
5. Instruct the patient to dilute carbonated beverages.	The fizz can foam in the back of the throat and cause vomiting.
6. Teach the patient's significant other which wires to cut and under what circumstances (i.e., if respiratory distress occurs). Send wire cutters home with the patient.	Health teaching is essential to ensuring safety in self-care at home.
7. Provide written self-care instructions and a written appointment for follow-up care.	Verbal instructions may be easily forgotten.

Systemic Lupus Erythematosus

There are three forms of lupus erythematosus: systemic, discoid, and drug-induced.

Systemic lupus erythematosus (SLE) is a chronic autoimmune disorder in which the body produces antibodies against its own tissue. These immune complexes circulate in the blood and stimulate inflammatory reactions in small blood vessels, connective tissue, and serous membranes throughout the body, thus giving rise to a wide variety of symptoms.

The cause of SLE is unknown. It is more prevalent in women of childbearing age (Whitney, 1989). SLE has a chronic unpredictable course, characterized by periods of remission and exacerbations. The average survival rate is ten years, with death most often occurring from renal failure secondary to infections (Whitney, 1989). Patients generally require hospitalization for treatment of severe problems such as anemia, pleurisy, pericarditis, and renal failure. The mean LOS for a DRG classification of systemic lupus erythematosus is 5.4 days without complications and 7.4 days with complications (Lorenz, 1991).

During exacerbations of the disease, menses will often be irregular. Pregnant women with SLE who are receiving treatment and have no renal damage have a better chance for successful delivery.

Discoid lupus affects only the skin. Its primary manifestation is a patchy, crusty rash on the face or other areas exposed to the sun. Occasionally, it may cause severe scarring, pigmentation changes, and alopecia (hair loss).

Drug-induced lupus can be caused by drugs such as hydralazine (Apresoline), methyldopa (Aldomet), chlorpromazine (Thorazine), and procainamide (Pronestyl). Patients have symptoms of SLE but there is no damage to the kidneys or central nervous system. Discontinuance of the causative drug corrects the problem.

There is no cure for SLE or discoid lupus.

General Medical Management

a. For drug induced lupus:
   • removal of causative agent
b. For discoid lupus:
   • avoid prolonged exposure to the sun

c. For SLE:

- Pharmacotherapy:
  - — nonsteroidal anti-inflammatory agents
  - — antimalarials
  - — steroids and cytotoxic agents (if steroids are ineffective)
- Measures to combat anemia:
  - — folic acid
  - — multivitamin and iron supplements
  - — in some cases where renal failure has developed, anabolic steroids also may be used. These agents stimulate erythropoietin production by the kidney, leading to increased production of RBCs. Periodic blood transfusions also may be required for severe anemia.
- Plasmapheresis:
  - — a procedure in which a blood cell separator removes abnormal components from the patient's blood

Integrative Care Plans

- Loss
- Arthritis

Discharge Considerations

- Follow-up care
- Measures to combat fatigue
- Protection of the skin

 # ASSESSMENT DATA BASE

1. History or presence of risk factors. Although SLE is not hereditary, the incidence is somewhat higher among individuals with a positive family history.

2. Physical examination based on a general survey (Appendix F) may reveal multisystem involvement, since SLE is an inflammatory disease of connective tissue that affects the skin, joints, pleural and pericardial membranes, kidney, bone marrow, and central nervous system. The American Rheumatism Association has identified 11 distinct physical characteristics and laboratory findings suggestive of SLE. A diagnosis of SLE is made by the coexistence of four or more of the following findings (Whitney, 1989):

   - malar rash — butterfly-shaped rash across nose and cheeks; may be unilateral or bilateral
   - pleurisy or pericarditis
   - polyarthritis — inflamed painful joints that is migratory and rarely results in joint deformity

- photosensitivity — development of a rash when exposed to intense sunlight
- discoid rash — patchy, red, crusty rash on areas exposed to the sun
- central nervous system changes such as seizures or psychosis
- ulceration of mucous membranes (mouth, nose, and vagina)
- hematologic abnormalities (anemia, thrombocytopenia, leukopenia)
- false-positive VDRL (serologic test for syphilis)
- elevated antinuclear antibodies (ANAs)
- proteinuria, cellular casts, or pus without bacteriuria reflected by urinalysis

   Additional symptoms may include:

- spleen and liver enlargement
- weight loss, fever, fatigue
- Raynaud's phenomenon (pallor-cyanosis-redness color changes in the fingers accompanied by pain and paresthesia)

3. Assess for factors that precipitate exacerbations:
   - excessive fatigue
   - prolonged exposure to ultraviolet rays (direct sunlight)
   - surgery
   - certain drugs such as penicillin, sulfonamides, and oral contraceptives

4. Assess the patient's feelings about condition and impact on lifestyle.

◣ NURSING DIAGNOSIS: PAIN

RELATED TO FACTORS: Joint inflammation secondary to SLE

DEFINING CHARACTERISTICS: Verbalizes joint aches, moaning and facial frowning with physical activity

PATIENT OUTCOME (collaborative): Demonstrates relief from discomfort

EVALUATION CRITERIA: Denies pain, performs activities without moaning or facial frowning

INTERVENTIONS	RATIONALE
1. See Nursing Diagnosis: Pain for arthritis (page 307).	

NURSING DIAGNOSIS: DISTURBANCE IN SELF-CONCEPT

RELATED TO FACTORS: Altered body image secondary to side-effects of steroids and rash secondary to lupus

DEFINING CHARACTERISTICS: May verbalize feelings of embarrassment, may report depression about having a chronic condition, may report withdrawal from social activities

PATIENT OUTCOME: Demonstrates acceptance of self in current situation

EVALUATION CRITERIA: Verbalizes acceptance of self, verbalizes realistic plans to accommodate limitations imposed by condition

INTERVENTIONS	RATIONALE
1. Allow the patient to express feelings. If concern is expressed about side effects of steroids, let the patient know that the moonface appearance and alopecia are minimized by having the physician adjust the dosage. Also let the patient know these changes are not permanent and subside after drugs are discontinued.	Expressing feelings helps facilitate coping. Knowing what to expect from prescribed treatments helps lessen anxiety.
2. Provide instructions for minimizing skin lesions: • Avoid prolonged exposure to direct sunlight between 10 a.m. and 4 p.m. (ultraviolet rays are strongest during this time). • Wear long sleeves and a wide-brimmed hat when in the sunlight. • Use a sunscreen lotion with a high protection rating of 15 or above. Allow 30 minutes for the lotion to absorb before swimming. Reapply after swimming.	Sunlight aggravates discoid lesions.

NURSING DIAGNOSIS: ACTIVITY INTOLERANCE

RELATED TO FACTORS: Complications secondary to SLE: anemia, pleurisy, pericarditis

DEFINING CHARACTERISTICS: Verbalizes increasing shortness of breath with activity, tachypnea and tachycardia with minimal exertion, may report being cold, CBC may reveal anemia (low hemoglobin, hematocrit, and RBC)

PATIENT OUTCOME (collaborative): Demonstrates increased tolerance to activities

EVALUATION CRITERIA: Fewer reports of fatigue and shortness of breath with exertion, absence of anemia by laboratory examination, lungs clear

INTERVENTIONS	RATIONALE
1. Evaluate the patient's daily routine. Assist with planning a daily schedule of activities that includes frequent rest periods.	Rest helps restore body energy. Balancing physical activity with rest helps control fatigue and increase endurance.
2. Encourage the patient to take prescribed medication for anemia and to keep follow-up appointments to have blood tests to monitor therapeutic effectiveness of the medication.	An inadequate supply of RBCs contributes to anemia and fatigue. A CBC is periodically done to evaluate effectiveness of medication.
3. Encourage the patient to monitor dietary intake: type of foods and quantity consumed. Have the patient record weight on a weekly basis. If dietary intake is inadequate, refer the patient to a dietitian for assistance in planning meals to combat anemia.	Foods high in iron are needed since iron is essential to erythropoiesis. Health teaching plays an important role in fostering patient compliance.

NURSING DIAGNOSIS: HIGH RISK FOR ALTERATION IN HOME MAINTENANCE MANAGEMENT

RELATED TO FACTORS: Knowledge about condition, treatment plan, and self-care preventive and maintenance activities

DEFINING CHARACTERISTICS: Verbalizes lack of understanding, requests information, reports history of repeated exacerbations or noncompliance

PATIENT OUTCOME (collaborative): Demonstrates willingness to comply with self-care maintenance and preventive measures

EVALUATION CRITERIA: Verbalizes understanding of condition and treatments, verbalizes realistic plans to incorporate preventive and maintenance measures into current lifestyle

• •

INTERVENTIONS	RATIONALE
1. Provide information about the nature of the condition. Emphasize there is no cure for SLE and that medical treatments are aimed at controlling discomfort and preserving joint function.	Compliance with prescribed treatments is enhanced when the patient understands the relationship between the condition and treatment program.
2. Refer the patient and significant others to the local Lupus Foundation or the Arthritis Foundation.	Information about all aspects of SLE can be obtained from the Lupus Foundation and the Arthritis Foundation.
3. Provide written instructions for self-care and information about prescribed drugs including name, dosage, schedule, purpose, and side effects that require medical attention.	Verbal instructions may be easily forgotten.

TABLE 4 - 1 Do's and Don'ts For Total Hip Arthroplasty

DO'S

1. For the first six weeks after surgery, sit or stand with the foot of the operated hip out in front of the other.
2. Keep a plump pillow between your legs when lying on your back or on your nonoperative side.
3. When lying on your back, keep the operated leg positioned so the toes and the kneecap point to the ceiling.
4. When walking or standing, you may put as much weight on the operated leg as is comfortable, unless instructed by your physician not to do so.
5. Use a toilet seat raiser for eight weeks when you go home.
6. You may take a shower but put a chair or stool in the shower for support or to sit on. Tub baths are not advised because they cause too much bending of the hip.
7. Follow the hip exercise program given to you by the physical therapist. These will strengthen your hip and improve your walking.
8. Always keep your knees apart when sitting.
9. When ascending stairs, advance the unaffected leg first, then the operated leg and your crutches or cane. When you descend stairs, advance the operated leg first with your crutches or cane, then the unaffected leg.
10. Walk as much as you like. Let your soreness be a guide as to how much you can tolerate. Do not be alarmed, for some pain and soreness is to be expected for few weeks.

DON'TS

1. Do not bend your hip past a 90-degree angle (which is the sitting position).
2. Do not sit in a low chair. Keep hips and knees level with each other. When sitting, slide the foot of the operated hip in front of the other.
3. Do not drive a car until your physician says you may do so.
4. Do not lie on your operated side. Lie on your back or your nonoperative side with a pillow wedged between your legs.
5. Do not pivot or the operative leg. Take small steps to turn.
6. Do not cross your legs at any time.
7. Do not run, jump, squat, or bend down.

BIBLIOGRAPHY

Arnett, F.C. Jr., Khan, M.A., & Willkems, R.F. (1989). A new look at ankylosing spondylitis. **Patient Care, 23,** 82–86, 91–92, 94–96.

Barrett, J.B., & Bryant, B.H. (1990). Fractures: Types, treatment, perioperative implications. **Journal of American Operating Room Nurses, 52,** 755–756, 758, 760–761.

Blair, K.A. (1990). Aging: Physiological aspects and clinical implications. **Nurse Practitioner, 15,** 14–16, 18, 23, 26–28.

Borden, R.M., & Sinkora, G.L. (1991). Bone stimulators for fusions and fractures. **Nursing Clinics of North America, 26,** 89–103.

Head, J.M. (1990). Multilevel spine fractures: Intraoperative nursing management. **Journal of Neuroscience Nursing, 22,** 370–374.

Hough, D., Crosat, S., & Nye, P. Patient education for total hip replacement. **Nursing Management, 22,** I–J, 80N, 80P.

Jones, I.H. (1990). Making sense of traction. **Nursing Times, 86,** 39–41.

Jones-Walton, P. (1991). Clinical standards in skeletal traction pin care. **Orthopaedic Nursing, 10,** 12–16.

Lorenz, E.W. (1991). St. Anthony's DRG Working Guidebook. Alexandria: St. Anthony's Publishing Company.

Rosa, D. (1991). Acute compartment syndrome. **Orthopaedic Nursing, 10,** 33–38.

Ruhl, J.M. (1991). Pelvic trauma. **RN, 54,** 50–55.

Slye, D.A. (1991). Orthopedic complications: Compartment syndrome, fat embolism syndrome, and venous thromboembolism. **Nursing Clinics of North America, 26,** 113–132.

Whitney, R. (1989). Unlock the mystery of lupus. **Today's Operating Room Nurse, 11,** 10–12, 30–32.

C

HAPTER FIVE
Problems of the Vascular System

Acute Peripheral Arterial Thrombosis

Acute peripheral arterial thrombosis is a medical emergency. The underlying pathology is a thrombus, which is often a blood clot but also may be an atherosclerotic plaque. The thrombotic emboli commonly originates in the heart, becomes dislodged, and travels through the bloodstream where it eventually occludes an artery in the leg. Untreated, this disorder can cause gangrene with amputation as the final outcome.

Patients experiencing this medical emergency commonly show extreme apprehension because of the severe pain caused by the interruption of arterial blood flow and the threat of possible loss of a limb. Treatment must be initiated within six hours of onset of symptoms to preserve the limb. The mean LOS for a DRG classification of acute peripheral arterial thrombosis is 4.5 days without complications and 6.1 days with complications (Lorenz, 1991).

General Medical Management

- Pharmacotherapy:
  - — thrombolytic agents (tissue plasminogen activator [tPA])
  - — anticoagulants (Coumadin is often prescribed for several weeks after discharge)
- Embolectomy:
  - —surgical removal of a blood clot if drug therapy fails

Integrative Care Plans

- Preoperative and postoperative care
- IV therapy

Discharge Considerations

- Activity limitations
- Medications prescribed for use at home
- Wound care and manifestations of wound infection if an embolectomy is performed

ASSESSMENT DATA BASE

1. History or presence of risk factors, for example, arteriosclerosis obliterans, polycythemia, trauma, cardiac surgery, myocardial infarction, atrial fibrillation

2. Physical examination based on a peripheral vascular assessment (Appendix E) reveals manifestations of abrupt ischemia distal to the occlusion:
   - pain
   - pallor with eventual cyanosis
   - absence of distal pulses (use a Doppler probe to confirm this finding)
   - coldness of the extremity
   - paresthesia

3. Diagnostic studies:
   - Arteriogram accurately confirms the presence and location of the thrombus.
   - Coagulation studies may reveal values below the normal range.

4. Assess emotional response to condition.

NURSING DIAGNOSIS: ALTERATION IN TISSUE PERFUSION: PERIPHERAL

RELATED TO FACTORS: Acute peripheral arterial thrombus

DEFINING CHARACTERISTICS: Pallor, verbalizes pain, cyanosis, absent pulse, coldness of extremity, paresthesia

PATIENT OUTCOME (collaborative): Demonstrates improved circulation

EVALUATION CRITERIA: Warm dry skin, presence of peripheral pulses, denies pain, normal skin color

INTERVENTIONS	RATIONALE
1. Monitor q15min peripheral vascular status: • peripheral pulses • skin color and temperature • pain level • sensation • mobility	To identify indications of progress toward or deviations from expected outcome.
2. Report all laboratory results to physician immediately.	Adequate hydration is essential to rapid distribution of medications. Thrombolytic

INTERVENTIONS	RATIONALE
Initiate prescribed IV therapy and monitor for complications (page 764). Administer thrombolytic agents and anticoagulants IV as ordered and evaluate their effectiveness.	agents dissolve blood clots. Anticoagulants prevent the formation of new blood clots.
3. Keep the patient NPO. Notify physician if symptoms persist or worsen during drug therapy. Prepare the patient for surgery as ordered.	Emergency embolectomy is required if drug therapy fails to reestablish circulation.
4. Maintain strict bedrest.	To reduce energy expenditure and prevent further progression of the embolism.
5. Keep the affected limb straight. Avoid hip and knee flexion. Do **not** elevate the limb. Do **not** apply heat to the affected limb.	In arteries, blood flows away from the heart. Elevating the limb causes increased accumulation of blood proximal to the occlusion, which increases pain. Heat increases metabolism that increases oxygen tissue demands. Flexion obstructs blood flow.

● ●

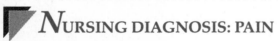

*N*URSING DIAGNOSIS: PAIN

RELATED TO FACTORS: Sudden obstruction of peripheral arterial blood flow

DEFINING CHARACTERISTICS: Verbalizes pain; frowning with tense facial expression; moaning; guarding of affected extremity; crying; changes in BP, pulse, and respiratory rates; restlessness

PATIENT OUTCOME (collaborative): Demonstrates less pain

EVALUATION CRITERIA: Verbalizes relief from pain, relaxed facial expression, less moaning, vital signs within normal range

● ●

INTERVENTIONS	RATIONALE
1. Use an overbed cradle to keep the linens off the feet or leave the feet uncovered.	Pressure from the weight of bed linens increases pain.
2. Administer low dose narcotic analgesia as ordered and evaluate its effectiveness. Suggest IV administration.	Low dose narcotic analgesia helps control severe pain without camouflaging symptoms. Medications given IV act rapidly.
3. Notify physician if pain persists or worsens. Prepare for emergency embolectomy as prescribed.	Surgery is the last resort to ensure preservation of the affected limb.

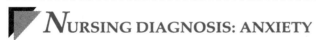

NURSING DIAGNOSIS: ANXIETY

RELATED TO FACTORS: Knowledge deficit about condition, diagnostic studies, treatment plan, fear of threat of loss of limb

DEFINING CHARACTERISTICS: Repetitive questioning, verbalizes fear of possible loss of limb, verbalizes lack of understanding, tense facial expression, overexcited, shakiness, quivering voice

PATIENT OUTCOME: Demonstrates less anxiety

EVALUATION CRITERIA: Relaxed facial expression, pulse rate between 60–100 beats per minute, respiratory rate between 12–24 per minute, BP between 90/60–140/90 mm Hg, calm steady voice tone, verbalizes feeling less nervous

INTERVENTIONS	RATIONALE
1. See Nursing Diagnosis: Anxiety (page 262).	
2. Reinforce physician's explanation about prescribed treatments. Inform the patient that frequent assessments of the affected limb will be made and necessary actions taken to guard against irreversible tissue damage.	Repetition facilitates learning. Providing frequent attention helps promote a feeling of security and reduce anxiety.

··

NURSING DIAGNOSIS: HIGH RISK FOR IMPAIRED HOME MAINTENANCE MANAGEMENT

RELATED TO FACTORS: Knowledge deficit about self-care on discharge, lack of adequate support system

DEFINING CHARACTERISTICS: Fails to request information or ask questions about follow-up care, verbalizes lack of understanding about need for continued treatment, refuses to set home care goals or participate in self-care

PATIENT OUTCOME: Demonstrates willingness to comply with discharge plan of care

EVALUATION CRITERIA: Verbalizes accurate understanding of home treatment regimen, participates in development of home care plan, requests instructions for home care

··

INTERVENTIONS	RATIONALE
1. Ensure the patient or significant other has a written appointment for follow-up care and written instructions for care at home activities. Provide written information about medications prescribed for home use, including name, purpose, dose, schedule, and reportable side effects.	Verbal instructions may be forgotten.
2. Instruct the patient to: • seek medical attention if symptoms of acute peripheral arterial occlusion recur (sudden onset of pain, pallor, cyanosis, paresthesia in the extremity) • take medication as prescribed and contact physician if adverse reactions occur • avoid crossing the legs	The patient is at risk for recurrence of the arterial occlusion. Effective anticoagulation is the key to preventing recurrences. Flexion of the extremities obstructs blood flow.

INTERVENTIONS	RATIONALE
3. If embolectomy was performed, advise the patient to a notify physician if manifestations of wound infection occur (redness, increased tenderness, purulent drainage, fever, swelling). Provide instructions for wound care. Emphasize using good handwashing technique when performing wound care at home.	Antibiotic therapy is required to resolve an infection. Basic aseptic technique helps reduce the risk of wound infection.
4. Emphasize the need for planned rest periods and for gauging activities to tolerance.	Discharge teaching helps improve patient compliance, promotes a gradual return to normal activity level, and increases patient involvement in assuming responsibility for own health.

Amputation

An **amputation** refers to removal of all or part of an extremity. When performing an amputation, the surgeon attempts to preserve as much of the limb as possible. The residual limb is commonly called the "stump."

An amputation may be open (guillotine) or closed. An open amputation is performed for severe infections. It involves cutting the bone and muscle tissue at the same level. The blood vessels are cauterized, and the wound is left open to drain. A bulky dressing is applied. To prevent skin retraction, often five pounds of skin traction are applied. The wound may be closed or left to heal by granulation when the infection clears.

For a closed amputation, the surgeon closes the wound with a skin flap created by cutting the bone about two inches shorter than the skin and muscles.

Preoperative preparation is the same for any patient undergoing surgery. Postoperatively, the patient returns to a medical/surgical unit with:

- IV infusion
- wound drainage device
- bulky dressing around stump

In some cases, a rigid plaster cast is applied to the stump in the operating room. A temporary prosthetic limb with prosthetic foot is later attached to the plaster cast, and the patient is allowed to ambulate with minimal weight bearing within a few days.

The physical therapist usually begins teaching transfer techniques and muscle-strengthening exercises after the wound drainage device is removed. Ambulation progresses as the patient learns how to balance on parallel bars in the physical therapy department. Use of an assistive device for ambulation is taught by a physical therapist.

Compression bandaging with either an Ace bandage or a shrinker sock begins following removal of the sutures. When the stump has healed completely and adequate shrinkage has occurred, a prosthetist fits the patient with a prosthesis and teaches proper application and care of the prosthesis.

Patients with lower limb amputation who are not candidates for a prosthesis can be mobile by using a wheelchair or crutches.

The major postoperative complications associated with amputation are infection, hemorrhage, contracture, and fat emboli. A common clinical event that is often a source of discomfort for most patients is phantom limb sensation. The reason for this phenomenon is unclear but is believed related to inflammation of cut nerve endings. Although rare, phantom limb sensation may become a chronic, severe problem requiring more aggressive interventions such as nerve blocks, psychotherapy, drug therapy, electrical nerve stimulation, or neuroma excision.

Lower extremity amputation may be below-the-knee (BKA) or above-the-knee (AKA). The mean LOS for a DRG classification of lower extremity amputation is 14.3 days (Lorenz, 1991).

Integrative Care Plans

- Loss
- Immobility
- Preoperative and postoperative care
- IV therapy

Discharge Considerations

- Follow-up care
- Wound care
- Stump wrapping
- Muscle-strengthening exercises
- Use of assistive device for ambulation
- Signs and symptoms of infection

THE PREOPERATIVE PERIOD

 # *A*SSESSMENT DATA BASE

1. Presence of factors contributing to the need for amputation:
   - chronic peripheral arterial disease (most common reason)
   - trauma
   - frostbite
   - bone cancer
   - severe infections (gas gangrene or osteomylitis)

2. Physical examination based on a peripheral vascular assessment (Appendix E) and a general survey (Appendix F) to establish baseline values.

3. Assess the patient's feelings about an amputation and its impact on lifestyle.

4. Assess muscle strength in unaffected extremities. Can the patient turn self and use arms to lift hips off the mattress? Disuse muscle weakness may be found in elderly patients, especially those who have been bedridden because of a disease process.

● ●

▼ **N**URSING DIAGNOSIS: ANXIETY

RELATED TO FACTORS: Knowledge deficit about preoperative and postoperative events

DEFINING CHARACTERISTICS: Verbalizes fear about some aspect of surgery, verbalizes lack of understanding, requests information

PATIENT OUTCOME: Demonstrates less anxiety

EVALUATION CRITERIA: Fewer reports of feeling nervous or anxious, verbalizes understanding of preoperative and postoperative events

● ●

INTERVENTIONS	RATIONALE
1. See Preoperative and Postoperative Care (page 738).	
2. Assist the patient with identifying the fears. If fear of loss of independence is expressed, remind the patient that a limb prosthesis allows resumption of independence with some adjustments. If fear of pain is expressed, explain that surgery allows greater freedom because a pain-free life is possible after complete healing has occurred. Explain that some pain after surgery is expected, and pain medication is available as needed. Explain phantom limb sensation. Let the patient know that phantom limb sensation gradually resolves as the incision heals.	Fear is an emotion arising from an unpleasant situation. Often the person has insight into the reason for the fears but has difficulty handling the fear. Providing accurate knowledge of the situation and focusing on the positive outcomes help reduce fear.
3. Ensure a trapeze bar is attached to the bed. Reinforce muscle-strengthening exercises taught by physical therapy. Encourage the patient to practice exercises at least four or more times a day or as instructed by physical therapy:	Strengthening muscles of the unaffected extremities is essential to prepare the patient for ambulation with assistive devices (crutches, walker) postamputation. A physical therapist is a specialist who can assist the patient in regaining as much physical independence as possible.

INTERVENTIONS	RATIONALE
a. Arm exercises — use overbed trapeze to lift hips off the mattress and then lower hips. If no trapeze is available, use hands to push against the mattress to lift and lower hips while in a sitting position. Repeat 10–15 times.	
b. Gluteal setting exercises — assume a supine position. Contract and relax gluteal muscles. Hold contraction for five seconds and then relax. Repeat 10–15 times.	
c. Quadriceps setting exercise — assume a supine or sitting position. Extend the leg and push popliteal space against the mattress while tightening thigh muscles. Repeat 10–15 times.	

NURSING DIAGNOSIS: ANTICIPATORY GRIEF

RELATED TO FACTORS: Perceived loss associated with amputation

DEFINING CHARACTERISTICS: Verbalizes fear of loss of independence, disfigurement, pain from amputation; may express helplessness, low self-esteem, or depression

PATIENT OUTCOME: Demonstrates awareness of impact of surgery on self-image

EVALUATION CRITERIA: Verbalizes feelings freely, reports awareness of need to make adjustments in current lifestyle

INTERVENTIONS	RATIONALE
1. Encourage the patient to express feelings about the impact of surgery on lifestyle. Ensure the patient about normalcy of feelings. Remind the patient that an active life is possible after surgery with some modifications. With patient permission, arrange a visit from someone who has successfully adapted to an amputation and prosthesis.	Often patients think an amputation means the end of life as they knew it. Interacting with someone who has made a successful adjustment to the same situation is a valuable strategy for promoting adaptation to alterations in body image.

INTERVENTIONS	RATIONALE
2. See Loss (page 733).	

THE POSTOPERATIVE PERIOD

 ## ASSESSMENT DATA BASE

1. See Preoperative and Postoperative Care (page 738).

 ## NURSING DIAGNOSIS: PAIN

RELATED TO FACTORS: Phantom limb sensation, surgical incision secondary to amputation

DEFINING CHARACTERISTICS: Verbalizes discomfort, frowning, moaning, guarding painful site, verbalizes feeling amputated limb is still present or pain from amputated limb can still be felt

PATIENT OUTCOME (collaborative): Demonstrates relief from discomfort

EVALUATION CRITERIA: Verbalizes absence of pain, no moaning, relaxed facial expression, fewer reports of phantom limb sensation

INTERVENTIONS	RATIONALE
1. See Pain (page 700).	
2. Evaluate the patient's pain to differentiate between phantom limb sensation and incisional pain. Explain phantom limb sensation: feeling limb is still present or feeling pain from amputated limb. If phantom limb sensation is the source of the discomfort: • administer prescribed analgesic • teach patient how to apply gentle pressure to the end of the stump by placing the stump in a towel and pulling up gently on the towel	Phantom limb sensation takes longer to resolve than incisional pain, which usually diminishes within a few days. Patients often confuse phantom limb sensation with incisional pain. Many patients may be reluctant to describe their pain and just report "pain in the stump" for fear the staff will label them as being "crazy" if they report feelings of phantom limb sensation.

Nursing Diagnosis: Disturbance in Self-Concept

RELATED TO FACTORS: Altered body image secondary to amputation

DEFINING CHARACTERISTICS: Verbalizes grief about loss of body part, may verbalize negative feelings about body and self-worth, may report depression

PATIENT OUTCOME: Demonstrates acceptance of self in current situation

EVALUATION CRITERIA: Verbalizes acceptance of physical changes, makes plans to continue lifestyle in view of current limitations

INTERVENTIONS	RATIONALE
1. See Loss (page 733).	
2. Consult physician about initiating a psychological consult if the patient has experienced a traumatic amputation or shows long-term maladaptive behaviors (statements of seeing self as having little value or worth, refuses to be involved in self-care).	Patients who experience traumatic amputation often take longer to work through the grief process than those who have elective amputation caused by a chronic painful disease process.
3. Encourage patient involvement. With each dressing change: • Explain what is done and why. • Describe the appearance of the incision. • Ask the patient to support the limb as the dressing is changed. • Have the patient open dressing packages. • Have the patient hold the dressing in place as the stump is wrapped.	Encouraging participation promotes adaptation to change in body image.
4. Refer the patient to a community based self-help group for amputees.	Support systems are used by individuals to strengthen their psychosocial defenses.

NURSING DIAGNOSIS: HIGH RISK FOR COMPLICATIONS: INFECTION, HEMORRHAGE, FLEXION CONTRACTURES, FAT EMBOLI

RELATED TO FACTORS: Amputation

DEFINING CHARACTERISTICS: Demonstrates early manifestations of infection, excess bleeding, flexion contractures, or fat emboli

PATIENT OUTCOME (collaborative): Demonstrates absence of permanent complications

EVALUATION CRITERIA: Absence of infection, hemorrhage, fat emboli, and flexion contractures

INTERVENTIONS	RATIONALE
Infection: 1. See Preoperative and Postoperative Care (page 738).	
Hemorrhage: 1. Monitor: • intake and output q8h • vital signs q4h • appearance of dressing q4–8h	To detect early signs of excess bleeding.
2. Place a tourniquet at the bedside.	For use in case of profuse bleeding.
3. Notify physician if the following occur: • output from the wound drainage device is bright red and continually increases, accompanied by a drop in urinary output in relation to intake, and hypotension accompanied by tachycardia and tachypnea	These findings signal excess bleeding. Normally, wound drainage output should diminish within 1–2 days.
Fat Emboli: 1. See Fat Embolism Syndrome (page 311).	

INTERVENTIONS	RATIONALE
Flexion Contractures: 1. Maintain continuous elevation of the stump during the first 24–48 hours as ordered; thereafter, avoid continuous elevation. Do **not** gatch the knee of the bed or place pillows beneath the residual limb. Raise the foot of the bed via blocks to elevate the stump.	Elevation reduces edema. Continuous elevation after 48 hours increases the risk of flexion contracture of the hip.
2. Place the patient in a prone position for 30 minutes 3–4 times daily after the prescribed period of continuous elevation ends.	The muscle normally contracts when cut. A prone position helps keep the residual limb in full extension.
3. Place a trochanter roll beside the thigh to keep the limb in adduction.	Abduction contractures may occur because flexor muscles are stronger than extensor muscles.
4. Initiate range-of-motion (ROM) exercises of the stump 2–3 times a day beginning on the first postoperative day. Consult physical therapist for appropriate exercises.	ROM exercises help maintain joint flexibility and muscle tone.

◣ NURSING DIAGNOSIS: HIGH RISK FOR IMPAIRED HOME MAINTENANCE MANAGEMENT

RELATED TO FACTORS: Knowledge deficit about care of stump at home, inadequate support system

DEFINING CHARACTERISTICS: Verbalizes lack of understanding, requests information, observation of incorrect care of stump, observation of inability to perform self-care of stump, reports lack or absence of support system at home

PATIENT OUTCOME (collaborative): Demonstrates willingness to comply with preventive and maintenance self-care activities on discharge

EVALUATION CRITERIA: Performs stump wrapping correctly, verbalizes understanding of discharge instructions, uses assistive device for ambulation safely, requests assistance when needed

INTERVENTIONS	RATIONALE

1. Explain the importance of stump care and stump wrapping. Provide instructions about:
 	
a. Proper care of the stump:
  • Use a 4–6 inch Ace bandage to wrap the limb.
  • Apply the Ace bandage firmly.
  • Use clean bandages. Replace bandages that are stretched out of shape.
  • Use proper limb wrapping technique.
  • Wash limb daily with mild soap and water. Rinse and dry thoroughly. Inspect the skin for irritation.
  • Avoid using any substances on the limb such as oils, ointments, powders, alcohol, and lotions unless prescribed by physician.
  • If limb stocking is worn with the prosthesis, change it daily. Clean the stocking by laundering in mild soap (Ivory) and lay flat to dry.
  • Continue with exercises taught by physical therapy to maintain muscle strength and toughen the end of the limb until fitted for a prosthesis, for example, pushing the end of the stump against a pillow for toughening, hamstring-setting and gluteal-setting exercises to increase muscle strength.
  • If a BKA was performed, avoid allowing the knee to hand over the edge of the bed or chair for long periods.
 	
b. Stump wrapping
	Compression bandaging helps control edema and molds the limb for a prosthesis. To ensure a good prosthetic fit, the stump must be well formed, firm, and have a smooth, round end.

INTERVENTIONS	RATIONALE
2. Evaluate the patient's level of independence with stump care and stump wrapping. Teach the patient and significant other stump wrapping and stump care. If unable to perform these activities, contact social services to make arrangements for home health care visits or placement in an extended care facility if significant other cannot help the patient.	Social services or discharge planning department are specialists concerned with ensuring continuity of care on discharge when a longer period of rehabilitation is required. Temporary assistance may be needed until the patient, especially if elderly, is capable of resuming independence.
3. Ensure the patient or significant other: • has a prescription for pain medication if needed • knows purpose of special care and wrapping of the residual limb • knows how to perform proper stump wrapping with an Ace bandage or how to apply a shrinker sock • has at least one week's supply of material for wound care • has necessary equipment for mobility (wheelchair, crutches, or walker) • knows to contact physician if signs and symptoms of wound infection occur (redness, drainage, fever, increased tenderness) • understands phantom limb sensation and how to control it: gentle pressure on the end of the stump and use of prescribed analgesics • knows exercises to maintain muscle strength and toughen the stump in preparation for a prosthesis	Discharge instructions are a safety measure that help patients know what to do to maintain health and how to care for themselves.

INTERVENTIONS	RATIONALE
• knows how to contact physician in the event of a problem • has a written list of available support services in the community	
4. Provide the patient with a written appointment for follow-up visit and written instructions for care of the stump.	Verbal instructions may be easily forgotten.

Chronic Peripheral Arterial Occlusive Disease

Chronic arterial occlusive disease can affect any artery in the body — aorta, carotid, coronary, cerebral, and major leg and feet arteries. When the disease process affects the arteries to the legs and feet, it is called chronic peripheral arterial occlusive disease or arteriosclerosis obliterans (ASO). The disease occurs bilaterally.

The primary cause of the disease is atherosclerosis. Atherosclerotic plaques accumulate along the lumen of the arteries causing narrowing or obstruction, eventually disrupting blood flow (Caswell, 1991).

ASO is a slow, insidious, progressive disease that eventually leads to severe tissue impairment. The presence of diabetes mellitus hastens the disease process. Because there is concomitant atherosclerotic involvement of the vascular network throughout the body (brain, coronary arteries), death commonly occurs from myocardial infarction or stroke.

Ischemic ulcers and dry gangrene are the major complications associated with ASO. The ulcers are painful and occur most often at pressure points (lateral malleolus). As arterial blood flow becomes increasing compromised, gangrene develops. The mean LOS for a DRG classification of ASO is 6.1 days (Lorenz, 1991).

General Medical Management

- Vasodilators may offer short-term benefits but do not halt the disease process. Intravenous infusions of 5% alcohol may be used because of its vasodilating effect. Anticoagulants and fibrinolytic agents are of no value because the disease process is not due to a blood clot.
- Surgery does not halt the disease. Surgical procedures are aimed at improving blood flow and vary depending on the site of the occlusion (see Table 5–1). Amputation is required for areas of gangrene.

Integrative Care Plans

- Loss
- Preoperative and postoperative care
- Amputation (if gangrene is present)

Discharge Considerations

* Follow-up care
* Foot care
* Measures to maximize peripheral circulation

 # ASSESSMENT DATA BASE

1. History or presence of primary risk factors: hypertension, hyperlipidemia, and cigarette smoking. Other predisposing factors include uncontrolled diabetes mellitus, obesity, family history of cardiovascular disease, and a sedentary lifestyle.

2. Physical examination based on a peripheral vascular assessment (Appendix E) of both lower extremities may reveal:
   * diminished or absent pedal pulses. A Doppler probe may be needed if pulses are nonpalpable.
   * cool feet with poor capillary refill
   * dependent rubor. The feet turn dusky red or reddish-blue when placed in a dependent position such as sitting or standing. For dark-skinned patients, examine the soles to detect dependent rubor.
   * elevational pallor. To assess, elevate the legs about 12 inches above the level of the heart for about 30 seconds. The foot or toes will become very pale.
   * trophic skin changes such as loss of hair on the legs, thickened toenails, and taut shiny skin
   * intermittent claudication (most prominent feature) refers to ischemic pain in the lower extremities with exercise, which is relieved by rest. It is generally described as tightness or cramping and occurs distal to the site of occlusion. The pain may occur in the buttocks, hip, thigh, calf, or arch of the foot. The amount of exercise that causes pain is constant for each patient. As the artery approaches complete occlusion, the pain begins to occur even at rest. Rest pain signals advance disease. Initially, rest pain occurs only when the patient is supine. The patient discovers pain can be relieved by placing the extremity in a dependent position such as dangling the legs over the side of the bed, sitting, or standing. As the disease progresses to total occlusion, the patient finds that no position gives relief from pain. Rest pain is often described as burning or gnawing.

3. Assess for Leriche's syndrome. This finding indicates involvement of the aortoiliac vessels:
   * muscle atrophy of the legs
   * impotence
   * intermittent pain in the lower back, buttocks, or thighs during activity, which is relieved by rest

4. Auscultate the abdominal aorta and femoral arteries for a bruit (swishing sound caused by blood flowing through narrowed vessels under high pressure).

5. Diagnostic studies:
   - Arteriography provides evidence of arterial narrowing or occlusion.
   - Doppler ultrasonography or plethysmography reveals diminished or absent blood flow through affected arteries.

6. Assess the patient's understanding of condition and its impact on lifestyle.

· ·

NURSING DIAGNOSIS: ALTERED TISSUE PERFUSION

RELATED TO FACTORS: ASO

DEFINING CHARACTERISTICS: Verbalizes pain accompanied by facial frowning, moaning, or guarding painful site; cool feet with absent or diminished pulses; dependent rubor; sluggish capillary refill; may show redden areas over bony prominences that do not blanch

PATIENT OUTCOME (collaborative): Demonstrates no further tissue impairment

EVALUATION CRITERIA: Verbalizes relief from pain, less moaning, relaxed facial expression, less guarding of extremities, absence of skin breakdown

· ·

INTERVENTIONS	RATIONALE
1. Administer prescribed narcotic analgesic and evaluate its effectiveness.	Analgesics block the pain pathway. Narcotic analgesics help control severe pain.
2. Apply a foot cradle to the bed to keep the weight of the linen off painful feet as needed. Drape the linen over the foot cradle to keep the feet warm.	Pressure increases pain.
3. Maintain a dependent position of the legs by placing the bed in a reverse Trendelenburg position. If the bed does not have controls to attain this position, place blocks beneath the head of the bed so the patient's legs are kept in a slight dependent position (20–30 degrees below waist level).	Gravity facilitates arterial blood flow.

INTERVENTIONS	RATIONALE
4. Rest if pain is present.	Muscle contractions with exercise compress blood vessels causing narrowing of vessels, thus decreasing blood flow. Rest allows muscle relaxation, hence improved blood flow. Also, activity demands more oxygen. When the narrowed vessels cannot meet this demand, ischemic pain occurs.
5. Prepare the patient for surgery as ordered.	Surgery is warranted if medical treatments fail to control the condition.

NURSING DIAGNOSIS: ANXIETY

RELATED TO FACTORS: Fear of uncertain outcome of condition

DEFINING CHARACTERISTICS: Verbalizes fear of threat of amputation, may express hopelessness

PATIENT OUTCOME: Demonstrates relief from anxiety

EVALUATION CRITERIA: Fewer statements of feeling nervous, anxious, or worried

INTERVENTIONS	RATIONALE
1. See Loss (page 733).	
2. See Nursing Diagnosis: Anxiety (page 262).	

NURSING DIAGNOSIS: HIGH RISK FOR ALTERATION IN HOME MAINTENANCE MANAGEMENT

RELATED TO FACTORS: Knowledge deficit about self-care measures to maximize circulation

DEFINING CHARACTERISTICS: Verbalizes lack of understanding, requests information, may report a history of noncompliance

PATIENT OUTCOME: Demonstrates willingness to comply with self-care preventive and maintenance measures to maximize circulation

EVALUATION CRITERIA: Verbalizes understanding of discharge instructions, observation of appropriate care of feet

• •

INTERVENTIONS	RATIONALE
1. Identify problem areas. Provide instructions on the proper care of feet and legs. Instructions should include: a. Avoid: — vigorous massage to the legs — direct application of hot water bottles and heating pads to the feet — smoking tobacco products. Refer the patient to a self-help, stop-smoking group, or hypnosis may be necessary — situations that interfere with circulation, such as crossing legs, wearing constrictive clothing, gatching the knee of the bed acutely, sitting or standing prolonged in one position — swimming in cold water — use of foot preparations unless prescribed by physician (plasters, corn removers, alcohol rubs)	Blood clots can be dislodged with rubbing and travel to the lungs causing pulmonary emboli. Compromised tissue is less sensitive to temperature changes. Burns can easily occur. Heat increases metabolic tissue demands. Nicotine and cold applications cause vasoconstriction. Flexion of the legs promotes venous stasis. Harsh chemicals can cause skin breakdown when circulation is compromised.
2. Help the patient plan an exercise program that will coincide with daily lifestyle. Suggest walking and swimming. Advise the patient to exercise ½ the claudication distance, then rest. For example, if pain occurs after walking one block (claudication distance), the patient should walk ½ block, then rest. Advise the patient to gradually increase exercise distance over several weeks.	Exercising to the point of pain causes further tissue damage. Exercise promotes development of collateral circulation and helps reduce cholestrol levels. Atherosclerosis is associated with a persistently elevated cholesterol level.

INTERVENTIONS	RATIONALE
3. Instruct the patient in proper care of the feet. • Consult a physician for treatment of cuts to the legs or feet. • Cut toenails straight across. Consult a podiatrist if needed. • Avoid going barefoot. Wear comfortable shoes that do not rub. • Use nonastringent soap for bathing. • Wash and thoroughly dry feet daily. Apply a skin lubricant afterward. • Wear socks to keep feet warm. Use cotton and wool because they retain heat better.	Compromised circulation increases the risk of skin breakdown. These activities are aimed at maintaining the suppleness and integrity of the skin.
4. Encourage the patient to adhere to prescribed treatments for controlling diabetes mellitus and hypertension if these are coexisting conditions.	These conditions are associated with atherosclerosis.
5. Assist the patient with identifying sources of stress. Help the patient learn relaxation techniques to control emotional tension.	The physiological mechanism by which the body responds to stress is the sympathetic nervous system. Epinephrine is released which causes vasoconstriction.
6. Refer the patient to a dietitian for assistance in planning a weight reduction diet if obese.	Obesity is associated with a high incidence of cardiovascular disease. The dietitian is a nutritional specialist who can assist the patient in planning a well-balanced diet that meets nutritional needs based on current health alteration.
7. Assist the patient in identifying ways to maintain lifestyle in view of current limitations imposed by chronic circulation problem.	Adaptation to a chronic illness can be eased when the changes can be easily incorporated into current lifestyle, causing minimal inconvenience.

INTERVENTIONS	RATIONALE
8. Teach the patient about prescribed drugs, including name, dosage, purpose, schedule, and reportable side effects.	Teaching helps promote safety in self-medication administration.
9. Provide wound care for leg ulcers, if present, as ordered (see Table 5–2).	Open lower extremity lesions coupled with impaired circulation are at great risk for infection.
10. Evaluate patient's understanding of condition. Correct any misconceptions. Explain purpose of all prescribed treatments. Emphasize: • There is no cure for atherosclerosis, which is the primary cause of ASO. • ASO is a progressive, irreversible disorder. • Medical treatments do not offer a cure but rather are aimed at controlling the disease process and minimizing complications.	Compliance is likely to be achieved when patients understand the condition and therapeutic plan.

Thromboangiitis Obliterans

Thromboangiitis obliterans, also called Buerger's disease, is an arterial occlusive disorder characterized by segmental inflammation with subsequent thrombus formation in the medium and small arteries and veins of the hands and feet. The feet are involved more often than the hands. Symptoms occur bilaterally in a symmetrical fashion.

The disease is a progressive disorder characterized by remission and exacerbation. It has an unknown etiology. Hospitalization is not required unless complications develop. The major complications are ulceration and gangrene. The mean LOS for a DRG classification of thromboangiitis obliterans is 4.5 days without complications and 6.1 days with complications (Lorenz, 1991).

General Medical Management

- Pharmacotherapy:
  — vasodilators and analgesics during exacerbations

Integrative Care Plan

- Raynaud's disease
- Chronic peripheral arterial disease

Discharge Considerations

- Follow-up care
- Measures to maximize peripheral circulation

ASSESSMENT DATA BASE

1. History or presence of risk factors:
   - family history of the disorder
   - history of recurrent thrombophlebitis and Raynaud's phenomenon

2. Inquire about factors that precipitate exacerbation of symptoms:
   - exposure to cold
   - heavy smoking

3. Physical examination based on a peripheral vascular assessment (Appendix E) during exacerbations may reveal:
   - migratory superficial thrombophlebitis (inflamed, tender, reddened segments of superficial leg veins)
   - elevational pallor. When feet are held about 12 inches above the level of the heart for 30 seconds, legs, feet, or toes become very pale.
   - edema of the feet (caused by disruption of blood flow from venous thrombosis)
   - diminished or absent pedal pulses. Use a Doppler probe to assess pulses if nonpalpable.
   - intermittent claudication
   - paresthesia
   - Raynaud's phenomenon (page 387)

4. See Chronic Peripheral Arterial Occlusive Disease for the reminder of this plan of care.

Aneurysm

An **aneurysm** is a localized dilation of the arterial wall at a weakened point. The aorta (thoracic and abdominal) and cerebral arteries are most commonly affected.

Aneurysms are commonly associated with hypertension. There are three types of aneurysms: sacular, dissecting, and fusiform. Dissecting aneurysms are the most dangerous type.

The patient is admitted to an ICU if in acute distress; otherwise, patient is admitted to a regular medical/surgical unit. Preoperative and postoperative care is the same for the patient undergoing cardiac surgery.

The major complication associated with an aneurysm is rupture, which leads to hemorrhage and possibly death. Severe hypertension increases the risk of rupture. The mean LOS for a DRG classification of aneurysm is 6.1 days (Lorenz, 1991).

General Medical Management

- Pharmacotherapy:
  - antihypertensives to maintain systolic pressure of 120 mm Hg or less
  - propranolol (Inderal) to reduce the pulsatile force within the aorta by reducing myocardial contractility
- Surgery when drug therapy fails to prevent enlargement of the aneurysm or the patient shows symptoms of acute distress. Surgery involves excision and removal of the aneurysm and replacement with a synthetic graft to restore vascular continuity.

Integrative Care Plans

- Cardiac surgery
- Preoperative and postoperative care

Discharge Considerations

- Follow-up care
- Measures to control hypertension

- Wound care
- Signs and symptoms of infection
- Activity limitations
- Medications to continue at home

THE PREOPERATIVE PERIOD

 *A*SSESSMENT DATA BASE

1. History or presence of risk factors associated with the development of aneurysms:
   - atherosclerosis (most common cause)
   - vessel trauma
   - pyogenic or syphilitic infections
   - congenital defects

2. Physical examination based on a general survey (Appendix F) and a cardiovascular assessment (Appendix G) may reveal:
   a. Clinical manifestations common to aneurysms, irrespective of the type and site:
      - hypertension with a widening pulse pressure
      - blood pressure in thigh lower than blood pressure in arm. Normally, BP in thigh is higher than that in arm.
      - weak or asymmetrical peripheral pulses
   b. Clinical manifestations specific to abdominal aortic aneurysms:
      - an abnormal pulsating abdominal mass (most prominent feature)
      - complaints of feeling "heartbeat" in the abdomen when supine
      - abdominal or low back pain
      - a bruit (swishing sound) on auscultation of the mass with the diaphragm of a stethoscope
   c. Clinical manifestations specific to thoracic aortic aneurysms (reflecting pressure of the mass against intrathoracic structures):
      - chest pain that radiates to the back and worsens when the patient is placed in a supine position (most prominent feature). In a dissecting aneurysm, the pain follows the direction in which the separation is progressing.
      - significant differences in BP readings between the arms
      - dyspnea and cough (reflects pressure against trachea)
      - hoarseness (reflects pressure against laryngeal nerve)
      - dysphagia (reflects pressure against the esophagus)
      - distended superficial veins on the chest, neck, or arms (reflects pressure against superior vena cava)
      - unequal pupils (reflects pressure against cervical sympathetic chain)

3. Diagnostic studies:
   • Radiological studies help define the location and confirm the presence and size of the aneurysm.
   • Aortogram confirms diagnosis of aneurysm.
   • EKG, cardiac enzymes, and echocardiogram done to rule out heart disease as a cause of chest pain.
   • Renal studies (creatinine, BUN) assess kidney function.
   • Pulmonary function studies assess lung function.

4. Assess the patient's understanding of condition, diagnostic studies, and treatment plan.

5. See Cardiac Surgery (page 486).

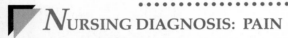

NURSING DIAGNOSIS: PAIN

RELATED TO FACTORS: Aortic aneurysm

DEFINING CHARACTERISTICS: Verbalizes pain in abdomen, low back, or chest; facial frowning; moaning; guarding painful site; shallow respirations

PATIENT OUTCOME (collaborative): Demonstrates relief from pain

EVALUATION CRITERIA: Reports reduction in intensity of pain, relaxed facial expression, absence of moaning

INTERVENTIONS	RATIONALE
1. Administer prescribed analgesic and evaluate its effectiveness prn. However, use narcotic analgesics sparingly.	Analgesics block the pain pathway. Large doses of narcotics may mask symptoms.
2. Notify physician if pain persists or worsens.	This could signal progression of the aneurysm and a need for immediate surgical intervention.

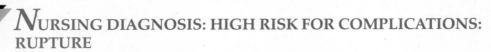

NURSING DIAGNOSIS: HIGH RISK FOR COMPLICATIONS: RUPTURE

RELATED TO FACTORS: Aortic aneurysm

DEFINING CHARACTERISTICS: Early manifestations of hypovolemic shock (falling BP, rising pulse rate, diminishing level of consciousness, cool and clammy skin)

PATIENT OUTCOME (collaborative): Demonstrates absence of complications

EVALUATION CRITERIA: BP remains between 90/60–120/80 mm Hg, absence of manifestations of hypovolemic shock

INTERVENTIONS	RATIONALE
1. Monitor: • intake and output qh if eight-hour urinary output is less than 240 mL, otherwise q8h • BP, pulse, and respiration hourly if in ICU, otherwise q2–4h • cardiovascular status (Appendix G), except weight, q4h • quality of pain q1–2h	To evaluate effectiveness of therapy and for early detection of complications.
2. Maintain bedrest in a semi-Fowler's position.	Bedrest reduces energy expenditure. An erect position facilitates breathing.
3. Maintain a quiet, stress-free environment.	The physiological mechanism by which the body responds to stress is the sympathetic nervous system. Epinephrine is released, which causes increased heart rate, cardiac output, and blood pressure. Maintaining a systolic pressure less than 120 mm Hg is essential to preventing rupture of the aneurysm.
4. Notify physician immediately if impending rupture is suspected. With a dissecting thoracic aortic aneurysm, suspect rupture if the patient suddenly experiences: • severe, tearing chest pain • shock (cool, clammy skin accompanied by hypotension, tachycardia, and pallor) • cardiac tamponade (page 497)	Immediate action is required to save the patient's life.

INTERVENTIONS	RATIONALE
Suspect impending rupture of an abdominal aortic aneurysm if the patient suddenly experiences: • constant, intense low back pain • absence of the pulsating abdominal mass • shock	
5. Initiate immediate action if rupture occurs: • Stay with the patient and have someone contact the physician immediately. • Place the patient in a supine position with legs elevated. • Obtain the crash cart for CPR and connect the patient to a cardiac monitor. • Activate emergency medical system for cardiac arrest if respirations or heart rate cease. • Obtain pericardiocentesis tray (for thoracic rupture). • Administer oxygen at 4 liters per minute. • Obtain diagnostic studies stat as ordered (chest x ray, CBC, electrolytes, cardiac enzymes, type and crossmatch for blood, and arterial blood gases). • Insert a Foley catheter and obtain a specimen for urinalysis if ordered.	Prompt intervention can reduce mortality.

INTERVENTIONS	RATIONALE
• Initiate an IV infusion (if not already present) and administer prescribed medication: — nitroprusside (Nipride) or trimethaphan camsylate (Arfonad) to reduce blood pressure — propranolol (Inderal) to reduce myocardial contractility and counteract the tachycardia caused by Nipride • Administer prescribed pain medication, such as morphine sulfate, which also helps slow respirations. • Prepare for emergency surgery.	

THE POSTOPERATIVE PERIOD

1. See Cardiac Surgery (page 486).

Hypertension

Hypertension is a persistent systolic pressure greater than 140 mm Hg or a diastolic pressure greater than 90 mm Hg. The diagnosis is confirmed by taking an average of two or more blood pressure measurements on two separate occasions. The primary pathology in hypertension is increased peripheral vascular resistance at the arteriole level.

Hypertension is asymptomatic. Symptoms indicate damage to target organs such as brain, kidney, eyes, and heart. Untreated, hypertension can lead to stroke, renal failure, blindness, and congestive heart failure.

Hypertension is classified as:

1. essential (primary or idiopathic) — unknown etiology; may become accelerated or malignant

2. secondary — caused by an underlying disease process

Hospitalization is not required for treatment of hypertension unless the patient experiences a hypertensive crisis. The mean LOS for a DRG classification of hypertensive crisis is 3.9 days (Lorenz, 1991). A hypertensive crisis, commonly called malignant hypertension, is a medical emergency characterized by a diastolic BP over 120 mm Hg accompanied by new or progressive target organ damage (Smith, 1991).

General Medical Management: (based on the Stepped Care Program) (Rodman, 1991)

• Step I. Conservative measures:

a. dietary modification:

— restricting sodium

— reducing intake of cholesterol and saturated fats

— reducing caloric intake to control weight

— reducing intake of alcoholic beverages

b. stop smoking

c. stress management

d. regular exercise program to decrease weight

- Step II. Pharmacotherapy if conservative measures fail to adequately control BP. One of the following may be used:
  - —diuretics
  - —beta-adrenergic blockers
  - —calcium channel blockers
  - —angiotensin converting enzyme (ACE) inhibitors
- Step III. Either the drug dose may be increased, a second drug from a different class may be added, or the drug substituted for another from a different class.
- Step IV. A third drug may be added or the second drug substituted for another from a different class.
- Step V. Further evaluation or referral to a specialist or a third or fourth drug may be added each from a different class.

General Medical Management for Hypertensive Crisis:

- Hospital admission to an ICU
- Pharmacotherapy with an IV infusion of a rapid acting antihypertensive agent such as nitroprusside (Nipride), diazoxide (Hyperstat), labetalol, nitroglycerin, or phentolamine

Integrative Care Plans

- Loss
- IV therapy

Discharge Considerations

- Follow-up care
- Medications prescribed for home use
- Signs and symptoms requiring medical attention

 # ASSESSMENT DATA BASE

1. History or presence of risk factors
   - obesity
   - positive family history
   - elevated serum lipid level
   - heavy cigarette smoking
   - renal disease
   - chronic hormonal therapy
   - heart failure
   - pregnancy

2. Inquire about compliance with prescribed antihypertensive management program.

3. Inquire about medications currently taken.

4. Assess BP in both arms — lying, sitting, and standing.

5. Physical examination based on a general survey (Appendix F) and neurological assessment (Appendix J) may reveal manifestations of organ damage:

   a. Brain — headache, nausea, vomiting, epistaxis, fleeting numbness or tingling in the extremities, hypertensive encephalopathy (drowsiness, confusion, convulsions, or coma)

   b. Eyes — retinopathy (can only be detected by use of an opthalmoscope, which would reveal retinal hemorrhage and exudates with papilledema), blurred vision

   c. Heart — heart failure (dyspnea on exertion, tachycardia)

   d. Kidneys — reduced urinary output in relation to fluid intake, sudden weight gain, edema

6. Diagnostic studies:

   • Chest x ray may show cardiomegaly.

   • EKG may reveal ventricular hypertrophy.

   • Urinalysis may show proteinuria, microscopic hematuria.

   • Chemistry survey may reveal elevated serum creatinine and blood urea nitrogen (BUN).

   • Lipid profile may reveal elevated cholesterol and triglycerides.

   • Serum electrolytes may reveal elevated sodium.

   • Catecholamine level is elevated if hypertension is caused by pheochromocytoma (tumor of adrenal medulla).

7. Assess patient's attitude about having a chronic condition. Look for clues that predispose to noncompliance (for example, statements such as "It can't be true. I don't feel sick." "I certainly don't want to have to take pills every day. It's such an inconvenience." "I can't afford medications." "I'm afraid of becoming addicted to drugs." "I didn't receive adequate instructions about my condition." "During clinic or office visits, I have to wait too long, and I never see the same doctor." "Health care staff don't seem to care.")

• •

◥ NURSING DIAGNOSIS: HIGH RISK FOR IMPAIRED HOME MAINTENANCE MANAGEMENT

RELATED TO FACTORS: Knowledge deficit about condition and treatment plan and difficulty adapting to a chronic condition

DEFINING CHARACTERISTICS: May report history of noncompliance, may verbalize concerns about side effects of medication, may verbalize lack of understanding, may verbalize statements indicative of possible noncompliance

PATIENT OUTCOME: Demonstrates willingness to comply with prescribed treatment plan

EVALUATION CRITERIA: Verbalizes understanding of condition and treatment plan, blood pressure remains below 140/90 mm Hg, verbalizes plans to make treatment program an integral part of lifestyle, verbalizes acceptance of chronic condition

• •

INTERVENTIONS	RATIONALE
1. Evaluate patient's understanding of hypertension: definition, significance of signs and symptoms. Correct any misconceptions. Emphasize that hypertension is a lifelong condition requiring continual treatment. It cannot be cured but can be controlled.	Many patients find it difficult to believe they have hypertension because it is asymptomatic initially until complications begin to develop secondary to organ damage. Compliance is enhanced when patients understand their condition.
2. See Loss (page 733).	
3. Teach the patient about prescribed medication, including dosage, schedule, name, purpose, and reportable side effects. See Table 5–3 for additional information to teach. Let the patient know that the physician may prescribe two or more antihypertensive drugs with different modes of action to effectively control blood pressure with minimal side effects. Encourage the male patient to report symptoms of sexual dysfunction.	An understanding of the relationship between drug therapy and hypertension is important to promoting compliance. Impotence is a major side effect of most antihypertensive agents, which can be easily corrected by adjusting the dosage or changing to another antihypertensive agent.
4. Assist the patient in planning a regular exercise routine (walking, swimming, tennis, bowling, bicycling). Provide a list of community support groups that focus on weight control and stop smoking if needed.	Exercise helps control weight and reduces stress and cholesterol levels. Support systems help strengthen an individual's psychosocial defenses. The nicotine in tobacco products causes vasoconstriction, which further promotes a rise in BP.
5. Assist the patient with identifying common sources of stress and planning ways to minimize those stressors. Suggest activities such as: • daily quiet periods alone	Epinephrine, a potent vasoconstrictor, is released during stress. It increases heart rate, cardiac output, and blood pressure. These activities help improve the individual's ability to counteract stress.

INTERVENTIONS	RATIONALE
• occasional long weekends involving some leisure activities • daily exercises after work • muscle relaxation exercises and relaxed breathing techniques such as yoga • biofeedback Consult an occupational therapist or recreational therapist for additional relaxation methods.	
6. Refer the patient to a dietitian for assistance in meal planning if dietary modification is prescribed (sodium restriction, reduced cholesterol, or weight reduction). Ensure the patient has written instructions about dietary modifications. Instructions may include: • Limit sodium intake (2–4 grams/day): — Do not add salt to food. — Avoid foods high in sodium (bacon, cold cuts, corned beef, sausage, canned-smoked-salted meats, olives, soy sauce). — Flavor foods with lemon or salt-free seasonings. — Increase intake of potassium-rich foods (fruits, vegetables), if taking a potassium-wasting diuretic. — Read labels for salt content. Some food labels reflect salt content by using the word "sodium" often listed as a compound, such as "disodium phosphate."	A dietitian is a nutritional specialist who can help the patient plan well-balanced meals within the context of prescribed dietary restrictions. Reducing dietary intake of sodium helps lessen water retention. Obesity and foods high in saturated fat and cholesterol are associated with a high incidence of cardiovascular disease.

●●●●●●●●●●●●●●●●●●●●●●●●●●●●●●●

NURSING DIAGNOSIS: HIGH RISK FOR IMPAIRED TISSUE PERFUSION

RELATED TO FACTORS: Organ damage secondary to uncontrolled hypertension

DEFINING CHARACTERISTICS: May demonstrate signs and symptoms of target organ damage (page 374)

PATIENT OUTCOME (collaborative): Demonstrates absence of target organ dysfunction

EVALUATION CRITERIA: BP maintained between 90/60–140/90 mm Hg, and absence of organ damage progression.

●●●●●●●●●●●●●●●●●●●●●●●●●●●●●●●

INTERVENTIONS	RATIONALE
1. Monitor: • BP q4h and prn • intake and output q8h, more often if output is significantly less than fluid intake • general status q8h	To evaluate effectiveness of therapy.
2. If the patient is admitted in hypertensive crisis, administer prescribed antihypertensive agents and evaluate their effectiveness.	Rapid reduction of BP is essential to offset extensive damage to the brain, kidneys, eyes, and heart.
3. Adhere to special precautions when administering emergency antihypertensive drugs intravenously: • Check BP every five minutes when beginning the infusion and every 15 minutes during maintenance. Use a flow sheet to record vital signs. Titrate dosage to maintain BP at prescribed level. • Discard IV solutions after 24 hours and hang a freshly prepared bag. • Wrap Nipride infusion (bag and tubing) with tinfoil. This drug is light sensitive. • Use an infusion pump to administer all continuous drips.	These measures ensure safe and effective drug therapy.

INTERVENTIONS	RATIONALE
• Gradually wean patient from continuous IV infusion of antihypertensive agent after oral antihypertensive is started. Do not discontinue the IV infusion abruptly. This can cause rebound hypertensive crisis.	
4. Notify physician if urinary output falls below 30 mL/hr.	This could signal renal insufficiency. Prompt intervention is required to prevent permanent renal damage.
5. Place on cardiac monitor while continuous infusion of antihypertensive medication is given.	Angina pectoris and possibly myocardial infarction may occur if the blood pressure drops too fast.
6. Maintain bedrest in semi-Fowler's position until BP is maintained at an acceptable level.	Bedrest helps reduce energy expenditure. A sitting position promotes arterial blood flow by gravity. Construction of the arterioles, as in hypertension, causes engorgement of blood in arteries.
7. Use a Dinamapp to monitor BP frequently.	This is a noninvasive device with an alarm that provides a continuous digital reading of BP.
8. Determine if hypertensive crisis is caused by noncompliance. If so, explore reasons for noncompliance. Assist the patient to explore ways to overcome perceived obstacles contributing to noncompliance. Reassess patient's knowledge of hypertension. Review basic principles of patient teaching for antihypertensive agents.	Noncompliance and failure to seek treatment for hypertension are common causes of hypertensive crisis.

Thrombophlebitis

Thrombophlebitis is an acute condition caused by thrombus formation in the veins, accompanied by inflammation of the vein wall. The thrombus is composed of RBCs, WBCs, and fibrin. One of the thrombi ends attaches to the vein wall and the other end flaps freely in the bloodstream (Caswell, 1991). The free end may dislodge and travel to other body parts and cause a potentially lethal complication.

Thrombophlebitis may develop in any vein but is more common in the deep veins (ileofemoral, popliteal, or calf veins) and the superficial (saphenous) veins of the legs.

Deep vein thrombosis carries the greatest risk of pulmonary embolism. For this reason, patients require hospitalization and aggressive therapy. Initially, the patient is given heparin IV for about 5–7 days. During the last 2–3 days of heparin therapy, warfarin (Coumadin) is given in conjunction with heparin because it takes about three days for Coumadin to begin acting. The major complication associated with anticoagulant therapy is bleeding.

The mean LOS for a DRG classification of thrombophlebitis is 7.4 days (Lorenz, 1991). Patients with deep vein thrombosis are often discharged on Coumadin therapy for about 1½ to 3 months. Permanent use of anticoagulant therapy may be required if the patient has a coexisting chronic condition commonly associated with thrombophlebitis (postphlebotic syndrome, heart disease).

Superficial thrombophlebitis is self-limiting, does not require hospitalization, and usually resolves in 3–5 days. Treatment is the same as for deep vein thrombophlebitis except aspirin is used as the primary anticoagulant.

Deep vein thrombosis may be more difficult to detect than superficial thrombosis. Many patients with deep vein thrombosis may not show the typical symptoms but may experience atypical manifestations, such as a sudden change in blood pressure without a concomitant change in pulse rate or respiration. Superficial thrombophlebitis produces visible and palpable manifestations.

When high-risk persons are hospitalized, preventive measures against thrombophlebitis should be initiated. These measures include low dose heparin therapy, aspirin, early postoperative ambulation, low molecular weight dextran, antiembolism stockings, ROM exercises for bedridden patients, or application of external limb compression devices.

General Medical Management

- Pharmacotherapy:
  — anticoagulants
  —thrombolytics
- Bedrest with affected leg elevated
- Continuous warm moist compresses
- Adequate hydration
- Antiembolism stockings
- Surgical implantation of a vena caval filter into the inferior vena cava for patients in whom long-term anticoagulant therapy is contraindicated

Integrative Care Plans

- Immobility
- IV therapy

Discharge Considerations

- Follow-up care
- Medications to continue at home
- Manifestations of recurrence
- Measures to prevent recurrence

 # ASSESSMENT DATA BASE

1. History or presence of risk factors. Three primary risk factors are:
   - venous stasis — heart disease, immobility, surgery, metastatic cancer, pregnancy
   - hypercoagulability of the blood — polycythemia, sickle cell anemia, hormone pills
   - injury to venous wall — extensive use of IV medications, infection, thromboangiitis obliterans (Buerger's disease)

2. Physical examination based on a peripheral vascular assessment (Appendix E) may reveal:
   - Swelling caused by increased hydrostatic pressure and fluid shift from veins to interstitial space as a result of obstruction of venous blood flow. The entire leg may be swollen with thrombosis of the iliac or femoral vein. **Measure the circumference of both legs (calf/thigh) if edema is present.** Mark area with an "X" so measurements are made at the same spot.
   - Redness or cyanosis of affected area
   - Cordlike nodule or lump along the affected vein on palpation
   - Normal pulses in the legs
   - Sluggish capillary refill

- Increased warmth, induration, and tenderness along the length of the affected vein caused by inflammatory reaction. (A cold extremity is characteristic of arterial occlusion not venous occlusion.)

- Pain, which typically occurs at the site of the thrombus with exercise, is aggravated by placing the extremity in a dependent position and is relieved by rest and elevation of the extremity. Pain also may be elicited on palpation of the area and by dorsiflexion of the foot (Homan's sign). Pain elicited on palpation is a more reliable sign of thrombophlebitis than the Homan's sign. A positive Homan's sign (pain in calf on foot dorsiflexion) indicates possible thrombophlebitis in the calf vein. Absence of calf pain when the foot is dorsiflexed is a negative Homan's sign.

3. Diagnostic studies:

- Venogram is the most definitive test that reveals the actual site of the thrombus.

- Doppler ultrasonography or plethysmography indicates sluggish blood flow through a vessel.

NURSING DIAGNOSIS: ALTERATION IN TISSUE PERFUSION

RELATED TO FACTORS: Thrombophlebitis

DEFINING CHARACTERISTICS: Verbalizes calf pain with exercise and palpation of the calf, positive Homan's sign, swelling

PATIENT OUTCOME (collaborative): Adequate circulation is restored

EVALUATION CRITERIA: Denies calf pain with exercise, absence of swelling, normal skin color

INTERVENTIONS	RATIONALE
1. Monitor peripheral vascular status (Appendix E) q8h.	To identify indications of progress toward or deviations from expected outcomes.
2. Keep affected leg elevated above the level of the heart.	To enhance venous return and reduce swelling.
3. Measure circumference of extremity daily and compare with unaffected extremity.	Measuring provides objective data to evaluate effectiveness of therapy.
4. Maintain bedrest until swelling and pain subside. Initiate measures to prevent complications of immobility while on bedrest (see Immobility, page 725).	Bedrest reduces energy expenditure.

INTERVENTIONS	RATIONALE
5. Apply knee-high antiembolism stockings as ordered. Follow package directions for measuring the stockings to ensure a correct fit. Refrain from applying the stockings to the affected leg if severe swelling exists. Remove the stockings in the morning and at bedtime to inspect, cleanse, and lubricate the skin. Explain that the stockings must always be worn.	Antiembolism stockings aid in venous compression and help prevent the formation of new clots.
6. Encourage intake of at least 2–3 liters of fluid, unless contraindicated. Initiate and maintain prescribed IV therapy.	To provide vascular access for administration of medication and to ensure adequate hydration to reduce blood viscosity.
7. Administer prescribed medication (anticoagulant, or thrombolytic, or both). Adhere to special precautions while the patient is receiving these drugs (see Tables 5–4 and 5–5).	Anticoagulants prevent the formation of new clots. Thrombolytic agents dissolve existing clots. The major problem with overmedication is bleeding.
8. Caution the patient against vigorous massage to the affected area.	Massage increases the risk of dislodging the clot.
9. Use a K-thermia pad to apply continuous warm, moist compresses to affected limb as prescribed. Adhere to facilities safety policy to ensure safe use of the K-thermia pad.	Heat enhances vasodilation and improves blood flow to the area.
10. Intervene appropriately and notify physician immediately if the patient develops manifestations of pulmonary embolism (page 47).	Pulmonary embolism is the major complication associated with deep vein thrombosis.

NURSING DIAGNOSIS: HIGH RISK FOR ALTERATION IN HOME MAINTENANCE MANAGEMENT

RELATED TO FACTORS: Knowledge deficit about condition and self-care preventive and maintenance measures on discharge

DEFINING CHARACTERISTICS: Verbalizes lack of understanding, requests information, may report a history of noncompliance

PATIENT OUTCOME: Demonstrates willingness to comply with treatment program for self-care prevention and maintenance

EVALUATION CRITERIA: Verbalizes understanding of information and home care instructions, seeks additional information

INTERVENTIONS	RATIONALE
1. Provide an explanation about: a. nature of the condition. Let the patient know the potential for recurrence. b. purpose of prescribed treatments c. prescribed diagnostic studies, including: • brief description of test • purpose • preparation required before test • care after test	A knowledge of what to expect helps lessen anxiety and promotes patient cooperation and compliance.
2. On discharge, provide instructions about prevention: • Wear support (antiembolism) stockings when engaging in activities that require prolonged standing. Change positions and flex and extend the legs and ankles at intervals when involved in an activity that requires standing in the same position. • Participate in a regular exercise program such as walking, bike riding, or swimming. • Avoid activities that constrict blood flow (crossing legs, constrictive clothing, prolonged sitting or standing in the same position).	Venous return is facilitated by support stockings and the pumping effect of muscle contraction and relaxation with exercise.

INTERVENTIONS	RATIONALE
3. Teach the patient about risk factors that predispose to recurrence. Discuss measures to eliminate or reduce risk factors, for example, stop smoking, better control of diabetes or hypertension (if present), weight control or reduction (if obese).	The incidence of recurrence is higher in persons at risk for thrombophlebitis.
4. Teach the patient about oral antico-agulation prescribed for home use.	Instructions about medications prescribed for home use help ensure safety in self-medication administration.
5. Ensure the patient has a written appointment for follow-up care and written instructions for self-care preventive measures.	Verbal instructions may be easily forgotten.

Vein Stripping and Ligation

Varicose veins are distended, tortuous superficial (saphenous) veins of the legs. The saphenous veins lie just beneath the skin and therefore do not have the support of muscles like the deep veins in the legs. Varicosities develop as a result of weakening of the valves in the veins. The weakened valves do not close properly, resulting in venous engorgement and stasis. Both extremities are often affected.

Vein stripping and ligation is the surgical procedure for varicose veins. It is indicated when the patient experiences persistent discomfort in the legs. General anesthesia is required.

The procedure involves ligation and removal of the saphenous vein through an incision made in the groin and ankle of the affected leg. Additional incisions may be made at various points along the affected limb to remove separate varicosities.

Patients often feel that their legs are unattractive and may report avoidance of social activities that entails wearing clothing that exposes the legs. Most patients express joy about the surgery because it means having legs that are cosmetically attractive and an end to chronic leg discomfort.

Preoperative preparation is the same for any patient undergoing surgery. Postoperatively, the patient returns to a medical/surgical unit with:

- IV infusion
- Ace bandages around operative leg
- thigh-high antiembolism stocking on nonoperative limb

Usually after 48 hours, the original dressing is removed and the patient is allowed to shower. The Ace bandage is then replaced with an antiembolism stocking. Low-dose heparin is often given as a prophylaxis against thrombophlebitis for a few days. The mean LOS for a DRG classification of vein stripping and ligation is 3.5 days (Lorenz, 1991).

Integrative Care Plans

- Preoperative and postoperative care
- IV therapy
- Immobility

Discharge Considerations

* Follow-up care
* Signs and symptoms of wound infection
* Measures to promote circulation

THE PREOPERATIVE PERIOD

 ASSESSMENT DATA BASE

1. History or presence of risk factors:
   * pregnancy
   * recurrent deep vein thrombophlebitis
   * prolonged standing
   * family history of varicose veins.

2. Physical examination based on a peripheral vascular assessment (Appendix E) and a general survey (Appendix F) may reveal:
   * dilated, tortuous superficial veins on the legs
   * complaints of dull aches, fatigue, cramps, and heaviness in the legs, especially after prolonged standing
   * brownish pigmentation of the skin
   * swelling, which generally subsides with elevation of the limb (also called orthostatic edema)

3. Diagnostic studies:
   * Venogram reveals exact location of varicosities both in superficial and deep veins.

4. See The Preoperative Period (page 739) for the remainder of this section.

THE POSTOPERATIVE PERIOD

 ASSESSMENT DATA BASE

1. See The Postoperative Period (page 741).
2. Assess neurovascular status (Appendix D) of the operative extremity.

NURSING DIAGNOSIS: HIGH RISK FOR ALTERATIONS IN TISSUE PERFUSION

RELATED TO FACTORS: Vein stripping and ligation

DEFINING CHARACTERISTICS: Edema, may report numbness and tingling, foot may be cool with sluggish capillary refill, may report Ace bandage too tight

PATIENT OUTCOME: Demonstrates adequate circulation

EVALUATION CRITERIA: Decrease in edema, warm extremities with rapid capillary refill, palpable pedal pulses, denies numbness and tingling, normal color

INTERVENTIONS	RATIONALE
1. Monitor neurovascular status (Appendix D) q2h x 24 hours, then q4h.	To detect early signs of circulatory problems.
2. Keep legs elevated when in bed and when sitting in a chair. Raise the foot of the bed. Do **not** gatch the knee of the bed.	Some swelling is expected after surgery. Elevating the extremity helps reduce swelling by promoting venous return. Gatching may promote stasis.
3. Encourage bed exercises until ambulation begins: flexion, extension, and rotation of the ankles. Ensure that pain medication is given at least 30 minutes before ambulation for the first two days.	To stimulate circulation. Patients are likely to be more cooperative with physical activities when they are not in pain.
4. Rewrap the Ace bandage prn if it becomes loose. Use a spiral wrapping technique, proceeding in a foot-to-head direction with the extremity elevated.	A compression bandage and wrapping in foot-to-head direction with the extremity elevated enhances venous return. This tight bandage also helps prevent bleeding. Less bandaging is required with a spiral wrap.
5. If the patient complains of sensory loss or "needles and pins" sensation or calf pain, loosen the Ace bandage and reposition the extremity higher. If no relief occurs in five minutes, notify physician.	Sensory loss may indicate temporary or permanent saphenous nerve damage from surgery. Calf pain may indicate thrombophlebitis.

INTERVENTIONS	RATIONALE
6. Keep antiembolism stockings on the nonoperative leg. Remove the stocking when providing hygienic care. Inspect, cleanse, and lubricate the skin, then reapply the stocking. Do **not** remove the Ace bandage as part of hygienic care until instructed to do so by physician.	Antiembolism stockings help prevent thrombophlebitis. Proper skin care helps maintain skin integrity. The Ace wrap acts as a compression bandage to reduce swelling and to maintain hemostasis.
See Nursing Diagnosis: Pain (page 741).	

. . . .

◤ NURSING DIAGNOSIS: HIGH RISK FOR COMPLICATIONS: INFECTION, HEMORRHAGE, THROMBOPHLEBITIS

RELATED TO FACTORS: Vein stripping and ligation

DEFINING CHARACTERISTICS: Fresh incisions, surgery on blood vessels, decreased physical activity

PATIENT OUTCOME (collaborative): Demonstrates absence of postoperative complications

EVALUATION CRITERIA: Absence of fever, excessive bleeding, and thrombophlebitis, postoperative recovery within DRG mean LOS

. . . .

INTERVENTIONS	RATIONALE
Infection, Hemorrhage, Thrombophlebitis: 1. See The Postoperative Period (page 743–745).	

NURSING DIAGNOSIS: HIGH RISK FOR ALTERATION IN HOME MAINTENANCE MANAGEMENT

RELATED TO FACTORS: Knowledge deficit about self-care activities on discharge

DEFINING CHARACTERISTICS: Verbalizes lack of understanding, requests information, observation of unsafe practices

PATIENT OUTCOME: Demonstrates willingness to comply with self-care activities on discharge

EVALUATION CRITERIA: Verbalizes understanding of discharge instructions, requests information, correct application of antiembolism stockings, correct performance of skin care to legs

INTERVENTIONS	RATIONALE
1. Allow the patient to express feelings about condition. Review underlying nature of varicose veins. After the bandages are removed, allow the patient to see the leg. Remind the patient that swelling must subside before the surgical outcomes can be judged.	Knowing what to anticipate helps promote adaptation.
2. Refer patient to the physical therapy department for exercise instructions. Encourage the patient to engage in a daily exercise program on discharge (walking or swimming).	A physical therapist can assist the patient in planning an exercise program that meets the patient's activity needs in view of current health status. Exercise promotes the development of collateral circulation.
3. Provide instructions about care of the extremities. Instructions should include: • Avoid activities that interfere with blood flow (wearing constrictive clothing, crossing legs). • Wear support stockings daily. Apply the stockings with legs elevated. Let the patient know that support stockings are available in various colors. • Elevate the feet above heart level a total of 10–18 hours daily for the first week and periodically thereafter.	These activities prevent circulatory compromise and maintain skin integrity.

INTERVENTIONS	RATIONALE
• Avoid sitting or standing in one position longer than 30 minutes. • Elevate feet when sitting. • Wash and thoroughly dry legs and feet daily. Apply a skin moisturizer.	
4. Provide written instructions about self-care activities and a written appointment for follow-up visit.	Verbal instructions may be easily forgotten.
5. Instruct the patient to contact physician if the following problems occur: • thrombophlebitis: calf pain with walking, increased swelling accompanied by numbness and tingling • infection: fever, increased redness and tenderness of the incisions, drainage from the incisions	Prompt medical attention and intervention can prevent further tissue damage.
6. If the patient is obese, explain the importance of reducing weight. Refer the patient to a dietitian for assistance in planning a weight reduction diet. Provide a list of community support groups that focus on weight loss.	Excess weight places undue stress on the cardiovascular system. A dietitian is a nutritional specialist who can assist the patient in planning a weight reduction diet that meets the patients needs in view of current health status.
7. Teach and allow the patient to practice correct application of the antiembolism stockings: lying on the bed with legs elevated. Explain the reason for the stockings. Instruct the patient to wear the stockings until all discoloration, swelling, and tenderness have subsided, usually about 2–3 weeks.	Individuals are more likely to comply with a health maintenance program when they understand the relationship between the activity and the health problem.

TABLE 5–1. Surgical Interventions For Chronic Peripheral Arterial Disorders

SYMPATHECTOMY

A resection of a portion of a specific sympathetic nerve chain (cranial, thoracolumbar, lumbar). It is performed under general anesthesia. A cervicothoracic sympathectomy is done for chronic arterial disorders of the upper extremities through an incision made over the third rib or above the clavicle. A lumbar sympathectomy is done for chronic arterial disorders of the lower extremities through a lower abdominal incision.

Permanent vasodilation is the outcome. In addition, the extremity no longer perspires. Effects are seen immediately after surgery—improved color and warmth. Mild discomfort and a sensation of heaviness are to be expected, caused by sudden increase of blood flow to the extremity. Periodic elevation of the extremity and application of antiembolism stockings relieve this discomfort. Patients should be cautioned against hot showers or baths, as these may cause generalized vasodilation thus precipitating orthostatic hypotension. Urinary retention may occur postoperatively and require catheterization until sphincter tone is regained. A nasogastric tube may be required to relieve paralytic ileus signaled by abdominal distention and absence of bowel sounds.

ENDARTERECTOMY

Surgical removal of obstructive intraluminal atheromatous plaques from an artery and the restoration of blood flow. It may be performed on the carotid artery to restore cerebral blood flow or the aortoiliac artery to restore blood flow to the lower extremity. A sympathectomy may be done in conjuction with peripheral endarterectomy.

VASCULAR BYPASS

Surgical anastomosis of a graft above and below the occluded section of an artery to restore blood flow using a saphenous vein from the patient's unaffected leg or a synthetic graft. Common bypass surgeries include coronary artery (for the heart), femoral-popliteal and aortofemoral (for the legs).

TABLE 5–2. Management of Leg Ulcers

1. Bedrest with leg elevated or limited ambulation.

2. Wet-to-dry dressings using Burrow's solution or normal saline solution.

3. Application of a Unna paste boot. Gauze strips impregnated with zinc oxide are wrapped around the leg. The bandage hardens into a semirigid boot. The boot is removed weekly and a new one reapplied. It takes about 2–3 weeks for the ulcer to heal.

4. Application of topical antibiotic ointment to treat infected ulcers.

5. Debridment, manually or using topical debriding agents (dextranomer, Carrington gel, Elase or Travase ointment).

6. Daily whirlpool cleansing.

7. Use of hyperbaric oxygen (HBO) therapy. The patient's entire body is placed into a special pressurized chamber and subjected to increased pressure (as much as three times the normal atmospheric pressure) and oxygen concentration. HBO treatments are painless, but some patients may experience a sensation of "fullness" in the ears, similar to what is felt when flying or driving down a mountain. Swallowing or yawning relieves this sensation. The average treatment time is two hours. No smoking is allowed during the therapy. Treatment is postponed if the patient has a cold, flu, fever, sore throat, runny nose, fever blisters, nausea, vomiting, diarrhea, or generalized malaise. There are no after effects from HBO therapy and no restrictions between treatments. Before each treatment:

   • makeup, hair spray, nail polish, perfume, deodorant, and shaving lotion containing an alcohol base must be removed.

   • all clothing, jewelry, dentures, and glasses must be removed. A gown made of 100% cotton is the only item that the patient is allowed to wear while in the chamber.

   • 400 units of vitamin E is given orally.

   • medications that are incompatible with HBO therapy must be withheld at least eight hours before therapy (aspirin, vitamin C, Talwin, morphine sulfate, alcohol).

8. Skin grafting is done for ulcers unresponsive to the above interventions.

TABLE 5–3. Antihypertensives: What the Patient Should Know and Why

INTERVENTIONS	RATIONALE
1. Take medication daily as prescribed.	The most common cause of severe hypertension is failure to take antihypertensive medication as prescribed. Hypertension treatment is for a lifetime.
2. Contact physician if adverse effects occur.	A trial-and-error period is anticipated. The physician will make adjustments in the dose, frequency, or change the drug to resolve adverse effects. It may take several months before the BP is well controlled with minimum side effects.

INTERVENTIONS	RATIONALE
3. Monitor own BP and record results in a booklet obtained from the physician's office. Periodic assessment of BP may be done by using an automatic BP device available in grocery or drug stores.	Continual BP measurements are essential for evaluating effectiveness of drug therapy.
4. If a dose is forgotten, do **not** take two doses the next time.	Doubling a dose can cause hypotension.
5. Change body position slowly. Sit first when moving from a supine to standing position.	To prevent orthostatic hypotension.
6. Weigh twice weekly and record weight in BP booklet.	Body weight is used to monitor fluid status.
7. Keep follow-up appointments and bring BP booklet to each visit.	So progress can be monitored.
8. Avoid hot baths, showers, and excess intake of alcohol.	These situations may cause further vasodilation and fainting.

TABLE 5–4. Discharge Instructions for Patients On Warfarin Therapy

1. Coumadin helps prevent the formation of new clots but does not dissolve existing clots.
2. Notify physician if pregnancy occurs while on therapy.
3. Do not take any other medications (including over-the-counter medicines) without checking with physician first.
4. Use an electic razor for shaving.
5. Avoid participating in contact sports.
6. Report signs of bleeding that do not stop after applying pressure for ten minutes.
7. Wear a Medic Alert bracelet or necklace.
8. If vegetarian, reduce intake of foods high in vitamin K, particularly green leafy vegetables, since vitamin K reduces the effectiveness of Coumadin.
9. Keep follow-up appointments to have blood level of the drug checked to ensure a safe therapeutic level is maintained.

10. Report signs of bleeding immediately: red or dark brown urine, black stools, unusual bleeding from gums, nose, or skin, severe pain in joints or stomach, severe headache, prolonged excessive menstrual flow.
11. Take the prescribed amount of medication at the same time each day in the evening.
12. When undergoing any type of invasive (medical, surgical, or dental) procedure, let the person know you are taking an anticoagulant.

TABLE 5–5. Thrombolytic Therapy

INTERVENTIONS	RATIONALE
1. Before administering streptokinase, assess the patient for a history of a streptococcal infection or history of receiving streptokinase with the last three months. Notify physician of positive findings.	Circulating streptococcal antibodies may reduce the effectiveness of the drug. One of the other types of thrombolytic agents may be used such as urokinase or alteplase (Activase) also called t-PA.
2. Assess time of onset of acute pain.	Thrombolytic agents given intravenously are most effective when given within six hours of acute thrombus occlusion, for intracoronary administration, within four hours after onset of chest pain.
3. Throughout drug administration, monitor: • peripheral vascular status (pedal pulses, skin color and temperature, sensation), vital signs, and neurological status (Appendix E) qh throughout therapy. • results of APTT, PT, hemoglobin, and hematocrit • intensity of pain • Hematest® all emesis, stools, and urine for blood	To evaluate effectivenss of therapy and to detect signs of bleeding, which is the major complication associated with thrombolytic agents. A decrease in pain intensity and resolution of S-T segment elevation on the EKG, with myocardial infarction, are desired therapeutic responses. Intracranial hemorrhage is the most dangerous side effect with thrombolytic therapy.
4. Use a volume controlled infusion pump when administering the prescribed thrombolytic agent by continuous IV drip.	Often a loading dose is given IV followed by a continuous IV drip. An infusion pump achieves better control of the flow rate.

INTERVENTIONS	RATIONALE
5. Take precautions against bleeding: • Use a soft bristle toothbrush. • Hold pressure on IV sites for 30 minutes after discontinuing the drug. • Do not give intramuscular injections for 24 hours. • Use acetaminophen for fever. Do not give aspirin or aspirin-containing products.	Thrombolytic agents act by converting plasminogen to plasmin, an enzyme that breaks down the clot. Bleeding is the major complication associated with thrombolytic therapy. Aspirin functions as an anticoagulant by inhibiting platelet adhesion.
6. Notify physician if the following occur: • neurological deficits (change in level of consciousness, change in pupillary response, headache, rising BP accompanied by a falling pulse rate) • abdominal pain • Hematest® positive stools, urine, or emesis	These findings signal bleeding and a need to discontinue drug therapy.
7. Stop the infusion immediately and notify physician if the following occur: • bronchospasms • dyspnea • cyanosis • convulsions • loss of consciousness	These findings signal anaphylaxis. This type of allergic reaction is most likely to occur with streptokinase since it is derived from bacteria. Allergic reactions rarely occur with urokinase since it is derived from the kidney.

BIBLIOGRAPHY

Becker, G., & Mose, K. (1991). High-tech options for leg ischemia. **Patient Care, 25,** 61–5, 68, 71–74, 80, 85.

Caswell, D. (1991). Vascular diseases. **Critical Care Nursing Clinics of North America, 3,** 491–558.

Fitzgerald, M. (1991). The physical exam. **RN, 54,** 34–38.

Lambert, W.C., & Doty, D.B. (1989). **Peripheral Vascular Surgery.** Chicago: Year Book Medical Publishers.

Lorenz, E.W. (1991). **St. Anthony's DRG Working Guidebook.** Alexandria: St. Anthony's Publishing Company.

North American Nursing Diagnosis Association. (1990). **Taxonomy I,** St. Louis, MO.

Rodman, M.J. (1991). Hypertension: First-line drug therapy. **RN, 54,** 32–39.

Smith, C., & Jones, L. (1991). Control of hypertensive emergencies. **Postgraduate Medicine, 89,** 111–6, 119, 237–242.

C

CHAPTER SIX
Problems of the Hematologic System

Lymphomas

Lymphomas are malignancies involving the lymphatic system. Hodgkin's disease and non-Hodgkin's disease are the most common lymphomas.

Hodgkin's disease originates in the lymphatics and metastasizes to other organs. It commonly affects young males most often between the second and fourth decades of life. With early diagnosis and treatment, the prognosis is good with an average survival rate of five years (Neely, 1989)

Non-Hodgkin's disease has a poor prognosis. It originates in extra nodal tissue and then metastasizes to the lymph nodes. By the time it is diagnosed, metastasis has already occurred (Neely, 1989).

Lymphomas have an unknown etiology. There are no risk factors or preventive measures. Lymphomas do not cause defects in the fetus if diagnosed during pregnancy or do not interfere with pregnancy. However, the treatments are harmful to the fetus. For this reason, pregnancy is discouraged until the disease is in remission.

A roman numeral (I, II, III, IV) is used in the staging classification to reflect the location and extent of metastasis of the disease. To indicate absence of symptoms, "A" is used; "B" indicates one or more symptoms.

When the staging classification of the disease has been established, a medical treatment plan then is developed. Nursing management for lymphomas primarily focuses on dealing with the side effects of therapy and the patient's and significant others psychosocial response to a diagnosis of cancer. The mean LOS for a DRG classification of lymphoma is 3.9 days without complication and 8.1 days with complications (Lorenz, 1991).

General Medical Management

- Radiation therapy
- Chemotherapy

Integrative Care Plans

- Loss
- Cancer

- Radiation therapy
- Chemotherapy

Discharge Considerations

- Follow-up care
- Community support systems
- Hospice care
- Medications to continue at home

 # ASSESSMENT DATA BASE

1. Physical examination based on a general survey (Appendix F) and palpation of the lymph nodes (axillary, cervical, and inguinal) may reveal:
   a. Hodgkin's disease:
      - firm, painless, asymmetrical enlargement of the cervical lymph nodes (most prominent finding). Tender nodes may suggest infection. Ingestion of alcohol causes the nodes to be tender.

      Secondary symptoms reflect metastasis to other body sites and a less favorable prognosis:

      - mediastinum—dysphagia, cough, shortness of breath, pleural effusion
      - bone marrow—anemia, bleeding tendencies, unexplained fever with night sweats, weight loss, anorexia
      - central nervous system—headaches
      - skin—nodules, pruritus
   b. Non-Hodgkin's disease:
      - generalized adenopathy involving more than one region accompanied by secondary symptoms
2. Diagnostic studies:
   - Lymph node biopsy confirms diagnosis. A finding of Reed-Sternberg cells is diagnostic for Hodgkin's disease.
   - Staging procedures are done to define the extent of the disease after the diagnosis has been confirmed. This may include:
     — CBC to assess bone marrow involvement.
     — Chemistry profile to access kidney and liver involvement.
     — Chest x ray may show pleural effusion or a mediastinal mass with metasteses.
     — Lymphangiogram reveals extent of lymph node involvement.
     — Staging laparotomy may be done to assess the extent of abdominal involvement.
3. See Integrative Care Plans to complete this plan of care.

Thrombocytopenia

Thrombocytopenia (low platelet count) may be antibody-mediated or acquired. Idiopathic thrombocytopenia purpura (ITP), also called autoimmune thrombocytopenia, is an antibody-mediated platelet destruction disorder. For unclear reasons, antibodies are produced that alter the structure of platelets subsequently triggering rapid platelet destruction by the reticuloendothelial system (liver and spleen).

ITP may be acute or chronic. The acute form is more common in children, generally follows a viral infection, and usually resolves spontaneously with therapy in less than six months. The chronic form is seen more often in adults and often has a poor prognosis. The mean LOS for a DRG classification of coagulation disorders is 5.5 days (Lorenz, 1991).

General Medical Management

- For ITP:
  - corticosteroids. An antacid should be given concurrently with steroids to prevent gastric ulcers
  - splenectomy if steroid therapy is ineffective in maintaining a platelet count greater than 50,000/mm^3
  - chemotherapy with vincristine (Oncovin) and cyclophosphamide (Cytoxan) if splenectomy ineffective
  - platelet transfusions only for life-threatening hemorrhages
- For acquired thrombocytopenia:
  - removal of causative agent
  - platelet transfusion if the platelet count falls below 20,000/mm^3

Integrative Care Plans

- Chemotherapy

Discharge Considerations

- Follow-up care
- Prevention of injury

 # Assessment data base

1. History or presence of causative factors:
   - ITP may be a secondary manifestation of other disorders such as leukemia, systemic lupus erythematosus, AIDS, and aplastic anemia.
   - Acquired thrombocytopenia may be caused by certain medications, radiation therapy, or chemotherapy.

2. Physical examination based on a general survey (Appendix F) may reveal bleeding, which may appear as:
   - petechiae (flat, red round spots that do not blanch when pressed) scattered over the extremities, trunk, and oral cavity
   - ecchymosis
   - bruising easily
   - bleeding gums
   - menorrhagia
   - spontaneous nosebleeds
   - oozing of blood from wounds and venipuncture sites
   - stools or emesis may be guaiac positive
   - hematuria (brownish or reddish urine)

3. Diagnostic studies:
   - platelet count is low (most significant finding).
   - coagulation times for PT and PTT are prolonged.
   - capillary fragility test is increased.
   - antibody screening is done to rule out ITP.
   - bone marrow aspiration reveals increased number of megakarocytes (precursors of platelets).

4. Assess understanding of the condition and its treatment.

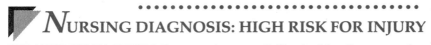

Nursing diagnosis: high risk for injury

RELATED TO FACTORS: Increased susceptibility for bleeding secondary to abnormal platelet function

DEFINING CHARACTERISTICS: Reports history of bruising easily, prolonged bleeding with minor injuries, observation of bruises or petechiae on the skin

PATIENT OUTCOME: Demonstrates no further injury

EVALUATION CRITERIA: No new ecchymotic areas or bruises, coagulation factors remain within normal range

• •

INTERVENTIONS	RATIONALE
1. Initiate bleeding precautions based on the platelet count (see Table 6–1).	To prevent further bleeding.
2. Advise the patient to wear a Medic Alert bracelet.	To ensure patient safety in case of an emergency.
3. Teach self-care measures to reduce the risk for bleeding at home. Instructions should include: • Avoid engaging in contact sports. • Avoid going barefoot. • Avoid aspirin and aspirin-containing products. Read product labels before buying over-the-counter medications. For pain, use acetaminophen or propoxyphene instead. • Inform health care professionals of condition before undergoing any surgery or dental extraction. • Wear heavy-duty gloves when gardening.	Blunt trauma may cause disruption of capillaries, hence bleeding. Aspirin prevents platelet adhesion. Health teaching enhances health status by improving the quality of life.
4. Teach first-aid measures for injuries: • Apply firm pressure for five minutes. • If bleeding continues, seek medical attention at closest emergency department.	First aid measures are essential to reduce the severity of injury.
5. See Nursing Diagnosis: Anxiety (page 262).	

Polycythemia

Polycythemia (erythrocytosis) refers to excess production of red blood cells (RBCs). It may be primary (polycythemia vera) or secondary.

Polycythemia vera is a neoplastic disorder of the bone marrow cells. It has an unknown etiology, an insidious onset, and has no known cure. It involves erythrocytosis, thrombocytosis, and leukocytosis. The platelets are dysfunctional.

Secondary polycythemia occurs as a compensatory mechanism when chronic hypoxia occurs. Hypoxia triggers the release of erythropoietin, a hormone produced by the kidney that stimulates erythropoiesis.

Secondary polycythemia produces no symptoms, except for laboratory examination, and requires no treatment. Polycythemia vera produces severe symptoms that require treatment. The mean LOS for a DRG classification of polycythemia vera is 4.0 days without complications and 6.6. days with complications (Lorenz, 1991).

General Medical Management

- Phlebotomy to reduce blood volume. The procedure is performed by a laboratory technician on an outpatient basis, usually every two months depending on the patient's hematocrit level. About 500 mL of blood is removed during each visit.
- Pharmacotherapy:
  — allopurinol to lower serum uric acid levels
  — myelosuppressive drugs, such as busulfan, may be given to reduce bone marrow hyperactivity. These drugs have caused acute leukemia in some patients. They are used during periods of exacerbation and discontinued while in remission.

Integrative Care Plans

- Loss
- Thrombophlebitis

Discharge Considerations

- Follow-up care
- Signs and symptoms requiring medical attention
- Medications for home use

 # ASSESSMENT DATA BASE

1. History or presence of diseases associated with hypoxia (chronic obstructive pulmonary disease [COPD], chronic heart disease, hemoglobinopathies).

2. Physical examination based on a general survey (Appendix F) may reveal:
   - increased skin color (often a ruddy, tanned appearance) caused by increased hemoglobin level
   - symptoms of circulatory overload (dyspnea, chronic cough, elevated BP, tachycardia, headache, dizziness) caused by increased blood volume
   - symptoms of thrombosis (angina, intermittent claudication, thrombophlebitis) caused by increased blood viscosity
   - splenomegaly and hepatomegaly
   - itching, especially following warm baths, resulting from hemolysis of immature RBCs
   - history of nosebleeds, ecchymosis, or GI bleeding from platelet dysfunction

3. Diagnostic studies:
   - CBC reveals elevated RBC, hemoglobin, hematocrit, WBC, and platelet counts. In secondary polycythemia, the WBC and platelet count remain normal.
   - Leukocyte alkaline phosphatase is elevated.
   - Serum B_{12} level is elevated.
   - Serum uric acid level is elevated.

4. Assess the patient's understanding of condition and treatment plan.

5. Assess the patient's feelings about having a chronic condition.

NURSING DIAGNOSIS: FLUID VOLUME EXCESS

RELATED TO FACTORS: Excess RBCs and blood volume

DEFINING CHARACTERISTICS: Reports easy fatigue with minimal exertion accompanied by tachycardia and tachypnea; RBC, hemoglobin, and hematocrit above normal limits; rales may be auscultated; BP above normal range; serum sodium below normal range

PATIENT OUTCOME (collaborative): Demonstrates relief from fluid volume excess.

EVALUATION CRITERIA: Participates in ADL without experiencing tachypnea, tachycardia, and fatigue; CBC and serum sodium within normal ranges; clear breath sounds; decreased weight; vital signs within normal range

INTERVENTIONS	RATIONALE
1. Before and after phlebotomy, monitor: • BP, pulse, and respiration • results of serum electrolyte reports, especially sodium • results of CBC report • weight	To evaluate effectiveness of therapy.
2. Arrange for phlebotomy as prescribed. Consult physician if vital signs, hemoglobin, hematocrit, and serum sodium remain elevated after the prescribed amount of blood has been drained.	Normally, postphlebotomy values should be lower than prephlebotomy values.
3. Limit fluid intake if symptoms of fluid excess are present: rales, hypertension, bounding pulse, increase respiratory rate.	To prevent further overload.
4. Administer prescribed medication to control proliferation of blood cells and evaluate its effectiveness.	Lifetime pharmacotherapy is required to effectively control polycythemia vera.

• •

 NURSING DIAGNOSIS:HIGH RISK FOR ALTERATION IN TISSUE PERFUSION: PERIPHERAL

RELATED TO FACTORS: Thrombus formation secondary to polycythemia

DEFINING CHARACTERISTICS: Elevated hematocrit, history of unusual excess bleeding with minor injury, reports bruising easily, may report history of thrombophlebitis

PATIENT OUTCOME: Peripheral tissue perfusion remains adequate

EVALUATION CRITERIA: Absence of excessive bleeding, no signs of thrombophlebitis

• •

INTERVENTIONS	RATIONALE
1. Monitor: • results of CBC reports, especially hematocrit • peripheral vascular status (Appendix E) q8h	To detect complications early.
2. Encourage active range-of-motion exercises if hospitalized and placed on bedrest.	Immobility predisposes patient to thrombus formation.
3. Encourage fluid intake in the absence of symptoms of fluid overload.	Fluids help reduce the blood viscosity.
4. Notify physician if thrombus formation occurs: a. angina pectoris (page 460) b. intermittent claudication (page 360) c. thrombophlebitis (page 381)	A common denominator for these three conditions is pain. Obstruction of a blood vessel by a thrombus (blood clot) interferes with blood flow to surrounding tissue. Ischemia occurs. If the thrombus obstructs blood flow to an area of the brain, neurological deficits are seen. Prompt intervention is required to relieve the thrombus to prevent permanent tissue damage.

NURSING DIAGNOSIS:HIGH RISK FOR ALTERATION IN HOME MAINTENANCE MANAGEMENT

RELATED TO FACTORS: Knowledge deficit about condition and treatment plan, difficulty adjusting to a chronic condition

DEFINING CHARACTERISTICS: Verbalizes lack of understanding, reports history of noncompliance, may verbalize feelings of depression

PATIENT OUTCOME: Demonstrates willingness to comply with treatment plan

EVALUATION CRITERIA: Verbalizes understanding of condition and treatment plan, verbalizes plans to incorporate treatment plan into current lifestyle

INTERVENTIONS	RATIONALE
1. Evaluate patient's understanding of condition. Provide information about: a. nature of the condition. Emphasize that polycythemia vera is a chronic condition that requires lifetime treatment. b. purpose of prescribed treatments c. prescribed medications, including name, dose, schedule, purpose, and reportable side effects d. signs of extremity thrombosis (page 381)	Compliance is enhanced when patients understand the relation between their condition and therapy.
2. Encourage the patient to express feelings about having a chronic illness. Provide correct answers to dispel any misconceptions.	Expressing feelings facilitates coping. An accurate knowledge of a given situation helps lessen anxiety.
3. Instruct the patient to seek medical attention if symptoms of circulatory overload or thrombus formation occur.	Prompt intervention is required to prevent permanent tissue damage.
4. Ensure the patient has written appointments for follow-up visits and written instructions for self-care activities.	Verbal instructions may be easily forgotten.
5. Keep the patient informed about results of CBC studies.	To promote patient involvement in assuming responsibility for maintaining own health.

Leukemia

Leukemia is a disorder characterized by excess proliferation of immature (blast cells) white blood cells (WBCs). It is classified by:

1. Cell maturity:
   - acute (poorly differentiated stem cells)
   - chronic (more mature cells)

2. Type of stem cell involved:
   - myelocytic (myeloblasts produced by bone marrow)
   - lymphocytic (lymphoblasts produced by lymphatic system)

Normally, stem cells (myoblasts and lymphoblasts) are not present in peripheral blood (Arena, 1991). Cell maturity and cell type are combined to form four types of leukemia:

- **acute myelocytic leukemia** (AML), also called acute myelogenous leukemia or acute granulocytic leukemia (AGL), characterized by excess production of myeloblasts
- **acute lymphocytic leukemia** (ALL) characterized by proliferation of lymphoblasts; found primarily in children
- **chronic lymphocytic leukemia** (CLL) characterized by proliferation of well-differentiated (easily recognized cells reflecting the tissue of origin) lymphocytes
- **chronic myleocytic leukemia** (CML), also called chronic granulocytic leukemia (CGL), prominent features are:
  — presence of Philadelphia chromosomes in blood cells. This is an abnormal chromosome found in bone marrow cells.
  — blast crisis. A phase characterized by the sudden proliferation of vast numbers of myeloblasts. This finding signals the conversion of CML to AML. Death often occurs within a few months as leukemic cells become resistant to chemotherapy during blast crisis.

The acute forms of leukemia have a rapid onset of symptoms that reflect infiltration of the bone marrow, whereas the chronic forms of leukemia have a gradual onset with organomegaly being a prominent clinical finding accompanied later by symptoms of pancytopenia (bone marrow suppression).

There is no known permanent cure for leukemia. The average survival rate varies from 2–5 years and longer with treatment, depending on the type of leukemia. Without treatment, it is less than a year (Konradi, 1989).

The goals of therapy are divided into two primary phases: induction remission and maintenance. During the induction phase, hospitalization is required. Large doses of chemotherapy agents are given, which cause the patient to be extremely ill. Maintenance therapy is done on an outpatient basis.

With treatment, leukemic patients experience periods of remission and exacerbation. The remission may range from 1–2 years or longer in some cases. Complete remission is defined as normal bone marrow, normal peripheral blood count with less than 5% stem cells (myeoloblast or lymphoblast), and absence of clinical manifestation of the disease (Arena, 1991). During remission, the patient feels well and can have a normal life. With each exacerbation (recurrence of symptoms), it becomes increasingly difficult to achieve remission.

The mean LOS for a DRG classification of leukemia is 8.1 days (Lorenz, 1991).

General Medical Management

- Chemotherapy
- Bone marrow transplant (in some cases)

Integrative Care Plans

- Loss
- Cancer
- Chemotherapy

Discharge Considerations

- Follow-up care
- Measures to protect against infection
- Community support services (hospice when death is imminent)
- Medications for home use

 # ASSESSMENT DATA BASE

1. History of exposure to predisposing factors, such as exposure to large doses of radiation, chronic use of certain drugs, and history of chronic viral infections
2. Physical examination based on a general survey (Appendix F) may reveal manifestations that reflect:

a. engorgement of the bone marrow with leukemic cells, subsequently suppressing bone marrow function causing:
  - anemia— weight loss, fatigue, pallor, malaise, weakness, anorexia
  - thrombocytopenia— bleeding gums, bruising easily, petechiae, ecchymosis
  - neutropenia— fever without evidence of infection, night sweats

b. infiltration of other organs with leukemic cells causing:
  - hepatomegaly
  - splenomegaly
  - lymphadenopathy
  - bone and joint pain
  - gingival hypertrophy

3. Diagnostic studies:

  - CBC shows decreased hemoglobin, hematocrit, red blood cell count, and platelets. WBC count is elevated with chronic leukemia but may be low, normal, or high with acute leukemia.
  - WBC differential count identifies which type of WBC is involved. With myelocytic leukemia, the neutrophils are involved. Lymphocytic leukemia reflects an elevated number of lymphocytes.
  - Bone marrow aspiration and biopsy provide the most definitive diagnostic data.
  - Serum uric acid is elevated because of release of oxypurines subsequent to rapid turnover of leukemic cells and use of cytotoxic drugs.

    Other studies are done to assess the extent of the disease and include chest x ray, chemistry profile, EKG, and specimen cultures (blood, throat, urine, sputum) to rule out infection as a cause of the fever, skin test (mumps, candida, and purified protein derivative (PPD)) to assess strength of the immune system.

4. Assess the emotional response of the patient and significant others to the illness and its impact on their lifestyles.

5. Assess the patient's understanding of the illness, treatment, and prognosis.

6. See Loss (page 733).

7. See Chemotherapy (page 707).

8. See Cancer (page 694).

Disseminated Intravascular Coagulation

Disseminated intravascular coagulation (DIC) is a thrombohemorrhagic disorder that occurs, not as a separate entity, but as a complication of certain disorders. DIC is characterized by acceleration of the coagulation process in which thrombosis and hemorrhage occur simultaneously.

For unclear reasons, increased amounts of thrombin are formed that activate the intrinsic clotting mechanisms causing the formation of excessive amounts of fibrin. The fibrin is deposited in small blood vessels throughout the body causing thrombi (Young, 1990). These fibrin thrombi obstruct circulation, leading to manifestations of impaired tissue perfusion. The brain, kidneys, lungs, skin, and GI tract are most commonly affected.

The fibrinolytic system is activated by fibrin thrombi, causing the release of large quantities of fibrin degradation products. These products consume clotting factors (fibrinogen, prothrombin, factors V and VII) and platelets, resulting in hemorrhage (Young, 1990).

The patient is seriously ill and requires constant monitoring in an ICU. After the bleeding has stopped and coagulation factors return to normal limits, the patient does not require lifetime follow-up. However, the patient continues to be at risk for recurring DIC if subjected to predisposing factors. Hemorrhage is the major cause of death.

The mean LOS for a DRG classification of coagulation disorders is 5.5 days (Lorenz, 1991).

General Medical Management

- Supportive measures such as supplemental oxygen and IV fluids to maintain BP
- Heparin therapy to prevent microthrombic formation
- Transfusion of platelets, fresh frozen plasma, or cryoprecipitate that must be given **after** heparin therapy to control increased bleeding caused by heparin. If given before heparin therapy, these products potentiate thrombi formation.
- Fibrinolytic inhibitors (Amicar) that block accumulation of fibrin degradation products and that must be given **after** heparin therapy and **only** if transfusions fail to stop bleeding. These agents enhance thrombus formation if given before heparin therapy.

Integrative Care Plan

• IV therapy

Discharge Considerations

• None

 # ASSESSMENT DATA BASE

1. Presence of predisposing factors:
    • septicemia (most common cause)
    • obstetrical complications
    • ARDS (adult respiratory distress syndrome)
    • extensive and severe burns
    • neoplasia
    • snake bites
    • hepatic disease
    • cardiopulmonary surgery
    • trauma
2. Physical examination based on a general survey (Appendix F) may reveal:
    a. Bleeding:
        • hematuria
        • oozing of blood from venipuncture sites and wounds
        • epistaxis
        • GI bleeding (guaiac positive stool and emesis)
    b. Impaired tissue perfusion:
        • cerebral: changes in the sensorium, restlessness, confusion, headache
        • kidney: decreased urinary output
        • lungs: dyspnea, orthopnea
        • skin: acrocyanosis (irregularly shaped cyanotic patches on periphery of arms or legs)
3. Diagnostic studies:
    • Platelet count is low.
    • PT and PTT are prolonged.
    • Fibrin degradation products are elevated.
    • Plasma fibrinogen level is low.

NURSING DIAGNOSIS: HIGH RISK FOR ALTERATION IN TISSUE PERFUSION

RELATED TO FACTORS: Hemorrhage secondary to DIC

DEFINING CHARACTERISTICS: Manifestations of shock, decreased sensorium, observation of persistent bleeding sites

PATIENT OUTCOME (collaborative): Demonstrates adequate tissue perfusion

EVALUATION CRITERIA: Absence of manifestations of shock, remains alert and oriented, no further bleeding normal lab values

INTERVENTIONS	RATIONALE
1. Monitor results of coagulation studies, vital signs, and current and potential sites of bleeding.	To identify indications of progress toward or deviations from expected outcome.
2. Initiate bleeding precautions (Table 6–1).	To minimize potential of further bleeding.
3. Administer prescribed medications and evaluate their effectiveness. With heparin therapy, watch for the formation of antiplatelet antibodies signaled by a sudden drop in the platelet count. Administer prescribed blood transfusions according to facility protocol and procedures. Evaluate closely for manifestations of a transfusion reaction (Table 6–2). Stop the transfusion if a reaction occurs and implement measures according to facility protocol and procedures.	When the primary disease is treated, the goal of additional treatment is to control the bleeding and restore normal levels of clotting factors. Blood transfusions may be required to replace clotting factors and to correct anemia that may occur with excess blood loss.
4. See Nursing Diagnosis: Anxiety (page 262).	

Hemophilia

Hemophilia is a recessive sex-linked hereditary bleeding disorder characterized by a deficiency of an essential clotting factor. It results from a mutation on the X chromosome. There are three forms of hemophilia:

- **hemophilia A** characterized by a deficiency of factor VIII; most common form; found exclusively in males
- **hemophilia B** characterized by a deficiency of factor IX; found exclusively in males
- **von Willebrand's disease** characterized by a defect in platelet adhesion and a deficiency in factor VIII; may occur in males and females

With hemophilia, the person experiences periods of exacerbations (hemorrhagic episodes) and remissions. The remission may last for several months. Often, when adolescence is reached, the frequency of hemorrhagic episodes begins to decline.

There is no cure for hemophilia. It is a chronic condition that requires lifetime adherence to safety precautions. The major cause of death with hemophilia is intracranial bleeding.

There is no screening test to detect carriers, hence the disease cannot be prevented. However, genetic counseling plays a significant role in controlling the incidence of the disease after it has been identified in a family member.

Females are carriers of the defective X chromosome. Carriers do not develop the disease but pass the disorder to all of their sons. Female offspring of male hemophiliacs are carriers, whereas the male offspring are normal. A female who is the offspring of a hemophiliac father and a carrier mother may develop hemophilia.

The mean LOS for a DRG classification of coagulation disorder is 5.5 days (Lorenz, 1991).

General Medical Management

- Periodic transfusions of fresh frozen plasma (FFP), cryoprecipitate, or lyophilized antihemolitic factor (AH7)

Integrative Care Plans

- Loss

420

Discharge Considerations

- Safety precautions
- Venipuncture technique for administration of clotting factor
- Signs and symptoms requiring medical intervention

 # ASSESSMENT DATA BASE

1. Inquire about a family history of bleeding disorders.

2. Inquire about unusual bleeding. Manifestations of hemophilia include persistent, slow bleeding following a minor cut or trauma (the most prominent finding). Spontaneous bleeding (bleeding without trauma) and petechiae do not occur in hemophilia. The disease is diagnosed early in the newborn when persistent prolonged bleeding occurs following a circumcision. Sometimes bleeding may stop, only to restart hours or days later.

3. Physical examination based upon a general survey (Appendix F) may reveal BLEEDING during periods of exacerbations:
   - hematoma formation (subcutaneous or intramuscular)
   - peripherial neuropathies — due to compression of a peripheral nerve from intramuscular hemorrhage. Look for severe pain, parasthesia, and muscle atrophy.
   - intracranial hemorrhage — headaches, visual disturbances, change in level of consciousness, rising BP and declining pulse rate, pupil inequality
   - hemarthrosis — bleeding into the joint. Look for severe pain, swelling, tenderness and stiffness of the affected joint.
   - hematuria
   - epistaxis

4. Diagnostic studies:
   - Factor assay studies are used to identify which clotting factor is deficient.
   - Partial thromboplastin time will be prolonged.

5. Assess the patient's and family's understanding of the condition and treatment.

6. Assess impact of condition upon current lifestyle.

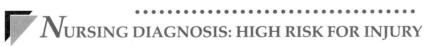 # NURSING DIAGNOSIS: HIGH RISK FOR INJURY

RELATED TO FACTORS: Uncontrollable bleeding secondary to hemophilia

DEFINING CHARACTERISTICS: May report history of hematoma formation, hemarthrosis, frequent bruising, prolonged bleeding, hematuria, or GI bleeding

PATIENT OUTCOME (collaborative): Demonstrates no further tissue injury

EVALUATION CRITERIA: Normal joint mobility, no further bruising, no permanent neurological deficits

INTERVENTIONS	RATIONALE
1. For head injury, monitor neurological status (Appendix J) q1–2h. Notify the physician at once if neurological deficits are detected, e.g headache, nausea, vomiting, inappropriate affect, impaired memory, dizziness, pupil changes, altered level of consciousness, impaired judgement or thought processes. Administer prescribed clotting factor and evaluate its effectiveness. Maintain bedrest in a semi-Fowler's or Fowler's position.	Head injury predisposes to intracranial hemorrhage. Clotting factors are required to stop bleeding. An erect position helps to reduce intracranial pressure associated with intracranial bleeding.
2. For hemarthrosis: • Monitor neurovascular status (Appendix D) of affected extremity. Notify the physician if joint swelling continues, or persistent pain or numbness and tingling occur once treatment has been initiated for 24 hours. • Maintain bedrest with affected joints elevated. Apply ice bag as ordered. Administer prescribed clotting factor and evaluate its effectiveness. • Initiate passive ROM exercises once swelling has subsided. Provide assistive device for ambulation. • Administer prescribed analgesic to control joint pain and evaluate its effectiveness.	Joint degeneration can occur with persistent bleeding into the joint. Clotting factors and cold application helps to halt bleeding. Immobility during bleeding episodes reduces circulation and hence helps to control bleeding. Exercise helps to maintain joint flexibility.
3. Avoid taking rectal temperatures. Administer oral medications when possible. Rotate injection sites and hold site for 5–10 minutes.	To reduce risk of bleeding.

INTERVENTIONS

4. For tissue swelling in or around the neck, nose, pharynx, or esophagus: • Monitor respiratory rate and breath sounds. • Keep oral airway and suction equipment at bedside. • Keep tracheostomy setup available. • Administer prescribed clotting factor and evaluate its effectiveness.	**RATIONALE** The risk of airway obstruction is great with severe neck injuries. Clotting factors are required to stop bleeding in or around the airway

NURSING DIAGNOSIS: HIGH RISK FOR ALTERATION IN HOME MAINTENANCE MANAGEMENT

RELATED TO FACTORS: Knowledge deficit about condition, treatment, and self-care measures

DEFINING CHARACTERISTICS: Verbalizes lack of understanding, requests information, may report history of noncompliance

PATIENT OUTCOME: Demonstrates a willingness to comply with therapeutic plan

EVALUATION CRITERIA: Verbalizes an understanding of condition and therapeutic plan

INTERVENTIONS

1. Evaluate patient and family's understanding of condition. Correct any misconceptions. Ensure that patient and family understand: a. Nature of the condition: what it is, how it is contracted, how to reduce the incidence in offspring. b. Purpose of prescribed treatments. Explain that cryopreciptate contains factor VIII and fibrinogen. It must be kept frozen, and then thawed when ready for use. Explain that the risk of contracting a blood-borne virus	**RATIONALE** Health teaching enhances patient compliance with prescribed therapeutic program.

INTERVENTIONS	RATIONALE
such as hepatitis or AIDS from cryopreciptate, lyophilized antihemolytic factor (AH7), or fresh frozen plasma (FFP) has been greatly reduced because all blood and blood products are now screened for these viruses.	
2. Refer the patient and family to the local chapter of the National Hemophilia Society.	This agency can provide written information about all aspects of hemophilia.
3. Teach the patient and family self-care measures to prevent injury. Instructions should include: • Avoid engaging in contact sports. • Avoid going barefoot. • Avoid aspirin and aspirin-containing products. Read product labels before buying over-the-counter medications. For pain, use acetominophen or propoxyphene instead. • Inform health care professionals of condition. Before undergoing any type of surgery or dental extraction, cryoprecipitate must be taken.	These measures are aimed at preventing bleeding.
4. Encourage the patient to wear a Medic Alert bracelet.	So that emergency personnel can readily identify condition in the event an emergency situation arises.
5. Teach first aid measures for injuries: a. Cuts and abrasions: Apply firm pressure for 5 minutes. If bleeding continues, administer cryoprecipitate. Report to emergency department for suturing if the cut is deep. Topical application of thrombin may be required to stop bleeding.	First-line intervention is essential to preventing permanent tissue damage. These measures help to control bleeding.

INTERVENTIONS	RATIONALE
b. Hemathrosis: Bedrest and immobilize the affected joint. Elevate the affected limb and apply ice. Administer cryo-precipitate. Report to emergency department if joint swelling and pain continues.	
6. Instruct the family and the patient to contact the physician or report to the hospital emergency department if either of the following occur: • severe pain and swelling of the joint unrelieved by first aid measures • head injury • swelling of tissue in the neck or the floor of the mouth • severe abdominal pain • hematuria • black, tarry stools	Hemophiliacs must learn which problems can be managed at home and which require immediate medical attention to offset permanent tissue damage.
7. Evaluate patient's and/or significant other's ability to administer clotting factors. Teach and have the patient and/or family member practice how to perform a venipuncture and administer the cryoprecipitate. Use a butterfly or wing-tip needle to teach venipuncture technique. Instruct the patient to carry a sup-ply of the concentrate with him at all times and to initiate the infusion as soon as possible if a bleeding episode occurs.	The quality and length of life can be enhanced by teaching the patient with a chronic illness how to live with it. Immediate infusion of cryoprecipitate with minor bleeding episodes can help prevent more serious bleeding.

▶ **NURSING DIAGNOSIS: HIGH RISK FOR DISTURBANCE IN SELF-CONCEPT**

RELATED TO FACTORS: Difficulty adapting to a chronic condition

DEFINING CHARACTERISTICS: Verbalizes negative feelings about lifetime limitations imposed by condition, may report history of non-compliance, may demonstrate behaviors consistent with grief

PATIENT OUTCOME: Demonstrates acceptance of self in current situation

EVALUATION CRITERIA: Verbalizes plans to incorporate limitations into current lifestyle, verbalizes an acceptance of condition, verbalizes fears and concerns freely

INTERVENTIONS	RATIONALE
1. Allow the patient and family to ventilate feelings. Encourage the family to avoid treating the person as an invalid. Emphasize the need to encourage participation in normal developmental activities which will not cause physical injury, e.g. swimming, golf, tennis.	Expressing feelings helps to facilitate coping. Normal developmental activities help to promote self-esteem.
2. Refer expressing difficulty making career choices to an occupational counselor for assistance in selecting an occupation/career which does not involve strenuous physical labor or pose a threat of physical injury.	Protection from physical injury is essential to controlling bleeding episodes.
3. See Loss (page 733).	
4. See Nursing Diagnosis: Anxiety, (page 262).	

- chronic blood loss
- history of chronic gastric ulcers or gastric resection
- presence of sickle cell disease
- currently taking chemotherapy
- renal failure
- chronic use of antibiotics
- nutritional deficiency
- extensive burns

2. Physical examination based on a general survey (Appendix F) may reveal:
   - fatigue, weakness (reflects tissue hypoxemia)
   - palpitations (reflects myocardial irritability because of hypoxemia)
   - light-headedness, irritability (reflects cerebral hypoxemia)
   - shortness of breath with exertion or tachypnea at rest (reflects impaired myocardial functioning because of hypoxemia)
   - pallor and complaints of being cold (reflects peripheral vascular vasoconstriction and shunting of blood to vital organs)

Additional symptoms may be present with severe nutritional deficiency anemias:

- iron deficiency— pica (craving of nonfood items such as clay, laundry starch)
- vitamin B_{12} deficiency— glossitis, neurological disturbances (symmetric paresthesia of hands and feet, disturbances in proprioception and vibratory sense, spastic ataxia)

3. Diagnostic studies:
   - CBC is below normal value (hemoglobin, hematocrit, and RBC).
   - Serum ferritin and iron levels are low in iron deficiency anemia.
   - Serum B_{12} level is low in pernicious anemia.
   - Direct combs test is positive indicating an autoimmune hemolytic anemia.
   - Hemoglobin electrophoresis identifies the type of abnormal hemoglobin in sickle cell diseases.
   - Schilling test used to diagnose vitamin B_{12} deficiency.

4. Assess patient's understanding of condition and treatment plan.

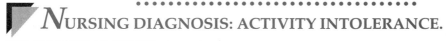

NURSING DIAGNOSIS: ACTIVITY INTOLERANCE.

RELATED TO FACTORS: Anemia

DEFINING CHARACTERISTICS: Reports persistent fatigue, exertional dyspnea; may report palpitations; may show tachycardia and tachypnea at rest

PATIENT OUTCOME (collaborative): Demonstrates increased tolerance to activities

EVALUATION CRITERIA: Fewer reports of fatigue and dyspnea when engaging in routine ADL, pulse rate 60–100 beats per minute, and respiratory rate 12–24 per minute at rest

• •

INTERVENTIONS	RATIONALE
1. Monitor: • results of CBC and arterial blood gases (ABG) reports • vital signs q4h • tolerance to physical activities	To identify indications of progress toward or deviations from expected outcomes.
2. Consult physician if the patient experiences irregular heart beats, persistent tachycardia, rales accompanied by diminished urinary output and increased blood pressure.	Cardiac abnormalities may develop with severe anemia because of myocardial hypoxemia. As a compensatory response to the low hemoglobin, heart rate increases to meet the body's demand for oxygen in the presence of a lower oxygen saturation of the blood. Body temperature may be lower than normal because of peripheral vasoconstriction and shunting of blood to central organs.
3. If the patient shows extreme hypoxia, perform prescribed treatments such as supplemental oxygen, blood transfusions, and bedrest in a semi-Fowler's position. If blood transfusion required, monitor for transfusion reaction (Table 6–2) per facility procedures. Implement facility protocol if a reaction occurs.	Supplement oxygen elevates the amount of oxygen available to RBCs. Bedrest reduces oxygen tissue demands. Transfusions of whole blood or packed RBCs provide a quick means of elevating the RBC count and hemoglobin and hematocrit values. An erect position allows fuller lung expansion.
4. Instruct the patient to engage in activities to tolerance and to avoid overexertion. Provide assistance as needed with ADL. Assist the patient in prioritizing activities and in planning rest periods throughout the day. Check pulse rate before and after physical activities.	Physical activity increases oxygen consumption. Rest reduces the body's energy demands. Physical endurance is enhanced when physical exertion is balanced with rest.
5. Encourage the patient to take antianemics as ordered, which may include supplements of iron, vitamin B_{12}, and folic acid. Explain purpose of prescribed supplements.	These nutrients are essential for erythropoiesis and synthesis of hemoglobin.

INTERVENTIONS	RATIONALE
6. If unable to take oral iron preparation and Imferon is prescribed, take appropriate steps to minimize discomfort from intramuscular injection of this drug: • Change the needle after withdrawing solution from the vial. • Use a Z-track method of injection. • Give deep intramuscular (IM) using the gluteal muscle. • Add 0.2 mL air to the medication-filled syringe.	Imferon is very irritating to subcutaneous tissue and can cause permanent staining. These measures ensure that the medication is deposited only into the musc
7. Encourage the patient to increase dietary intake of organ meats (especially liver), egg yolk, nuts, seafood, green leafy vegetables, whole grain breads and cereals.	These foods are excellent sources of iron, vitamin B_{12}, and folic acid.

• •

▶ NURSING DIAGNOSIS: HIGH RISK FOR IMPAIRED HOME MAINTENANCE MANAGEMENT

RELATED TO FACTORS: Knowledge deficit about condition and treatment plan

DEFINING CHARACTERISTICS: Verbalizes lack of understanding, requests information, reports history of noncompliance

PATIENT OUTCOME: Demonstrates willingness to comply with therapeutic plan

EVALUATION CRITERIA: Verbalizes understanding of condition and treatment plan, resolution of anemia

• •

INTERVENTIONS	RATIONALE
1. Discourage use of hot water bottles or heating pad to resolve cold sensitivity. Provide instructions about measures to conserve body heat to relieve cold sensitivity: • increasing room temperature • using extra blankets • wearing extra clothing	Application of a heat source directly to the body could result in burns. Cold sensitivity is a reflection of the body's attempt to compensate for chronic hypoxemia by lowering metabolic rate and shunting blood to vital organs. These heat conservation measures help prevent additional heat loss from the body.

INTERVENTIONS	RATIONALE
2. Provide information about the primary condition causing the anemia. Explain how it leads to anemia. Define anemia and its signs and symptoms. Explain purpose of prescribed therapy.	Health teaching promotes patient cooperation and compliance with the therapeutic plan.
3. If iron therapy is to be continued at home, provide the following instructions: • The medication turns stools dark green. • If constipation or diarrhea occurs, notify physician. A change in the dosage or interval can correct bowel problems. • Take the iron supplement with citrus juice because vitamin C and an acid medium enhance iron absorption. • Avoid taking iron with milk. An alkaline medium inhibits the absorption of iron. • Take after meals to minimize gastric discomfort. • If a liquid preparation is used, dilute with citrus juice and drink through a straw to prevent staining the teeth. • Keep follow-up appointments to have hemoglobin and hematocrit checked. • Report signs of iron toxicity to the physician: headache, metallic taste, joint stiffness.	Health teaching is essential to promoting safety in self-care at home.
4. Explain that it may take several weeks before results are noticed from oral iron supplements.	Depleted iron stores have to be replenished before evidence can be seen in serum studies, usually about two months.

TABLE 6–1. Bleeding Precautions

PRECAUTIONS WHEN RISK FOR BLEEDING EXISTS (PLATELET COUNT LESS THAN 50,000/CU MM^3)

1. Place a sign "Bleeding Precautions" above the patient's bed so other healthcare workers know of precautions.
2. Hold all venipuncture sites for five minutes.
3. Avoid intramuscular injections if possible.
4. Instruct the patient to avoid excessive physicial activity.
5. Administer platelet transfusions as ordered.
6. Use an electric razor for shaving instead of a blade.
7. Use a soft bristle toothbrush for brushing teeth.
8. Guaiac all stools and emesis for blood.
9. Avoid rectal temperatures and enemas.
10. Avoid aspirin and aspirin-containing products.
11. Inspect urine for gross hematuria.
12. Check color and consistency of stools. Black tarry stools reflect GI bleeding.
13. Instruct the patient to avoid going barefeet.
14. Inspect the skin, oral cavity, and conjunctiva daily and record extent of petechiae and bruising if present.
15. During menses, record the number of sanitary pads used.
16. Monitor results of coagulation studies (prothrombin time, partial thromboplastin time) and CBC.

PRECAUTIONS WHEN RISK FOR SPONTANEOUS HEMORRHAGING EXISTS (PLATELET COUNT LESS THAN 20,000/CU MM^3)

1. All of the above.
2. Administer stool softeners (if stool guaiac is negative).
3. Instruct the patient to avoid forceful nose blowing and coughing.
4. Maintain bedrest to avoid unecessary trauma.
5. Use toothettes for mouth care instead of a toothbrush.
6. Every 2–4 hours, encourage turning, deep breathing, and gentle range-of-motion exercises.
7. Avoid use of commercial mouthwashes. Use a saline solution or a mixture of sodium bicarbonate and hydrogen peroxide.
8. Keep skin lubricated with an emollient lotion or cream.

9. Keep head of bed elevated to reduce intracranial pressure and the risk of intracranial hemorrhage.

10. Monitor intake and output q2h. If output falls below 30 mL/hr, notify physician.

11. Monitor vital signs, skin color and temperature, pedal pulses, mental status, and lung sounds q4h.

TABLE 6–2. Types of Transfusion Reactions

TYPE	CAUSE	MANIFESTATIONS
Hemolytic	Infusion of incompatible blood, either ABO or Rh factor	back or chest pain, fever, chills, flushing
Febrile	Antileukocyte antibodies	fever, chills, headache, tachycardia
Allergic	Hypersensitivity to plasma antigens	urticaria, pruritus, erythematous rash, fever, chills
Anaphylactic	Most likely to occur in persons who lack IgA. RBCs without IgA must be given to prevent this reaction.	wheezing, hypotension, tachycardia, tachypnea

TABLE 6–3. Types of Sickle Cell Crisis

THROMBOLYTIC CRISIS (INFARCTIVE OR VASO-OCCLUSIVE CRISIS)

• Caused by obstruction of small blood vessels by sickle-shaped RBCs causing tissue hypoxia

• Primary manifestations:
  — severe pain that can occur anywhere in the body, but most often the chest, bones, and abdomen
  — fever with signs of obvious infection
  — severe anemia
  — hematuria (if infarct occurs in kidney)

• Primary complications:
  — priapism (painful, persistent penile erection); often requires surgical intervention to resolve this complication; permanent impotence is the surgical outcome
  — organ failure or dysfunction, (myocardial infarction, stroke, kidney failure, leg ulcers)

APLASTIC CRISIS

- Life-threatening condition characterized by suppression of the bone marrow due to engorgement by sickled RBCs
- Primary manifestations:
    - CBC reveals below normal WBC, RBC, and platelets
    - bleeding tendencies (reflecting thrombocytopenia)
    - activity intolerance, pallor, tachycardia (reflecting anemia)
    - fever (reflecting leukopenia)

HEMOLYTIC CRISIS

- Caused by rapid destruction of RBCs by the spleen; splenectomy may ultimately be required
- Primary manifestations:
    - hemoglobinuria
    - jaundice (caused by release of bilirubin from destroyed RBCs)
- Primary complication:
    - gallstones may develop with repeated attacks

BIBLIOGRAPHY

Arena, F.P. (1991). Update on acute lymphocytic leukemia. **Hospital Medicine, 27,** 33–36.

Herring, W.B., Romanan, S.V., & Reed, R.E. (1989). When the hematocrit rises. **Patient Care, 23,** 176–80, 185–188, 191.

Konradi, D. (1989). A close-up look at leukemia. **Nursing, 19,** 34–41.

Martinelli, A.M. (1991). Sickle cell disease: Etiology, symptoms, patient care. **Journal of Association of Operating Room Nurses, 53,** 716–720, 722–724.

Neely, S.M. (1989). Non-Hodgkin's lymphomas: Classification and staging as guides to therapy. **Consultant, 12,** 102–112.

Schneiderman, E. (1990). Thrombocytopenia in the critically ill patient. **Critical Care Nursing Quarterly, 13,** 1–6.

Weborn, J.L. (1991). A three point approach to anemia. **Postgraduate Medicine, 89,** 179–183, 186, 221–223.

Young, L.M. (1990). DIC: The insidious killer. **Critical Care Nurse, 10,** 2–28, 30, 32–33.

CHAPTER SEVEN

Problems of the Cardiovascular System

Myocardial Infarction

Acute myocardial infarction (AMI), also called a heart attack, refers to regional destruction of myocardial tissue when blood supply is suddenly impaired by either chronic narrowing of a coronary artery from atherosclerosis or complete occlusion from an embolus or thrombus. The infarcted tissue is permanently destroyed resulting in loss of contractile function.

The major complications associated with AMI are heart failure, arrhythmias, and cardiogenic shock. With extensive blockage, large areas of the myocardium are destroyed and death can occur. Elderly patients are at increased risk for developing complications because of the normal physiological changes that occur with the aging process, such as thickening of medial layer of the blood vessels that causes vessel narrowing and fibrous tissue buildup in the myocardium, resulting in reduced contractility and reduced cardiac output (Gawlinski & Jensen, 1991).

The most critical time for the patient with AMI is the initial 48 hours. The patient is placed in a coronary care unit (CCU) for about 3–5 days and then transferred to a telemetry unit until discharged. The mean LOS for a DRG classification of AMI is 8.2 days (Lorenz, 1991).

All patients experiencing an AMI do not experience chest pain. Some persons, approximately 10% of mostly middle-aged men, may experience a silent MI (Gawlinski & Jensen, 1991). For years these persons may experience silent ischemia, their heart disease progressing without symptoms, until a severe MI occurs. Persons having three or more risk factors for heart disease are at risk for silent ischemia. It can be detected by any of the following tests: stress test, Holter monitoring, or cardiac imaging (thallium scans, stress echo test, or cardiac catheterization).

General Medical Management

- Pharmacotherapy:
  - anticoagulants (to prevent formation of new clots)
  - nitrates (to maintain vasodilation, thus reducing afterload and preload)
  - calcium channel blocking agents (to promote vasodilation and reduce myocardial contractility)
  - beta-adrenergic blocking agents (to reduce myocardial contractility, thus oxygen consumption)

445

— thrombolytic agents such as tissue plasminogen activator (tPA), urokinase, or streptokinase (to dissolve existing blood clots); may be given intravenously within 4–6 hours from onset of chest pain.

• Surgery:

— for persistent, chronic, incapacitating chest pain: coronary artery bypass graft (CABG) or percutaneous transluminal coronary angioplasty (PTCA). PTCA involves insertion and inflation of a balloon-tip catheter into the occluded coronary artery to compress the atheromatous lesion and spread it over the vessel wall, thus improving blood flow to the myocardium. Patients with single-vessel disease and whose anginal attacks have been occurring less than one year are the best candidates for PTCA. Patients must continue drug therapy as before the procedure and continue lifestyle changes, reflecting risk factor modification since this is a treatment modality not a cure. The procedure for PTCA is the same for coronary arteriography, except that the CABG team is on standby in case of complications. Also, laser angioplasty may be done. Although does not cure angina it helps lessen the intensity of chest pain.

• Dietary modification:

— reduced sodium and cholesterol

Integrative Care Plans

• IV Therapy
• Loss
• Coronary artery disease
• Immobility

Discharge Considerations

• Follow-up care
• Dietary modifications
• Exercise program
• Community support groups
• Medications to continue at home
• Signs and symptoms requiring medical attention
• Activity limitations

*A*SSESSMENT DATA BASE

1. History or presence of risk factors:
   • coronary artery disease
   • previous heart attack
   • positive family history of heart disease or heart attacks
   • high serum cholesterol level (above 200 mg/dL)

- excessive cigarette smoking
- routine high-fat diet
- obesity
- a sedentary lifestyle
- postmenopausal female on estrogen therapy
- middle-aged male (especially one with a type A personality)

2. Physical examination based on a cardiovascular assessment (Appendix G) may reveal:
- Chest pain that is unrelieved by rest or nitrates (most significant finding). It is often accompanied by:
  — feelings of impending doom and/or death
  — diaphoresis
  — nausea and sometimes vomiting
  — dyspnea
  — shock syndrome in varying degrees (ashen, cool, clammy skin, falling BP, rapid pulse, diminished peripheral pulses, poor capillary refill, diminished heart sounds)
  — fever (within 24–48 hours)

3. Assess chest pain in relation to:
- Provoking factors. Ask the patient, "What provokes the pain?" or "What were you doing just before the chest pain started?" Chest pain begins spontaneously and is not associated with any precipitating factor.
- Quality. Ask the patient, "What does the pain feel like?" The pain is often described as a heavy tightening, constricting, or choking sensation.
- Region. Ask the patient, "Where does the pain occur? Does it move or remain in the same place?" Often the pain occurs substernally and radiates to the neck, jaw, back, shoulder, or down the left arm. Or the pain may occur in the epigastric region. The patient often interprets this as indigestion and takes antacids without relief.
- Severity. Ask the patient, "How bad is the pain—mild, moderate or severe? What relieves the pain?" Often the pain is severe and incapacitating. It is not relieved by rest or nitrates.
- Time. Ask the patient, "How long ago did the pain start? How often does the pain occur?" The pain often persists for hours or days. Typically during an attack the patient clenches the fist over the chest or rubs the left arm.

4. After chest pain has subsided, assess the patient's feelings and concerns about current condition and perceptions about impact on current lifestyle.

5. Diagnostic studies:
- EKG reveals ST segment displacement, Q waves, and T wave changes.
- Chest x ray rules out cardiac enlargement and pulmonary congestion.

- CBC reveals leukocytosis.
- Cardiac enzymes (Gawlinski, 1989):
  — creatine kinase (CK)–isoenzyme MB begins to rise in six hours, peaks in 18–24 hours, and returns to normal within 3–4 days, unless new necrosis occurs. The CK–MB enzyme is the most reliable indicator of an AMI because it is produced only by damaged myocardial tissue.
  — lactic dehydrogenase (LDH) begins to rise in 6–12 hours, peaks in 3–4 days, and remains elevated for 6–12 days.
  — Serum aspartate aminotransferase (AST) begins to rise in 8–12 hours and peaks in 1–2 days. This enzyme rises with severe damage to any muscles in the body.
- Additional testing include serum electrolytes, serum lipids, urinalysis, arterial blood gases (ABG).

◢ NURSING DIAGNOSIS: PAIN

RELATED TO FACTORS: Cardiac tissue ischemia

DEFINING CHARACTERISTICS: Verbalizes chest pain, clenched fist over chest, rubbing left arm, moaning and frowning accompanied by tachypnea and tachycardia

PATIENT OUTCOME (collaborative): Demonstrates relief from chest pain

EVALUATION CRITERIA: Denies chest pain, relaxed facial expression, respiratory rate 12–24 per minute, pulse rate 60–100 beats per minute

INTERVENTIONS	RATIONALE
1. Administer oxygen via nasal annula at 6 L/min if no history of chronic lung disease; 2 L/min if history is positive.	The myocardium requires a constant supply of oxygen. Supplemental oxygen increases arterial oxygen tension.
2. Initiate prescribed IV therapy and perform maintenance activities (page 764).	To provide vascular access for administration of medications.
3. Administer prescribed medication for chest pain prn and evaluate effectiveness. Withhold the analgesic and notify physician if respirations fall to less than 12 per minute, pulse rate is greater than 100 beats per minute, and BP is less than 90/60 mm Hg.	Morphine sulfate, a narcotic analgesic, helps block the pain pathway. It also produces systemic vasodilation thus reducing afterload. With effective pain control, anxiety can also be lessened. These vital sign values represent early stages of shock, an indication of impending heart failure.

INTERVENTIONS	RATIONALE
4. Give stool softeners as ordered and high-fiber foods to prevent constipation.	Straining with defecation and using a bed-pan triggers the Valsalva maneuver, increases intrathoracic pressure, and compresses the coronary arteries, which could trigger angina or arrhythmias.
5. Administer prescribed nitrates, beta-adrenergic blocking agent, or calcium channel blocking agents and evaluate their effectiveness. Withhold the drug if hypotension or bradycardia occurs and notify physician.	Nitrates act directly on the smooth muscles to cause generalized vasodilation. Beta-adrenergic blocking agents act by blocking sympathetic impulses to the heart, thus reducing heart rate, blood pressure, and myocardial contractility and ultimately reducing myocardial oxygen consumption. Calcium channel blocking agents act by blocking the influx of calcium in the smooth muscles of the coronary arterioles, resulting in vasodilation, reduced myocardial contractility, and reduced systemic vascular resistance.
6. Maintain bedrest in a semi-Fowler's position until chest pain subsides.	Physical exertion increases tissue demands for oxygen, placing an additional strain on damaged myocardium. To meet increased oxygen demands, myocardial contractility and heart rate have to increase. These physiological responses increase chest pain.

◤ NURSING DIAGNOSIS: ACTIVITY INTOLERANCE

RELATED TO FACTORS: Decreased cardiac output secondary to AMI

DEFINING CHARACTERISTICS: Verbalizes fatigue and recurring chest pain with ADL , tachycardia and tachypnea with minimal physical exertion

PATIENT OUTCOME: Demonstrates improved tolerance to activities

EVALUATION CRITERIA: Fewer reports of palpitations, chest pain, fatigue, and shortness of breath when performing ADL

INTERVENTIONS	RATIONALE
1. Monitor: • vital signs q2h while in CCU; less often if stable • cardiovascular status (Appendix G) on each shift • bowel elimination daily • results of cardiac enzyme studies • intake and output on each shift • ECG recording frequently	To identify indications of progress toward or deviations from expected outcome.
2. Maintain bedrest 24–48 hours after AMI.	To reduce myocardial oxygen demand. Within a few days, collateral circulation develops to supply blood to areas of diminished perfusion.
3. Plan nursing activities to allow for long periods of uninterrupted rest.	Rest allows the body to restore energy.
4. Assist with ADL. Allow the patient to participate more in performing daily hygienic care if cardiac enzyme levels begin to fall. Report cardiac enzymes that persist past the expected peak period.	Cardiac enzyme levels that are 4–8 times the normal values are associated with complications of AMI such as arrhythmias, congestive heart failure, and cardiogenic shock.
5. Keep the patient in semi-Fowler's or Fowler's position.	Fuller lung expansion is attained in an erect position. This position also helps reduce venous return and thus cardiac workload when heart failure is imminent.

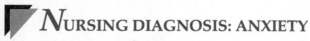

NURSING DIAGNOSIS: ANXIETY

RELATED TO FACTORS: Fear of threat of sudden death and knowledge deficit about condition, diagnostic studies, and treatment plan

DEFINING CHARACTERISTICS: May verbalize fear of sudden death, may verbalize concerns about role changes in the family, verbalizes lack of understanding, may express concerns about impact of condition on sexual functioning, may report insomnia

PATIENT OUTCOME (collaborative): Demonstrates relief from anxiety

EVALUATION CRITERIA: Verbalizes understanding of condition, diagnostic studies, treatment plan; fewer reports of feeling anxious or nervous; relaxed facial expression

• •

INTERVENTIONS	RATIONALE
1. See Nursing Diagnosis: Anxiety (page 262).	
2. Encourage involvement of significant others in the patient's rehabilitation program.	Support systems, such as significant others, help reinforce the person's coping mechanisms.
3. Maintain effective pain control. Administer prescribed antianxiety agents, such as diazepam (Valium), prn and evaluate their effectiveness.	Severe anxiety increases heart rate, thus placing an additional strain on an already weakened heart.
4. Provide simple explanations of all treatments during painful episodes. Reserve more detailed teaching until after pain is controlled.	Patients retain less information when they are anxious, and too much information increases their worries. Pain interferes with learning.

• •

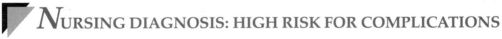

NURSING DIAGNOSIS: HIGH RISK FOR COMPLICATIONS

RELATED TO FACTORS: Myocardial tissue damage

DEFINING CHARACTERISTICS: May demonstrate arrhythmias (irregular heart rate and rhythm) or congestive heart failure (dependent edema, rales, tachycardia, BP greater than 140/90 mm Hg)

PATIENT OUTCOME (collaborative): Cardiac function remains stable

EVALUATION CRITERIA: Absence of symptoms of congestive heart failure and regular heart rate and rhythm, LOS does not exceed DRG classification

• •

INTERVENTIONS	RATIONALE

Arrhythmias:
 	
1. Monitor:
  • ECG tracings frequently
  • results of serum electrolyte studies, especially serum potassium
	To identify indications of progress toward or deviations from expected outcome. A potassium imbalance can precipitate arrhythmias.

2. Connect to ECG monitor. Administer appropriate medication to treat the specific arrhythmia. Place a strip of the ECG tracing on the chart each shift and prn when an arrhythmia is observed.	ECG monitoring allows for early detection of arrhythmias and prompt treatments. Persistent arrhythmias predispose patient to diminished cardiac output. A strip provides a permanent record of the patient's medical history.
3. Report abnormal heart rates and rhythms to the physician immediately. Treat arrhythmias immediately according to facility protocol and procedures.	Arrhythmias predispose patient to diminished cardiac output by increasing preload–venous return. This places an additional strain on an already compromised myocardium.
Congestive Heart Failure: 1. See Congestive Heart Failure (page 462).	

NURSING DIAGNOSIS: HIGH RISK FOR IMPAIRED HOME MAINTENANCE MANAGEMENT

RELATED TO FACTORS: Inability to accept lifestyle changes imposed by chronic condition, knowledge deficit about self-care activities on discharge

DEFINING CHARACTERISTICS: May deny seriousness of condition, may verbalize hopelessness or depression over perceived losses, verbalizes lack of understanding, requests information, may report history of noncompliance

PATIENT OUTCOME: Demonstrates willingness to follow prescribed plan for home maintenance and prevention

EVALUATION CRITERIA: Verbalizes acceptance of responsibility for required self-care activities, verbalizes realistic plans relative to present situation

INTERVENTIONS	RATIONALE
1. See Loss (page 733).	
2. Explore patient's concerns about sexual activity after AMI and provide sexual counseling. A simple statement like the following may be used: "After a heart attack, many patients have concerns about when to resume sexual activity or even fear that sexual activity may cause another heart attack. Would you like to discuss this area of concern?" Encourage the patient to ask the physician when sexual activity can be resumed. Let the patient know that in most cases sexual activity can be resumed within 2–4 weeks, depending on the severity of the attack. Advise the patient to take the following precautions when sexual activity is resumed: • Take nitroglycerin (NTG) prophylactically if angina is experienced during sexual intercourse. • Avoid engaging in sexual activity when tired, after eating a heavy meal, or after alcohol intake. • Contact physician if dyspnea during sexual intercourse, palpitations or increased heart rate lasting more than 15 minutes after intercourse, or insomnia after intercourse occurs.	Sexuality is an important component of self-concept. A sudden illness requiring alterations in one's lifestyle often causes concern about one's sexuality. Nitroglycerin allows dilation of coronary vessels, thus improving blood flow to the myocardium. Certain activities place additional strain on weaken heart. These symptoms signal myocardial ischemia.

INTERVENTIONS	RATIONALE
3. Initiate cardiac rehabilitation program per facility protocol. Refer the patient to the local chapter of the American Heart Association.	A cardiac rehabilitation program begins with admission. It is a program, supervised by a nurse and/or physical therapist, that allows the patient to gradually return to a level of physical independence beginning with activities of daily living (ADL) and progressing to a regular exercise program that continues on discharge. The American Heart Association provides information about heart disease, preventive and maintenance self-care activities, and local support groups. Continued support is essential to help individuals adapt to lifestyle changes.
4. Provide information about the nature of heart disease and prevention. Instruction should include: a. Stop smoking. Explain that nicotine causes vasoconstriction. b. Reduce weight if obese. Refer to dietitian for assistance in planning a weight reduction diet. Explain that excess body fat places additional strain on damaged myocardium. c. Adhere to a fat-controlled diet to control serum cholesterol levels and reduce sodium intake. • Avoid fried foods. • Remove skin from chicken. • Use lean meats without visible fat. • Use skim milk and cheeses instead of whole milk. • Limit intake of egg yolks to no more than three per week. • Use polyunsaturated oils and margarine instead of butter, lard, or shortening.	The risk of recurrence of an AMI is decreased by reducing exposure to those factors contributing to atherosclerosis.

INTERVENTIONS	RATIONALE
• Limit intake of red meat, luncheon meats, bacon, and sausage. • Eat more fish, chicken, turkey, and veal. d. Follow prescribed antihypertensive diet and take prescribed antihypertensive medication if hypertensive. Explain that hypertension increases workload of the heart. e. Participate in a planned exercise program to exercise the heart. Encourage regular walking if a community rehabilitation program is not available. Avoid exercising immediately after eating. Instruct the patient to do mild stretching for five minutes before and after exercising to "warm up" and "cool down." Explain that exercise helps improve circulation, increases the production of high-density lipoprotein (HDL), and exercises the heart muscle. Low-density lipoproteins (LDL) carry the greatest risk for coronary artery disease (CAD).	
5. Ensure the patient has a written appointment for follow-up care and written instructions for preventive and maintenance activities.	Verbal instructions may be easily forgotten.
6. Teach the patient how to assess pulse rate. If treadmill testing is not available or not done, instruct the patient to monitor pulse rate before beginning exercises and during exercises until maximum exercise level is attained. Explain that maximum exercise level would be 20 beats per minute over the resting pulse.	Pulse rate is a good indicator of activity exercise tolerance. Usually a treadmill test is performed to determine a patient's maximum exercise level before an exercise program is started. If treadmill testing is not available, pulse rate can be used to monitor exercise tolerance.

INTERVENTIONS	RATIONALE
7. If hypertension or diabetes mellitus coexist, emphasize the importance of taking prescribed medication and following prescribed treatment program.	These conditions are associated with a high incidence of atherosclerosis.
8. Teach the patient how to minimize anginal attacks. **Instructions should include:** • reassess priorities in view of current health needs and learn ways to cope with unavoidable stress. Explain that excess stress causes vasoconstriction, which increases cardiac workload. • plan time for rest periods to allow the body to replenish energy lost with activity. • eat smaller portions of food and avoid hurried eating. Explain that an increased blood supply is needed to digest large meals, which places additional stress on the heart to increase cardiac output. • reduce intake of caffeine beverages because they increase the heart rate. • wait at least two hours after eating before engaging in physical exercises to allow food to digest. • wear warm clothing in cold weather since exposure to cold causes vasoconstriction, which reduces blood flow to the heart muscle. • avoid constipation since straining with stools initiates the Valsalva maneuver, which increases intrathoracic pressure and compresses the coronary arteries.	An understanding of the relationship between the therapeutic plan and the condition helps promote compliance.

INTERVENTIONS	RATIONALE
9. If NTG tablets are prescribed, instruct the patient to take one before engaging in activities that precipitate angina.	NTG produces vasodilation, which allows for increased blood flow to the myocardium. Chest pain occurs when blood flow to the myocardium is inhibited.
10. If nitroglycerin is prescribed for prn use, provide the following information and instructions: • NTG dilates blood vessels to allow more blood to the heart muscle. • Expect a slight headache and a sensation of warmth that lasts only briefly, until the body adjusts to the dosage. Contact the physician if headache and palpitations persist because these findings indicate a need for reducing the dosage. **For tablets:** • Carry NTG tablets always. • Keep the bottle in a cool, dry place. • Keep tablets tightly capped in its dark-colored glass bottle because they are light-sensitive. • Discard unused tablets after six months and replace with new ones. • At first sign of chest pain, place one tablet under the tongue. Do not swallow the saliva until the tablet has dissolved to allow complete absorption of the drug. Rest until pain has subsided. If chest pain is not relieved in five minutes, take another tablet. If no relief occurs in five minutes after the second tablet, take a third tablet. If no relief occurs in five minutes after the third tablet, contact the physician or go to the nearest emergency facility. • NTG tablets are not addictive and may be taken as often as needed for chest pain.	Health teaching is essential to safety in self-medication administration.

INTERVENTIONS

RATIONALE

For topicals:

- Do not rub the ointment into the skin.
- Topical agent may be applied anywhere on the body.
- Remove the old ointment or patch after applying the new one.
- Topicals must be applied at prescribed intervals to maintain a consistent blood level of the drug. Unlike NTG tablets, they cannot be used prn.

Coronary Artery Disease

The underlying disease process in coronary artery disease (CAD) is atherosclerosis. In atherosclerosis, fatty fibrous plaques adhere to the lumen of the coronary arteries causing them to become hard, rigid (arteriosclerosis), and narrow. Blood flow through the narrowed lumen is reduced which often causes myocardial ischemia. Plaque formation predisposes one to thrombosis, which can lead to acute myocardial infarction. For unclear reasons, the aorta and arteries in the brain, kidney, and heart are more susceptible to atherosclerotic changes.

Patients with CAD often remain asymptomatic for years and initially seek medical attention because of severe angina pectoris (chest pain). An anginal attack is not indicative of a heart attack; however, it does signal heart disease and an increased risk for a heart attack. Angina pectoris is believed to occur from spasms of the coronary artery. It does not result in permanent damage to the myocardium as does acute myocardial infarction (Shoemaker et al, 1989).

When a patient presents with symptoms of CAD, a thorough assessment must be done to rule out other conditions associated with chest pain, such as thoracic aortic aneurysm, pleurisy, pericarditis, AMI, pneumothorax, or hiatal hernia. The patient is usually kept in an ICU until it is determined that an acute myocardial infarction is not being experienced and until arrhythmias, if present, are controlled.

There is no cure for coronary artery disease because the underlying disease process is atherosclerosis. Medical therapy is aimed at controlling the progression of the disease.

General Medical Management

- Pharmacotherapy:
  - nitrates
  - first drug of choice in relieving angina pectoris
  - beta-adrenergic blocking agents and calcium channel blocking agent if nitrates fail to control attacks
  - dietary modification (reducing fat content to lower cholesterol level)
  - medications that reduce serum lipids if dietary measures fail to maintain a serum cholesterol level less than 200 mg/dL):
    a. agents that restrict lipoprotein production:
      - nicotinic acid (niacin)
      - clofibrate (Atromid-S)

   b. agents that speed the removal of lipoproteins:
      — cholestyramine (Questran)
* Surgery if above measures fail to control angina:
   — percutaneous transluminal coronary angioplasty (PTCA)
   — coronary artery bypass graft (CABG)

Integrative Care Plans

* Loss

Discharge Considerations

* Follow-up care
* Medications to continue at home
* Signs and symptoms requiring medical attention
* Dietary modifications
* Preventive and maintenance activities

ASSESSMENT DATA BASE

1. History or presence of risk factors. The three most significant risk factors in the development of atherosclerosis are elevated serum lipids, hypertension, and cigarette smoking. Other associated factors include stress, a positive family history, obesity, sedentary lifestyle, estrogen therapy in postmenopausal women, birth control pills, and diabetes mellitus.

2. Physical examination based on a cardiovascular assessment (Appendix G) may reveal:
   * angina pectoris (chest pain) (most prominent finding) that may be accompanied by:
      — feelings of apprehension
      — urge to void
      — diaphoresis
      — nausea
      — dyspnea
      — cool extremities

3. Assess the chest pain to identify the type of angina:
   * Stable angina — chest pain occurring intermittently with a predictable pattern of onset, duration, and intensity. It is relieved by rest and lasts less than 15 minutes.
   * Unstable angina — unpredictable chest pain that occurs at any time, even at rest or during sleep. The attacks generally last over 20 minutes and progressively increase in frequency, intensity, and duration. This type often leads to a myocardial infarction within 3–18 months.

- Nocturnal angina — chest pain occurs at night, usually during sleep. It can be relieved by sitting.

- Angina decubitus — chest pain precipitated by lying and relieved by sitting.

- Prinzmetal's angina — chest pain occurring at rest with sudden onset. Increased risk for myocardial infarction.

4. Assess chest pain in relation to:

- Provoking factors. Ask the patient, "What provokes the pain?" or "What were you doing just before the chest pain started?" Generally, any event that places a severe strain on the heart rate or reduces myocardial blood flow can precipitate angina:

   — cigarette smoking

   — excessive physical exertion

   — eating a heavy meal

   — emotional stress

   — sexual activity

   — drinking cold beverages or exposure to cold

- Quality. Ask the patient, "What does the pain feel like?" The pain is often described as a burning, squeezing, or choking sensation.

- Region. Ask the patient, "Where does the pain occur? Does it move or remain in the same place?" Often the pain occurs in the substernal or midanterior chest and radiates to the neck, jaw, shoulder blade, or down the left arm.

- Severity. Ask the patient, "How bad is the pain — mild, moderate, or severe? What relieves the pain?" The chest pain may be mild, moderate, or severe and is relieved by rest.

- Time. Ask the patient, "How long ago did the pain start? How often does the pain occur?"

- Typically during an attack of chest pain, the patient clenches the fist over the chest or rubs the left arm. The onset of pain may be gradual or sudden and last 15 minutes or longer.

5. Assess the patient's feelings and concerns about condition and perceived impact on lifestyle.

6. Diagnostic studies:

- EKG may show ST segment depression during the actual painful attack; otherwise, the EKG is normal when the patient is pain-free.

- Chest x ray determines if there is cardiac enlargement or pulmonary congestion.

- Cardiac enzymes (CK–MB, AST, LDH) rule out myocardial infarction. Usually, these enzymes are normal.

- Serum lipid level is usually elevated. Cholesterol and triglycerides are the predominant elevated lipids in CAD.

   Later when the patient is stabilized, additional testing may include treadmill exercise test, nuclear imaging, or coronary angiography.

7. See Myocardial Infarction (page 445) for the remainder of this plan of care.

Congestive Heart Failure

Heart failure, more commonly called **congestive heart failure** (CHF), refers to the inability of the heart to meet the oxygen and nutrient demands of the body. CHF is sequelae of myocardial dysfunction. It is characterized by diminished cardiac output and increased intravascular volume. Any condition that results in damage to the myocardium, thus impairing the ability of the heart to contract, can cause CHF.

The ventricles are most commonly affected. Either the left or right ventricle may be affected initially, most often the left. Right ventricle failure is seen as cor pulmonale secondary to chronic lung disease. Eventually, both ventricles are affected.

When myocardial damage occurs gradually, the heart attempts to compensate by an increased rate (tachycardia), enlarging muscle mass (hypertrophy), and by enlargement of the chamber (dilation). As these compensatory mechanisms are exhausted, the patient becomes symptomatic.

Excess fluid retention by the body is the underlying basis for the symptoms that occur in CHF. As compensatory mechanisms fail, cardiac output falls, causing a reduction in renal perfusion, hence glomerular filtration. The body responds to this reduced renal blood flow by generalized vasoconstriction, secretion of aldosterone from the adrenal cortex, and by releasing antidiuretic hormone from the hypothalamus (Shoemaker et al, 1989). The result is increased sodium and water reabsorption in the renal tubules, hence increased intravascular volume.

CHF may be acute (develops quickly) or chronic (develops slowly). A patient in acute CHF fears that death is imminent, is restless, has reduced powers of concentration, and is often lethargic due to hypoxia. Hypoxia occurs when fluid extravasates from the pulmonary capillary bed into the alveoli, thus impairing gas exchange.

General Medical Management

• Pharmacotherapy:
  — digitalis preparations (to slow heart rate and increase the force of ventricular contractions thus increasing cardiac output)
  — diuretics (to help rid the body of excess fluid, thus reducing pulmonary venous pressure)
  — vasodilators (to reduce afterload [peripheral vascular resistance] thereby improving cardiac output)

- Low-sodium diet
- Supplemental oxygen
- Bedrest

Digitalis is one of the major drugs used to treat CHF. For acute CHF, the physician usually prescribes a loading or digitalizing dose given intravenously. This involves giving a large dose within 24–48 hours. Serum digitalis levels are assessed daily during digitalization to determine when a therapeutic level has been reached. The patient then is placed on a maintenance dose (usually 0.125 mg or 0.25 mg) when the therapeutic level has been reached.

Drug therapy is not curative but helps to control the symptoms. Drug therapy and diet therapy must be followed for life. Often a potassium supplement is prescribed for patients taking maintenance doses of a potassium-wasting diuretic (thiazide or loop diuretics). Providing a supplement is the preferred alternative to eating potassium rich foods because these foods also add calories. Moreover, to be effective potassium-rich foods must be eaten daily. High-potassium foods are bananas, oranges, orange juice, and dried fruits.

Integrative Care Plan

- Loss
- Myocardial infarction
- Immobility

Discharge Considerations

- Follow-up care
- Medications to continue at home
- Signs and symptoms of increasing heart failure
- Dietary modifications
- Activity limitations
- Community support agencies

 # ASSESSMENT DATA BASE

1. History or presence of causative factors such as hypertension, valvular or congenital heart disease, myocardial infarction, or renal failure.
2. Physical examination based on a cardiovascular assessment (Appendix G) and a general survey (Appendix F) may reveal pulmonary edema (outstanding clinical feature in left ventricular failure).

Left ventricular failure is characterized by:

- rales
- dyspnea on exertion
- narrowing pulse pressure
- orthopnea

- productive cough (may be frothy or blood-tinged sputum)
- paroxysmal nocturnal dyspnea (sudden awakening from sleep in acute respiratory distress caused by extravasation of fluid into the alveoli while in a supine position)
- Cheyne-Stokes respirations, with severe CHF

Right ventricular failure is characterized by systemic venous congestion and peripheral edema:

- jugular vein distention (JVD) when in a sitting position
- anorexia
- anasarca

Clinical findings common to both left and right ventricular failure:

- fatigue and weakness
- tachycardia
- cyanosis, with severe heart failure
- pale, dusky, sweaty skin
- weight gain
- systolic murmur
- diastolic gallop rhythm (third heart sound during diastole)
- oliguria
- increased pulmonary artery and capillary wedge pressures
- increased right atrial pressure (also called central venous pressure, CVP)

3. Assess the patient's feelings and concerns about having a chronic condition and its perceived impact on lifestyle.

4. Diagnostic studies:
   - Chest x ray reveals cardiomegaly, interstitial edema, or pleural effusion. These findings confirm a diagnosis of CHF.
   - EKG reveals tachycardia, chamber hypertrophy, and ischemia (if caused by AMI).
   - Serum electrolytes reveal low sodium level resulting from hemodilution of the blood from excess fluid retention.

▶ NURSING DIAGNOSIS: ACTIVITY INTOLERANCE

RELATED TO FACTORS: Decreased cardiac output

DEFINING CHARACTERISTICS: Verbalizes fatigue, palpitations, and shortness of breath with physical exertion; may report chest pain with physical exertion

PATIENT OUTCOME: Demonstrates improved tolerance to activity

EVALUATION CRITERIA: Fewer reports of shortness of breath, palpitations, weakness, and fatigue when engaging in activities of daily living (ADL); denies chest pain, absence of tachypnea with minimal physical exertion

INTERVENTIONS	RATIONALE
1. Monitor tolerance to activities. During the acute phase, check pulse rate before and after activity. Begin activities progressively when allowed. Plan activities to allow for long periods of uninterrupted rest. Reduce activity if the patient experiences a pulse rate 20 beats per minute (bpm) above the resting pulse, shortness of breath, or chest pain.	Physical endurance can be increased when activities are performed in increments. These findings indicate the patient has reached maximum activity limit.
2. Assist with ADL as needed. Maintain bedrest as ordered and perform measures to prevent complications of immobility (page 725).	Rest reduces cardiac workload by reducing energy requirements of the body.

NURSING DIAGNOSIS: FLUID VOLUME EXCESS

RELATED TO FACTORS: Heart failure

DEFINING CHARACTERISTICS: Peripheral edema, pulmonary rales, weight gain, increased BP accompanied by tachycardia and tachypnea, anasarca, jugular vein distention, serum sodium below normal range

PATIENT OUTCOME (collaborative): Demonstrates fluid and biochemical balance

EVALUATION CRITERIA: Decreasing weight, clear breath sounds, vital signs within normal limits, urinary output greater than 30 mL/hr, serum electrolytes within normal limits, absence of edema, strong pedal pulses, improved skin color

INTERVENTIONS	RATIONALE
1. Monitor: • weight daily • cardiovascular status (Appendix G) q2h, less often when stable • vital signs q2h • intake and output q8h • results of laboratory studies, for example, digitalis level, serum electrolytes, ABG • hemodynamic values every hour if a pulmonary artery catheter is in place	To evaluate effectiveness of therapy.
2. Administer prescribed cardiac glycoside safely and evaluate its effectiveness:. • Check apical pulse for one full minute before giving the drug. Withhold the drug if pulse rate is less than 60 bpm. Wait one hour, then reassess pulse. If pulse rate is still below 60 bpm, check BP and consult physician. • Report factors that predispose patient to digitalis toxicity: — acidosis — hypokalemia — hypomagnesemia — hypercalcemia — renal or hepatic dysfunction — serum digitalis level above normal range • Report manifestations of digitalis toxicity: — GI disturbances (nausea, vomiting, anorexia, diarrhea). — visual disturbances (halo vision, double vision, blurred vision) — cardiac disturbances (bradycardia, arrhythmias)	Digitalis increases the force of myocardial contractions and slows heart rate. If toxicity occurs, the drug is discontinued and the underlying predisposing factor corrected.

INTERVENTIONS	RATIONALE
3. Maintain the patient in a semi-Fowler's or Fowler's position.	To reduce venous return to the heart.
4. Initiate prescribed IV therapy. Perform preventive and maintenance measures for IV therapy (page 764). Use a volume-control pump for all IV fluids.	Vascular access is needed to administer urgent medications. The risk of fluid overload is controlled by using an infusion pump for IV fluids.
5. Administer oxygen at 2 L/min or as prescribed based on the results of the ABG report.	To increase arterial oxygen tension thereby relieving dyspnea and fatigue.
6. Administer prescribed vasodilators. Use a volume-control pump to administer these drugs when ordered intravenously. Check BP q15–30min. Titrate flow rate to maintain BP at the level prescribed by physician.	Vasodilators decrease afterload (vascular resistance), thereby reducing the workload of the heart. Hypotension is a major side effect of these drugs.
7. Administer prescribed diuretic and evaluate its effectiveness. Let the patient know to expect an increased urinary output with diuretic therapy.	Diuretics rid the body of excess fluid.
8. Provide a low-sodium diet as ordered. Before discharge, have the dietitian visit to assist the patient in meal planning for a low-sodium diet.	Sodium is an osmotic electrolyte that attracts water. A dietitian is a nutritional specialist and can make a comprehensive assessment of the person's nutritional needs and outline a mutually accepted diet plan.
9. Restrict fluid intake, usually 1–2 liters per day, as ordered.	To reduce venous pressure.
10. Consult physician if symptoms persist or worsen.	Extensive myocardial damage is unresponsive to medical therapy. If this is the case, the only viable alternative for the patient is a heart transplant.

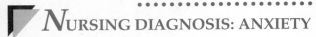

NURSING DIAGNOSIS: ANXIETY

RELATED TO FACTORS: Feeling a sense of suffocation and knowledge deficit about condition, diagnostic studies, treatment plan

DEFINING CHARACTERISTICS: Verbalizes lack of understanding, reports feeling a sense of suffocation with dyspnea, tense facial expression, irritable, demanding, verbalizes fear of being left alone, requests information

PATIENT OUTCOME: Demonstrates less anxiety

EVALUATION CRITERIA: Fewer reports of feeling nervous or anxious, relaxed facial expression, verbalizes understanding of instructions

INTERVENTIONS	RATIONALE
1. Administer prescribed morphine sulfate prn if chest pain is present and evaluate its effectiveness.	This drug relieves pain and helps reduce respirations and anxiety.
2. Explain all procedures in a calm reassuring voice. During the acute stage, provide simple, brief explanations. Begin thorough teaching when respiratory distress has subsided. Reassure the patient that after the body is rid of excess fluid, breathing difficulties should subside.	Anxiety and discomfort interfere with learning.
3. See Nursing Diagnosis: Anxiety (page 262).	

NURSING DIAGNOSIS: HIGH RISK FOR IMPAIRED HOME MAINTENANCE MANAGEMENT

RELATED TO FACTORS: Knowledge deficit about self-care on discharge, ineffective coping with lifestyle changes imposed by a chronic condition

DEFINING CHARACTERISTICS: May verbalize lack of understanding, requests information, may deny seriousness of condition, may verbalize hopelessness or depression over perceived losses associated with a chronic illness, may report a history of noncompliance

PATIENT OUTCOME: Demonstrates willingness to adhere to prescribed therapeutic plan for home maintenance and prevention.

EVALUATION CRITERIA: Verbalizes acceptance of responsibility for self-care, verbalizes understanding of condition and therapeutic plan, verbalizes realistic plans with respect to current situation

• •

INTERVENTIONS	RATIONALE
1. Teach the patient or significant other how to assess a radial pulse and explain its significance in managing prescribed drug therapy.	The patient will be required to continue digoxin at home. An abnormal pulse rate or rhythm signals digitalis toxicity and a need for medical attention.
2. Instruct the patient to contact the physician if signs and symptoms of increasing heart failure develop: • persistent fatigue • increasing shortness of breath • swelling of feet • decreasing urinary output • daily weight gain	The patient needs reevaluation for possible adjustment in drug therapy.
3. Instruct the patient to weigh daily, preferably early morning, wearing the same amount of clothing each time, and to keep a record of results. Explain that body weight is one of the best indicators of fluid status.	In addition to providing information about the effectiveness of prescribed therapies in restoring fluid equilibrium, body weight also provides the patient with objective data that can help promote compliance.
4. Review all prescribed medications. Let the patient know to anticipate more frequent voiding while taking the diuretic. Caution the patient that orthostatic hypotension (dizziness, light-headedness) may be experienced when moving abruptly from a supine position to a standing position. Advise the patient to sit upright for a few minutes before standing to prevent orthostatic hypotension. Instruct the patient to report adverse reactions:	Dosage adjustment, potassium supplement, or both (for hypokalemia) is required. A potassium imbalance may potentiate the effect of digitalis preparations and cause arrhythmias.

INTERVENTIONS	RATIONALE
• hypokalemia (with loop diuretics) —persistent weakness, irritability, reduced powers of concentration • dehydration — thirst, concentrated urine, persistent orthostatic hypotension • hyperkalemia (with potassium-sparing diuretics) — irregular pulse, nausea, diarrhea, muscle spasms • digitalis toxicity — irregular pulse, blurred vision, GI disturbances.	
5. Advise the patient to take the diuretic in the morning.	To avoid having sleep disrupted during the night from voiding.
6. Provide a written appointment for follow-up care and written self-care instructions.	Verbal instructions may be easily forgotten.
7. Ensure the patient understands dietary restrictions and can identify foods high in sodium.	Restricting sodium intake is essential to control fluid retention.

Integrative Care Plans

* Cardiac surgery if valves have to be replaced
* Congestive heart failure
* Loss
* Immobility

Discharge Considerations

* Follow-up care
* Signs and symptoms of increasing heart failure
* Medications to continue at home
* Self-care measures to protect against recurring infections

ASSESSMENT DATA BASE

1. History or presence of risk factors;
   * congenital heart disease
   * history of open heart surgery
   * user of intravenous street drugs
   * previous invasive cardiovascular diagnostic procedure
2. Physical examination based on an assessment of cardiovascular status (Appendix G) and a general survey (Appendix F) may reveal:
   * the classical triad—anemia, intermittent fever, and either a systolic murmur (with aortic stenosis, tricuspid insufficiency, or mitral insufficiency), or a diastolic murmur (with aortic insufficiency, tricuspid stenosis, or mitral stenosis)
   * arthralgia
   * anorexia and weight loss
   * fatigue
   * splenomegaly
   * vascular lesions:
     — Osler's nodes (tender, red nodules in the skin).
     — Janeway lesions (flat, nontender, red spots found on the soles and palms that blanch with pressure)
   * petechiae
   * symptoms of congestive heart failure (page 462)
3. Diagnostic studies:
   * Blood culture is positive for the infective organism.
   * CBC shows eukocytosis, and hemoglobin, hematocrit and RBC below normal range.
   * Erythrocyte sedimentation rate (ESR) is elevated, reflecting inflammation.

- Urinalysis UA displays hematuria and proteinuria.
- Rheumatoid factor is positive.
- Chest x ray detects congestive heart failure and cardiac hypertrophy.
- EKG assesses for heart failure and arrhythmias.
- Echocardiogram determines extent of valve damage.

4. Assess patient's feelings and concerns about condition after cardiopulmonary distress is under control.

NURSING DIAGNOSIS: ACTIVITY INTOLERANCE

RELATED TO FACTORS: Diminished cardiac output secondary to infective endocarditis

DEFINING CHARACTERISTICS: Persistent fatigue, tachypnea and tachycardia with minimal exertion

PATIENT OUTCOME: Demonstrates tolerance to activities.

EVALUATION CRITERIA: Fewer reports of fatigue, tachycardia, and shortness of breath with physical exertion

INTERVENTIONS	RATIONALE
1. See Nursing Diagnosis: Activity Intolerance (page 464).	

NURSING DIAGNOSIS: ANXIETY

RELATED TO FACTORS: Threat of sudden death, knowledge deficit about condition, diagnostic studies, and treatment plan

DEFINING CHARACTERISTICS: Verbalizes lack of understanding, may report feeling nervous fearful of being left alone, may report feeling of doom

PATIENT OUTCOME (collaborative): Demonstrates less anxiety

EVALUATION CRITERIA: Fewer reports of feeling nervous or anxious; relaxed facial expression; verbalizes understanding of condition, diagnostic studies, and treatment plan

INTERVENTIONS	RATIONALE
1. See Nursing Diagnosis: Anxiety (page 262).	
2. Consult physician if the patient continues to appear extremely anxious. If not already assessed, suggest arterial blood gases (ABG) analysis.	An antianxiety agent may be required. Anxiety creates an additional stress on an already compromised heart. Hypoxia also can cause restlessness.

 # NURSING DIAGNOSIS: SLEEP PATTERN DISTURBANCE

RELATED TO FACTORS: Chills and sweats secondary to infection

DEFINING CHARACTERISTICS: Reports insomnia and inability to rest due to wet linen from sweating, fever, WBC greater than 10,000/mm^3

PATIENT OUTCOME: Demonstrates relief from insomnia

EVALUATION CRITERIA: Fewer reports of insomnia, reports feeling rested and comfortable, temperature 98.6°F, WBC between 5,000-10,000/mm^3

INTERVENTIONS	RATIONALE
1. Monitor: • temperature q4h • results of CBC reports, especially WBC	To identify indications of progress toward or deviations from expected outcome.
2. Change linen and gown daily and when wet from perspiration. Provide a bed bath in morning, at bedtime, and prn during diaphoretic episodes.	To promote comfort.
3. Administer prescribed antibiotic and evaluate its effectiveness.	To resolve the infection.
4. Administer prescribed antipyretic prn. Consult physician if temperature remains greater than 101°F despite intervention.	This may signal a need for repeat blood cultures because patient may have developed an infection at another site.

INTERVENTIONS	RATIONALE
5. Provide hydration as ordered. Notify physician if the patient shows increasing intolerance of fluids: • rising central venous pressure • pulmonary artery pressure and blood pressure • persistent rales accompanied by shortness of breath at rest	Fluids help cool the body. A compromised heart may be unable to tolerate additional fluid volume necessary to maintain cooling of the body.
6. When fever is present, apply light covers over the patient.	To allow cooling of the body via evaporation.
7. Adhere to universal precautions (good handwashing technique before and after patient contact and wearing gloves when contact with blood or body fluid is likely to occur) when providing direct care.	To prevent nosocomial infection. Healthcare workers are the most common source of nosocomial infections.

· ·

NURSING DIAGNOSIS: HIGH RISK FOR IMPAIRED HOME MAINTENANCE MANAGEMENT

RELATED TO FACTORS: Ineffective coping with lifestyle changes imposed by chronic illness, knowledge deficit about self-care activities on discharge

DEFINING CHARACTERISTICS: May verbalize hopelessness and depression, may verbalize difficulty coping with perceived losses, may report history of noncompliance

PATIENT OUTCOME: Demonstrates willingness to comply with therapeutic plan for self-care on discharge

EVALUATION CRITERIA: Verbalizes acceptance of responsibility for own self-care, requests information about available community resources, discusses feelings and concerns about lifestyle changes required in view of current situation

· ·

INTERVENTIONS	RATIONALE
1. See Loss (page 733).	
2. Ensure the patient: • knows signs and symptoms of increasing heart failure and to contact the physician if these occur: — persistent fatigue — daily weight gain — peripheral edema — diminished urinary output — increasing shortness of breath • understands the need for prophylactic antibiotic therapy when undergoing any surgical or dental procedure. Explain that one episode of infective endocarditis increases susceptibility to repeat infections. Emphasize the need to inform physicians of history of valvular heart disease when undergoing any medical or dental care. Let the patient know that lifetime treatment is required.	Compliance with a therapeutic plan is enhanced when patients understand the relationship between their condition and treatments.
3. Advise the patient to obtain a Medic Alert bracelet through a local chapter of the American Heart Association.	To provide emergency medical personnel ready access to information about the patient in the event of an emergency.
4. Provide the patient or significant other with a written appointment for follow-up visit and written instructions for self-care measures. Explain that repeat blood cultures are part of follow-up evaluation for about two months after prescribed antibiotic therapy is completed.	Verbal instructions may be easily forgotten. Bacteria may exist in the vegetative lesions for months, or the patient may be reinfected by a different organism.

Cardiac Surgery

Cardiac surgery may involve a coronary artery bypass graft (CABG), heart transplant, replacement of defective heart valves with artificial valves, or repair of congenital defects. Surgery is performed through a midline sternotomy. Because intractable chest pain, arrhythmias, or severe heart failure are often present, the patient may be admitted to a coronary care unit (CCU) before surgery.

Cardiac surgery may take five hours. To ensure systemic circulation during open heart surgery, the surgeon inserts a catheter into the ascending aorta and the superior and inferior vena cava for connection to a cardiopulmonary bypass machine. Venous blood flows through the machine where it is filtered and oxygenated, then pumped back into the body through a catheter in the aorta. To arrest the heart (making it motionless) for surgery, a cold cardioplegic solution is infused into the mediastinum and the coronary arteries. When surgery is completed and warmed blood is allowed to flow through the chambers and coronary arteries, the heart begins to contract again. If it fails to contract, the surgeon delivers a small shock directly to the myocardium to initiate electrical activity.

Preoperative preparation is the same for any patient undergoing surgery. Postoperatively, several operating room staff and a respiratory therapist transport the patient directly to the (ICU) with:

- an endotracheal tube connected to a mechanical ventilator
- peripheral IV lines
- pulmonary artery catheter (Swan-Ganz catheter) to provide a direct means to monitor hemodynamic status
- Foley catheter
- intra-arterial line to provide a direct means to monitor blood pressure
- mediastinal chest tubes (often connected to an autotransfusion device for reinfusion of the patient's own blood)
- temporary pacemaker wires that can be connected to an external pacemaker in case heart block develops
- midsternal dressing
- dressing along the lower extremity from which the vein was taken if a CABG was performed using the patient's own vessel instead of a synthetic vessel

The respiratory therapist connects the patient to the ventilator, obtains arterial blood gases (ABG), and adjusts the ventilator settings according to the ABG results. The endotracheal tube is removed when the gag reflex returns and the ABG are within an acceptable range. Two ICU nurses are often needed to receive the patient and connect all of the different lines to the monitoring devices.

The mean LOS for a DRG classification of a cardiac valve procedure is 18.1 days with cardiac catheterization and 12.1 days without; 13.6 days for coronary bypass with cardiac catheterization and 11.3 days without (Lorenz, 1991).

Patients are placed in a cardiac rehabilitation program on discharge, which includes educational classes, discussion sessions, a planned physical exercise program (in which the heart rate and BP are monitored by a physical therapist or nurse). Sexual activity is usually permitted in 2–3 weeks.

THE PREOPERATIVE PERIOD

1. See Preoperative and Postoperative Care (page 738).

THE POSTOPERATIVE PERIOD

 # *A*SSESSMENT DATA BASE

1. Obtain readings from all hemodynamic monitoring devices to ensure proper functioning. This is the first priority.
2. Perform a cardiovascular assessment (Appendix G), a routine postoperative assessment (Appendix L), and a neurological assessment (Appendix J).

*N*URSING DIAGNOSIS: ALTERATIONS IN FLUID VOLUME: EXCESS

RELATED TO FACTORS: Diminished cardiac output secondary to cardiac surgery

DEFINING CHARACTERISTICS: Hemodynamic monitoring devices show readings above normal range, cardiac output measurement below normal range, tachycardia, decreased urinary output in relation to fluid intake, rales

PATIENT OUTCOME (collaborative): Demonstrates fluid and biochemical balance

EVALUATION CRITERIA: Hemodynamic parameters within normal range, BP between 90/60–140/90mm Hg, heart rate between 60–100 beats per minute, absence of edema, clear lung sounds

INTERVENTIONS	RATIONALE

1. Monitor:
  • cardiovascular status (Appendix G) hourly until stable
  • hemodynamic parameters hourly:
    — central venous pressure (CVP); normal range 2–8 mm Hg or 3–11 cm of water
    — cardiac output (CO); normal range 3–5 L/min
    — pulmonary capillary wedge pressure (PCWP); normal range 6–12 mm Hg
    — cardiac index (CI); normal 2.5–3.5 L/min/m^2
    — systemic vascular resistance (SVR); normal 600–1400 (dynes xcm/sec^5), and mean arterial pressure (MAP); normal 70–100 mm Hg
  • intake and output hourly
	To evaluate effectiveness of therapy. Many parameters are needed to adequately evaluate cardiovascular function because none alone provides sufficient evidence.

2. If hemodynamic readings reveal high preload (PCWP and diastolic pressure above normal range), administer prescribed rapid acting diuretic, vasodilator, inotropic agent, and reduce flow rate of IV fluids as prescribed.	These agents help rid the body of excess fluid. Fluid volume excess places an additional strain on an already compromised heart.
3. If hemodynamic readings reveal a low preload (below normal range for CVP, PCWP, SVR, and CO accompanied by a urinary output less than 0.5 mL/kg/hr), increase IV flow rate. Administer prescribed vasoactive agents and/or blood transfusions if hemoglobin, hematocrit, and RBC are below normal range. Perform autotransfusions if an autologous collection chamber is in place.	Renal function can be threatened if fluid deficit is severe and is allowed to persist.

INTERVENTIONS	RATIONALE
4. Titrate prescribed vasoactive agent, such as dobutamine (Dobutrex) and nitroprusside (Nipride), to maintain hemodynamic parameters within prescribed range. Report adverse drug effects.	Dopamine increases myocardial contractility, hence cardiac output, while Nipride lowers BP by reducing afterload. Collectively, these agents increase SVR and renal perfusion thus helping rid the body of excess fluid.

· ·

 # NURSING DIAGNOSIS: HIGH RISK FOR COMPLICATIONS

RELATED TO FACTORS: Cardiac surgery

DEFINING CHARACTERISTICS: Manifestations of bleeding, atelectasis, infection, emboli, arrhythmias, or postpump psychosis.

PATIENT OUTCOME (collaborative): Absence of postcardiac surgery complications

EVALUATION CRITERIA: Mean LOS for assigned DRG is not exceeded; absence of infection, arrhythmias, bleeding, emboli, atelectasis, and postpump psychosis

· ·

INTERVENTIONS	RATIONALE
Infection: 1. See Preoperative and Postoperative Care (page 738).	
Arrhythmias: 1. Monitor: • ECG recordings frequently • laboratory tests of serum drug levels • results of ABG and serum electrolyte reports	To detect arrhythmias. Drug toxicity, acid-base imbalances, and electrolyte imbalances can precipitate cardiac arrhythmias.
2. If heart block occurs, connect the cardiac pacing wires to the external pacemaker to initiate cardiac pacing and notify physician. Set the pacing and sensing limits on the pacemaker unit according to physician orders. Follow facility ICU protocol and procedures for treatment of arrhythmias.	Untreated, arrhythmias can lead to congestive heart failure by placing additional strain on an already compromised heart.

INTERVENTIONS	RATIONALE
3. Place an ECG strip on the patient's medical record on each shift and when any type of arrhythmia is detected.	To provide a permanent record of the effectiveness of interventions.
Bleeding: 1. Monitor: • results of prothrombin time (PT) and partial thromboplastin time (PTT) • volume of drainage from the mediastinal tube hourly • heart sounds q4h	Large doses of anticoagulant are used with a cardiopulmonary bypass machine that increases the risk for postoperative bleeding.
2. Notify physician immediately if: • cardiac tamponade is detected: — faint heart sounds accompanied by a sudden decrease in the amount of mediastinal drainage — jugular vein distention — pulsus paradoxus — narrowing pulse pressure — tachycardia — elevated pulmonary artery pressure (PAP), CVP, and PCWP • 200 mL or more mediastinal drainage is obtained for two consecutive hours accompanied by a falling BP, PCWP, and tachycardia	These findings signal hemorrhage and a need for protamine sulfate (if PT and PTT prolonged), blood transfusion, or pericardiocentesis (if cardiac tamponade is confirmed).
Emboli: 1. Monitor neurological status (Appendix J) and neurovascular status of both lower extremities (Appendix D) q4h. Notify physician of any deficits such as alteration in level of consciousness; diminished reflexes, motor function, or sensation or complaints of pain with dorsiflexion of the foot.	The patient is at risk for stroke, which could occur as a result of an air or thrombotic emboli or reduced cerebral perfusion during cardiopulmonary bypass.

INTERVENTIONS	RATIONALE
2. Apply midthigh support hose as prescribed. Remove daily for cleansing and inspection of the skin.	These stockings help prevent venous stasis.
3. Assist with ambulation when allowed. Encourage active range-of-motion (ROM) exercises, until ambulation is allowed.	To promote circulation.
Atelectasis:	
1. See Preoperative and Postoperative Care (page 738).	
Postpump Psychosis: 1. Monitor for personality changes each shift (confusion, disorientation, paranoid statements, combative behaviors). If these occur, use reality orientation, keep siderails up at all times, use restraints, and administer prescribed tranquilizer prn. Perform measures to promote rest: • reducing environmental noise • ensuring a comfortable room temperature • providing effective pain management • planning for periods of uninterrupted rest	Alterations in physiologic status due to cardiopulmonary bypass, sleep deprivation, sensory overload, and emotional stress of surgery predispose patient to psychotic reactions.

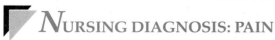

NURSING DIAGNOSIS: PAIN

RELATED TO FACTORS: Cardiac surgery

DEFINING CHARACTERISTICS: Verbalizes pain, frowning, moaning, guarding painful site

PATIENT OUTCOME (collaborative): Demonstrates relief from pain

EVALUATION CRITERIA: Denies pain, relaxed facial expression, absence of moaning

INTERVENTIONS	RATIONALE
1. Administer prescribed analgesic prn and evaluate its effectiveness.	Analgesics block the pain pathway.
2. Assist the patient with splinting the chest when coughing.	To reduce strain on the suture line.

· ·

◤ NURSING DIAGNOSIS: HIGH RISK FOR IMPAIRED HOME MAINTENANCE MANAGEMENT

RELATED TO FACTORS: Knowledge deficit about self-care measures on discharge, ineffective coping

DEFINING CHARACTERISTICS: Verbalizes lack of understanding, requests information, may report history of noncompliance, may express difficulty coping with required lifestyle changes imposed by chronic illness

PATIENT OUTCOME (collaborative): Demonstrates willingness to comply with self-care preventive and maintenance activities at home

EVALUATION CRITERIA: Verbalizes understanding of home care instructions, verbalizes satisfaction with discharge plans to meet home needs, demonstrates ability to meet home care needs

· ·

INTERVENTIONS	RATIONALE
1. Ensure the patient or significant other has a written appointment for follow-up care and written instructions for self-care activities.	Verbal instructions may be easily forgotten.
2. Evaluate the patient's and significant other's plans for resuming a normal lifestyle within the context of current condition. Refer the patient to a community based program for cardiac surgery patients such as the Mended Heart Club, if available.	Often, expectations about cardiac surgery may be unrealistic. Some patients may view the surgery as a cure and assume they no longer have to follow any limitations. A support system consisting of persons who have experienced the same or similar surgery can assist the patient to cope with required lifestyle modifications.

INTERVENTIONS	RATIONALE
3. Instruct the patient to report manifestations that signal cardiac dysfunction: • sudden severe chest pain unrelieved by nitrates • increasing dyspnea, fever, or persistent chest pain with minimal exertion • persistent fatigue, palpitations	Patients are prone to recurring chest pain, especially if it occurred before surgery. Postpericardiotomy syndrome, an inflammatory delayed response, may occur 2–3 weeks or as late as one year after surgery. Anti-inflammatory drugs and corticosteroids may be required to resolve this complication.
4. Encourage participation in a regular exercise program. Suggest walking. Teach the patient and significant other how to assess a radial pulse. Advise the patient to check pulse before beginning exercises, halfway through, and on completion of exercises. Advise the patient to slow the exercise if pulse rate exceeds 20 beats per minute above the pre-exercise pulse rate.	Exercise is essential for promoting circulation and maintaining muscle tone. Pulse rate in the absence of a stress test can serve as a guide to exercise tolerance.
5. Inform the patient that incisional discomfort may continue until the sternum has healed completely, usually about 6–12 weeks. Ensure patient has a prescription for a mild analgesic.	A knowledge of what to expect helps lessen anxiety.
6. Provide the patient with sufficient materials to do dressing changes. Let the patient know that drainage of serosanguineous fluid from the incision and drain sites may occur and to cover the sites with a sterile dressing. Advise the patient to shower instead of taking tub baths. Wash hands thoroughly before and after wound care.	A clean, dry wound retards infection. A shower provides a continuous flushing of the wound.

INTERVENTIONS	RATIONALE
7. Review prescribed medications, including name, purpose, dosage, schedule, and reportable side effects.	To ensure safety in drug self-administration.
8. If a CABG was performed using the patient's own saphenous leg vein, instruct the patient to: • elevate the legs when possible • wear support stockings until swelling has subsided • walk in moderation Let the patient know that edema of the graft donor leg is expected and usually resolves in about 12 weeks.	Exercise helps promote collateral circulation.
9. Remind the patient that cardiac drugs prescribed before surgery need to be continued after surgery. Cardiac surgery does not cure heart disease. Chest pain may still be experienced but with less intensity.	To correct unrealistic expectations most patients have about cardiac surgery.

BIBLIOGRAPHY

Bayer, A.S., Hutler, A.M., & Wilson, W. R. (1991). Current management of infective endocarditis. **Patient Care, 25,** 15–8, 21–23, 28.

Braun, A.E. (1991). What to do when a patient needs defibrillation or cardioversion. **Nursing, 21,** 50–54.

Edwards, N.L. (1990). Recognizing valvular heart disease. **Emergency Medicine, 22,** 56–60, 62, 65.

Gawlinski, A. (1989). Nursing care after AMI: A comprehensive review. **Critical Care Nursing, 12,** 64–72.

Gawlinski, A., & Jensen, G. (1991). The complications of cardiovascular aging. **American Journal of Nursing, 91,** 26–30.

Jacobsen, W.K. (1992). **Manual of Post Anesthesia Care,** Philadelphia: W. B. Saunders Company.

Jacobson, C. (1991). Mechanisms of arrhythmia formation. **Critical Care Quarterly, 14,** 1–9.

Lorenz, E.W. (1991). **St. Anthony's DRG Working Guidebook.** Alexandria: St. Anthony's Publishing Company.

Pelter, M.A. (1989). Thrombolytic therapy in acute myocardial infarction. **Critical Care Nursing, 12,** 55–65.

Poterfield, L., & Poterfield, J.G. (1989). What you need to know about today's pacemakers. **RN, 52,** 48–52.

Solomon, J. (1991). Managing a failing heart. **RN, 54,** 46–51.

Shoemaker, W.C., Ayres, S., Grenvik, A., Holbrook, P.R., & Thompson, W.L. (1989). **Textbook of Critical Care,** Philadelphia: W.B. Saunders Company.

Teplitz, L. (1991). Classification of cardiac pacemakers. **Journal of Cardiovascular Nursing, 5,** 1–8.

C

HAPTER EIGHT

Problems of the Sensory System

Cataracts

A **cataract** is an opacity or clouding of the lens. The lens is normally transparent and allows light to pass through to the retina. As clouding develops, visual impairment occurs. Cataracts are usually bilateral; however the degree of visual impairment is often different in each eye.

Surgery is the only treatment for a cataract. However, the mere finding of a cataract is not an indication for surgery. Surgery is indicated when significant vision loss has occurred. When the lens is removed (aphakic), the patient may have lens replacement by three means:

1. Cataract glasses — these prescribed glasses have thick heavy lenses. They do not provide perfect vision but do offer significant precataract improvement. The patient requires an adjustment period because these glasses magnify images thus creating distortions in depth perception (objects may suddenly pop in view, patient may under reach for objects, and steps and walls may appear curved). These glasses can be worn immediately after surgery.

2. Contact lens — there is less magnification with these lenses so depth perception is normal. The patient must wait at least six months after cataract extraction before contact lenses can be worn. Extended-wear soft lenses are available that can be worn for up to six months, then removed and cleaned. Temporary cataract glasses must be worn until contact lenses are allowed.

3. Intraocular lens implant — replacement of the diseased lens with a clear polymer lens. Patients can expect at least a visual acuity of 20/40 with this type of lens. Glasses are no longer required. It takes about one year for complete healing and formation of fibrous tissue to hold the lens securely in place.

General Medical Management

- Cataract extraction, with or without lens implantation

Integrative Care Plans

- Eye Surgery

Discharge Considerations

- See Eye Surgery

 # ASSESSMENT DATA BASE

1. History or presence of causative factors:
   - senile cataracts — commonly seen in the elderly
   - congenital cataracts — occurs in infants
   - traumatic cataracts — occurs in individuals who have sustained a severe eye injury
   - secondary to certain systemic diseases characterized by metabolic derangements (diabetes mellitus) and chronic eye disease (uveitis)
   - high dose of steroid therapy

2. Physical examination based on a general assessment of the eye (Appendix H) may reveal:
   a. Reports of reduced visual acuity that may include:
      - glare when looking at lights, especially with night driving
      - blurred vision
      - double vision
      - altered color perception
   b. A "white pupil" on inspection of the eye, a characteristic finding of a "mature cataract" indicating significant vision loss

3. Diagnostic studies:
   - Ophthalmoscopic and biomicroscopic examinations performed by an ophthalmologist are most diagnostic because they allow direct visualization to evaluate the degree of lens opacity. These examinations are performed in an ophthalmologist's office.

4. See Eye Surgery (page 499) for the remainder of this care plan.

Eye Surgery

Eye surgery can be performed for various eye conditions. The types of Surgical procedures for the most common eye conditions are:

a. for errors of refraction — radial keratoplasty, corneal transplant

b. for diabetic retinopathy — photocoagulation, vitrectomy

c. for glaucoma — peripheral iridectomy, laser trabeculoplasty, trabeculectomy, cyclocryotherapy

d. for cataracts — cataract extraction (either intracapsular or extracapsular), phacoemulsification and aspiration, intraocular lens implant

e. for retinal detachment — scleral buckling

Most eye surgery is done on an outpatient basis under local anesthesia. General anesthesia can be used at the patient's request and for patients who are extremely anxious, deaf, or mentally retarded. Local anesthesia generally requires a facial and retrobulbar injection of lidocaine and bupivacaine HCL to block nerves. A preanesthetic such as diazepam (Valium) is often given to reduce anxiety when receiving injections on the face and around the eye.

Preoperatively, the patient can receive several types of eye medications to prepare the eye for surgery:

• mydriatic and cyclopedgic eye drops

• antibiotic eye drops as a prophylaxis against infection

• intravenous infusion of an agent to lower intraocular pressure (mannitol or a carbonic anhydrase inhibitor)

The patient is instructed to have a driver available to provide transportation postoperatively because driving is restricted for a few days. After the anesthesia wears off, the patient is discharged.

Postoperatively, the patient has a patch over the eye. The patch is removed and reapplied on the first postoperative day when eye drops are begun (mydriatics, steroids, antibiotics, or miotics). Mild discomfort and scratchiness are expected. Atropine sulfate eye drops and cold compresses can be ordered to relieve these discomforts.

Integrative Care Plans

- Preoperative and postoperative care

Discharge Considerations

- Follow-up care
- Signs and symptoms requiring medical attention
- Self-administration of eye drops
- Activity limitations

THE PREOPERATIVE PERIOD

 # ASSESSMENT DATA BASE

1. Physical examination based on a general assessment of the eye (Appendix H) to establish baseline values.

2. Assess vital signs.

3. Assess understanding of preoperative and postoperative events for eye surgery.

4. Assess ability to self-administer eye medication. If patient cannot self-administer eye medication, inquire about availability of someone to provide assistance with instillation of eye medication at home.

5. Assess for the presence of other coexisting health problems, medications currently taken, problems with constipation, and coughing or sneezing.

6. Inquire about availability of a driver to provide transportation home postoperatively.

7. Assess for drug allergies, especially sulfa drugs. Sulfa agents are commonly prescribed as a prophylaxis against infection.

8. See Preoperative and Postoperative Care (page 738).

NURSING DIAGNOSIS: ANXIETY

RELATED TO FACTORS: Knowledge deficit about preoperative and postoperative events, fear of some aspect of surgery

DEFINING CHARACTERISTICS: Verbalizes lack of understanding, may report fear of possible loss of vision or some other aspect of surgery, tense facial expression

PATIENT OUTCOME: Demonstrates relief from anxiety

EVALUATION CRITERIA: Fewer reports of feeling anxious or nervous, verbalizes understanding of preoperative and postoperative events, relaxed facial expression

INTERVENTIONS	RATIONALE
1. Explain preoperative and postoperative events. Inform the patient that activities that increase intraocular pressure (IOP) (sneezing, coughing, bending over with head below waist level, straining) should be avoid postoperatively until approved by the opthalmologist.	A knowledge of what to expect helps alleviate anxiety and promotes patient cooperation.
2. Answer questions. Refer specific questions about the surgery to physician. Provide time for the patient to express feelings. Inform the patient that improvement in vision may not occur immediately after surgery but should gradually improve as swelling subsides. If a corneal transplant is performed, vision improvement may take six months or longer.	Honesty promotes trust and cooperation. Sharing feelings helps relieve tension.
3. See Preoperative and Postoperative Care (page 738).	

THE POSTOPERATIVE PERIOD

 # *A*SSESSMENT DATA BASE

1. On return from surgery:
   - Assess for pain and nausea.
   - Obtain vital signs.
   - Check status of eye patch/shield. There should be no drainage on the eye patch/shield.
   - Assess level of consciousness.
2. See Preoperative and Postoperative Care (page 738).

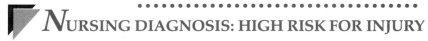

*N*URSING DIAGNOSIS: HIGH RISK FOR INJURY

RELATED TO FACTORS: Temporary loss of peripheral vision and depth perception secondary to eye surgery

DEFINING CHARACTERISTICS: Observation of patch or shield over one eye, may bump into furniture, may verbalize difficulty seeing

PATIENT OUTCOME: Demonstrates no injury

EVALUATION CRITERIA: Absence of bruising on legs, denies falls, absence of manifestations of increased intraocular pressure or bleeding

• •

INTERVENTIONS	RATIONALE
1. Keep bed in low position, siderails elevated, and call bell at bedside. Reorient patient to structural layout of the room. Instruct the patient to signal for assistance when getting out of bed until able to ambulate without assistance.	Some momentary loss of balance can occur when the eye is covered, especially in the elderly.
2. Instruct the patient to turn head completely to the operated side when walking to ensure pathway is clear. Keep eye patch/shield on as directed to prevent accidental injury to the eye.	Peripheral vision is lost when the eye is covered with a patch or shield.
3. Initiate measures to prevent increased IOP: • Keep head of bed elevated approximately 45 degrees for the initial 24 hours. • Remind the patient to avoid coughing, sneezing, bending over with head lower than waist, and straining. • Administer prescribed antiemetic for complaints of nausea. • Administer prescribed stool softener if history of constipation. Allow to use regular bathroom rather than bedpan because using the bathroom results in less increased IOP.	An elevated IOP increases pain and the risk for disruption of sutures used in eye surgery.

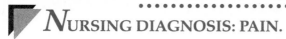

NURSING DIAGNOSIS: PAIN.

RELATED TO FACTORS: Eye surgery

DEFINING CHARACTERISTICS: Verbalizes mild pain and scratching sensation in operative eye, frowning, moaning

PATIENT OUTCOME (collaborative): Demonstrates relief from eye discomfort

EVALUATION CRITERIA: Denies eye discomfort, absence of moaning, relaxed facial expression

INTERVENTIONS	RATIONALE
1. Administer prescribed analgesic as ordered and evaluate effectiveness. Notify physician if eye pain persists or worsens after medication.	Analgesics block the pain pathway. Severe eye discomfort indicates the development of complications and a need for prompt medical attention. Mild discomfort is expected.
2. Administer prescribed anti-inflammatory and anti-infective ophthalmic agents.	To reduce swelling and to prevent infection.
3. Apply cold compresses as ordered using aseptic technique. Adhere to universal precautions (good hand-washing technique before and after wound care, wearing gloves when contact with blood or body fluid is likely to occur). Teach the patient how to apply the compresses using aseptic technique in preparation for discharge. Emphasize the importance of handwashing before eye care at home. Explain purpose of the compresses.	Cold helps reduce swelling. Disruption of tissue predisposes patient to bacterial invasion.

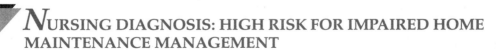

NURSING DIAGNOSIS: HIGH RISK FOR IMPAIRED HOME MAINTENANCE MANAGEMENT

RELATED TO FACTORS: Knowledge deficit about self-care on discharge, inadequate support system

DEFINING CHARACTERISTICS: Verbalizes lack of understanding, may report difficulty with self-administration of eye drops, requests information, may report nonavailability of significant other to assist with home care needs

PATIENT OUTCOME (collaborative): Demonstrates willingness to comply with prescribed self-care measures to safeguard operative eye on discharge

EVALUATION CRITERIA: Verbalizes understanding of discharge instructions, correctly performs eye care, verbalizes satisfaction with arrangements made for home care assistance

• •

INTERVENTIONS	RATIONALE
1. Provide written instructions for eye care and follow-up appointment.	Verbal instructions may be easily forgotten.
2. Instruct the patient in eye care at home: **Eye Safety:** • Wear the eye patch/shield when sleeping and avoid sleeping on the affected side for at least one month or as prescribed to prevent inadvertent rubbing of the eye. To prevent injury to the eye, wear eyeglasses during waking hours when the eye shield or patch is not worn . • Wear prescription sunglasses with a high UV rating when exposed to prolonged sunlight because some photosensitivity occurs after eye surgery. More sun rays are blocked by sunglasses with a high UV rating. • Avoid vigorous activities that cause jarring of the body (contact sports, running), bending over, heavy lifting, and straining for six months or as ordered because these activities can disrupt sutures or implants.	Discharge teaching and practice with self-care procedures are important to ensure safety with home care activities and to promote compliance.

INTERVENTIONS	RATIONALE
Medications and Treatments:	
• Explain the purpose of prescribed eye drops, including name, dosage, schedule, purpose, and reportable side effects.	
• Teach and have the patient practice:	
a. How to apply eye shield/patch	
b. How to prepare and apply cold compresses to the eye, using aseptic technique	
c. How to self-administer eye drops	
Complications:	
• Instruct the patient to inspect the eye daily in front of a mirror for signs of infection (or graft rejection if corneal transplant was done). Contact physician if increased redness, swelling, irritation, pain or drainage or decreased vision persist over 24 hours because these findings indicate infection or corneal graft rejection and a need for prompt medical attention.	
3. Contact social services or discharge planning department if the patient cannot perform self-care skills and there is no significant other to help the patient.	These departments are responsible for planning continuity of care for patients requiring home care assistance during the recovery period. Assistance can involve temporary placement in an extended care facility or home visits by a visiting nurse.

Glaucoma

Glaucoma is an eye disease characterized by increased intraocular pressure (IOP). Increased pressure causes ischemic damage to the optic disc and nerve cells of the retina, with progressive loss of peripheral vision (Martinelli, 1991).

Increased IOP occurs when the outflow of aqueous humor in the anterior portion of the eye is restricted. Aqueous humor is continuously secreted by the ciliary body to provide nutrients for the lens. It exits the anterior chamber via the trabecular meshwork and the canal of Schlemm.

There are two primary forms of glaucoma:

1. **Primary angle-open glaucoma** (chronic simple glaucoma) caused by degeneration of the trabecular meshwork; bilateral involvement; gradual onset of symptoms

2. **Primary angle-closure glaucoma** (acute glaucoma) caused by blockage of the trabecular meshwork by peripheral iris tissue; unilateral involvement; symptoms occur suddenly

Primary angle-closure glaucoma may be acute or chronic. The acute form is a medical emergency. The patient should be referred to the nearest medical facility and receive prompt treatment by an ophthalmologist to prevent blindness. Hospitalization is required. The mean LOS for a DRG classification of glaucoma is 3.5 days (Lorenz, 1991).

Chronic angle-closure glaucoma is caused by a narrow angle of the anterior chamber. Persons with this type of glaucoma experience mild symptoms of acute glaucoma when exposed to situations that dilate the pupil, for example, when mydriatic drugs are used, during excitement, in darkness, or when eyes are closed for an extended period such as sleeping.

Glaucoma is treated without hospitalization, unless surgery is required.

General Medical Management

- Pharmacotherapy:
  - miotics and cholinesterase inhibitors such as pilocarpine nitrate, carbachol, demecarium bromide (Humursol)
  - beta-adrenergics such as timolol maleate (Timoptic Solution)
  - osmotic agents such as mannitol, glycerin (Osmoglyn)

— carbonic anhydrase inhibitors such as acetazolamide (Diamox)

— adrenergics such as epinephrine bitartrate (Epitrate)

• Surgery, especially for acute glaucoma

Integrative Care Plans

• Eye Surgery

Discharge Considerations

• See Eye Surgery

 # ASSESSMENT DATA BASE

1. History or presence of risk factors:
   • positive family history (believed to be a link in primary angle-open glaucoma)
   • eye tumor
   • intraocular hemorrhage
   • intraocular inflammation (uveitis)
   • contussion of the eye from trauma during cataract surgery

2. Physical examination based on a general assessment of the eye (Appendix H) may reveal:
   For primary angle-open:
   • reports slow loss of peripheral vision (tunnel vision)
   For primary angle-closure:
   • sudden onset of severe pain in the eye often accompanied by headache, nausea, and vomiting
   • complaints of rainbow halo around lights, blurred vision, and decreased light perception
   • fixed, moderately dilated pupil with inflamed red sclera and steamy cornea

3. Diagnostic studies:
   • Tonometry is used to measure IOP. Glaucoma is suspected if IOP is greater than 22 mm Hg.
   • Gonioscopy allows the ophthalmologist to directly visualize the anterior chamber to differentiate between angle-closure glaucoma and angle-open glaucoma.
   • Ophthalmoscopy allows the examiner to directly visualize the optic disc and other internal eye structures.

4. Assess the patient's understanding of condition and emotional response to condition and treatment plan.

◥ NURSING DIAGNOSIS: PAIN

RELATED TO FACTORS: Acute glaucoma

DEFINING CHARACTERISTICS: Verbalizes pain in eye, guarding painful site, frowning, moaning

PATIENT OUTCOME (collaborative): Demonstrates relief from discomfort

EVALUATION CRITERIA: Denies pain, relaxed facial expression, no moaning

INTERVENTIONS	RATIONALE
1. Monitor: • BP, pulse, and respiration q4h if not receiving osmotic agent intravenously, q2h if receiving osmotic agent • degree of eye pain q30min during the acute phase • intake and output q8h while receiving intravenous osmotic agent • visual acuity each time before instillation of prescribed ophthalmic agent. Ask if objects are clear or blurred. Determine if the patient can read printed material when held at arm's length.	To identify indications of progress toward or deviations from expected outcome.
2. Administer prescribed ophthalmic agent for glaucoma. Notify physician of the following: • hypotension • urinary output less than 240 mL for eight hours • no relief in eye pain within 30 minutes of drug therapy • continual diminishing visual acuity	Intravenous osmotic agents cause rapid reduction of IOP. Osmotic agents are hyperosmolar and can cause dehydration. Mannitol can precipitate hyperglycemia in diabetic patients. Miotic eye drops provide better drainage of aqueous humor and reduce its production. Controlling IOP is essential to preserving vision.
3. Prepare the patient for surgery as ordered (see Eye Surgery, page 499).	After IOP is under control with angle-open glaucoma, surgery must be performed to permanently relieve pupillary block.

INTERVENTIONS	RATIONALE
4. Maintain strict bedrest in a semi-Fowler's position. Initiate measures to prevent increased IOP: • Advise the patient against coughing, sneezing, straining, or placing head lower than waist.	Pressure in the eye is increased when the body is flat and when the Valsalva maneuver is activated, such as with these activities.
5. Provide a quiet, dark environment.	Stress and light raise IOP that triggers pain.
6. Administer prescribed narcotic analgesia prn and evaluate effectiveness.	To control pain. Severe pain triggers the Valsalva maneuver, raising IOP.

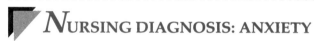

NURSING DIAGNOSIS: ANXIETY

RELATED TO FACTORS: Fear of permanent blindness, knowledge deficit about treatment

DEFINING CHARACTERISTICS: Verbalizes feelings of nervousness or being afraid, repetitive questioning, quivering voice, acknowledges lack of understanding

PATIENT OUTCOME: Demonstrates relief from anxiety

EVALUATION CRITERIA: Fewer reports of feeling nervous and worried, verbalizes an understanding of treatment plan, relaxed body position

INTERVENTIONS	RATIONALE
1. Although blindness before starting treatment is likely to be permanent because of destruction of retinal nerve cells subsequent to increased IOP, do **not** tell the patient that impaired vision or vision loss will be permanent.	Visual acuity only reflects sharpness of vision. **Only** the ophthalmologist can determine if vision loss will be permanent after a thorough examination of internal eye structures.
2. Allow the patient to express feelings about the condition. Maintain a calm, efficient manner. Explain the purpose of all prescribed treatments.	Expressing feelings helps the patient identify the source of anxiety and use coping responses. A calm approach by the caregiver conveys confidence and control. A knowledge of what to expect helps lessen anxiety.

INTERVENTIONS	RATIONALE
3. Keep call bell at bedside and instruct the patient to signal for assistance as needed. Keep siderails up to remind the patient not to get out of bed.	Anxiety increases when patients feel they are alone and without help.
4. Maintain effective pain control.	Pain is a source of anxiety.

NURSING DIAGNOSIS: HIGH RISK FOR IMPAIRED HOME MAINTENANCE MANAGEMENT

RELATED TO FACTORS: Knowledge deficit about self-care on discharge, lack of adequate support system

DEFINING CHARACTERISTICS: Verbalizes lack of understanding, requests information, reports nonavailability of significant other to assist with required home care, inability to perform home care activities safely

PATIENT OUTCOME (collaborative): Demonstrates willingness to comply with measures for proper eye care on discharge

EVALUATION CRITERIA: Performs required eye care safely, verbalizes understanding of condition and instructions, verbalizes satisfaction with plans for home care assistance

INTERVENTIONS	RATIONALE
1. When acute symptoms are under control, provide information about the condition. Emphasize that glaucoma requires lifetime treatment. Instruct the patient to seek medical attention if eye discomfort and symptoms of increased IOP recur while taking medication. Remind the patient that the risk of glaucoma occurring in the unaffected eye is always present.	To promote patient cooperation.

INTERVENTIONS	RATIONALE
2. Teach and have the patient practice self-administration of eye drops if surgery is not performed. If patient cannot administer eye drops, teach significant other. Consult social services discharge planning department to arrange for home health care visits if patient cannot perform self-care activities and if support system is inadequate. Provide information about the dose, name, schedule, purpose, and reportable side effects of all medications prescribed for home use.	Health teaching is essential to safety in self-care. Usually, daily administration of antiglaucoma eye drops to control IOP is the goal of therapy, unless surgery has been performed to permanently relieve obstruction of the outflow of aqueous humor. Social services discharge planning department is responsible for ensuring continuity of care for patients on discharge when continued care is needed for recovery and health maintenance.
3. Ensure all instructions and information about prescribed medication are in writing.	Verbal instructions may be easily forgotten.
4. Review general practices for eye safety: • When using spray cans, make sure the opening is facing away from the face before spraying. • Avoid spraying insecticides and other lawn and garden chemicals on windy days. • When applying chemicals outside, stand with the back against the wind so the wind blows the substance away. • Wear sunglasses with a high UV rating for prolonged exposure to the sun. Never look directly at the sun for prolonged periods. • Ensure good light when reading. • Wear goggles when using a lawn mower or lawn edger.	To guard against eye injury.

Retinal Detachment

With **retinal detachment,** the retina separates from the pigmented epithelium and the choroid. The detached portion becomes blind because it no longer receives nourishment from its primary source of nutrition, the choroid. A tear or hole in the retina can extend the separation as fluid from the vitreous cavity seeps through the opening and runs behind the retina, further elevating it away from the pigment epithelium and choroid. At the time of the tear, blood cells and pigment are released into the vitreous. There is no pain or redness in the affected eye. Retinal detachment may be unilateral or bilateral, depending on the causative factor. Surgery is required to reattach the retina (page 499).The mean LOS for a DRG classification of retinal detachment is 2.9 days (Lorenz, 1991).

General Medical Management

• Strict bedrest and eye patch to both eyes
• Surgery: scleral buckling

Integrative Care Plan

• Eye Surgery

Discharge Considerations

• See Eye Surgery

 ## ASSESSMENT DATA BASE

1. History or presence of causative factors:
    • diabetic retinopathy or recent penetrating intraocular injury
    • recent cataract surgery, uveitis, eye tumor

2. Physical examination based on a general assessment of the eye (Appendix H) may reveal:
    • complaints of sudden appearance of flashing lights (photopsia) followed by floating spots (caused by bleeding into the vitreous cavity)

- complaints of progressive loss of vision or a sensation of a veil over a portion of the eye (vision loss occurs in the area of the detachment)

3. Diagnostic studies:

- Ophthalmoscopic examination confirms the diagnosis. It provides direct visualization and may reveal a gray, opaque retina in folds. Normally, the retina is pink. A ballooning of the retina can be seen if subretinal fluid collection is large.

4. Assess the patient's understanding of condition and emotional response to condition and treatment plan.

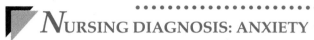

NURSING DIAGNOSIS: ANXIETY

RELATED TO FACTORS: Knowledge deficit about condition, threat of permanent loss of vision, sensory deprivation associated with covering both eyes

DEFINING CHARACTERISTICS: Reports feeling anxious or nervous, verbalizes fear of permanent blindness, verbalizes fear of some aspect of surgery, repetitive questioning, verbalizes lack of understanding, tense body posture

PATIENT OUTCOME: Demonstrates relief from anxiety

EVALUATION CRITERIA: Fewer reports of feeling anxious or nervous, relaxed body posture, verbalizes understanding of therapeutic plan

INTERVENTIONS	RATIONALE
1. Allow the patient to express feelings. Explain purpose of all prescribed treatments. Remind the patient the extent of residual visual impairment (if any) is best determined after surgery.	Expressing feelings helps lessen anxiety. A knowledge of what to expect also helps allay fear.
2. While both eyes are covered: • Provide auditory stimulation (radio or reading) to the patient. • Explain activities occurring in the room. • Call patient by name on entering the room and identify self during each visit. Never touch the blind patient without speaking first.	These measures provide the patient with some degree of independence with little danger of injury. Keeping the patient informed about events occurring in the room helps lessen anxiety.

INTERVENTIONS	RATIONALE
• Place items on the overbed table within the patient's reach. Explain where items are located. Place the item in the same place each time it is removed and returned to the table. To prevent spills, place a straw in the water pitcher so the patient can drink directly from the pitcher instead of pouring the water into a cup or glass. • Tell the patient when you are leaving the room. • Orient patient to the room. • Visit frequently to assess needs. • Arrange items on the meal tray and explain where each food item is located using a clock-rotation description, for example, milk is at 12 o'clock, bread is at 3 o'clock.	

◣ NURSING DIAGNOSIS: HIGH RISK FOR INJURY

RELATED TO FACTORS: Visual impairment secondary to retinal detachment

DEFINING CHARACTERISTICS: Observation of eye patch or shield over both eyes, retinal separation confirmed by ophthamologic examination, reports visual impairment consistent with retinal detachment

PATIENT OUTCOME (collaborative): Demonstrates no further injury

EVALUATION CRITERIA: Reports no further vision loss, no falls

INTERVENTIONS	RATIONALE
1. Keep call bell at bedside and siderails elevated. Instruct the patient to signal for assistance.	To provide a sense of security.

INTERVENTIONS	RATIONALE
2. Maintain strict bedrest as ordered in the prescribed supine position: • right lateral position (if the retinal tear is in the nasal position of the left eye or the temporal position of the right eye) • left lateral position (if the retinal tear is in the nasal position of the right eye or the temporal position of the left eye)	To allow the vitreous humor to act as a hemostatic force to control bleeding.
3. Avoid moving the patient. Delay full hygienic care until the tear has been surgically repaired. Instruct the patient to avoid sudden movements of the head and coughing. Admininster prescribed antiemetic, cough suppressant, and analgesic prn	Jarring the body places additional stress on an already weakened retina, which can cause further separation.
4. Keep both eyes covered until surgery is performed.	Even though retinal detachment may be unilateral, movement of one eye causes movement of the other eye (consensual movement). Eye movement increases the risk of further separation.
5. Prepare the patient for surgery as ordered. See Eye Surgery (page 499).	Surgery is the only treatment to resolve retinal detachment.

E ar Surgery

Most **ear surgery** for adults is done as treatment for:

1. otosclerosis — condition in which the stapes becomes fixated to the oval window as a result of bony overgrowth of the labyrinth. Both ears are affected, but at different rates.

2. Ménière's disease — disorder of the membraneous labyrinth in which there is hydropic distention of the endolymphatic system. It has an unknown etiology, and usually affects only one ear.

3. Improving sensorineural hearing loss.

Types of ear surgery include:

1. **Cochlear implantation** — electrode-type device is surgically implanted in the cochlea to allow some degree of hearing for persons who suffer from sensorineural deafness. The device is attached to an external microphone that the patient wears behind the ear. The quality of speech heard by the patient is equated with that spoken by the cartoon character Donald Duck. Intensive rehabilitation is required for the patient to learn how to use the device.

2. **Stapedectomy** — procedure in which the stapes is removed and replaced with a prosthesis to restore hearing in patients who suffer from otosclerosis. It is generally performed through a transtympanic approach.

Before surgery the patient has a complete audiological analysis and laboratory studies to rule out metabolic disorders and infection as causes of the severe hearing loss. Preoperative preparation is the same for any patient undergoing surgery.

Postoperatively with a transtympanic approach the patient usually returns to a medical/surgical unit with a cotton wick in the ear that is removed on the first postoperative day. Bedrest in a semi-Fowler's position is usually followed for the first 24 hours. Mild pain is expected. Some dizziness and light-headedness may be experienced when getting out of bed for the first time. Cracking and popping sounds may be experienced but should resolve as healing progresses. Hearing is diminished but gradually improves as swelling subsides.

Integrative Care Plans

• Preoperative and postoperative care

516

Discharge Considerations

- Follow-up care
- Activity limitations
- Signs and symptoms requiring medical attention
- Medications for home use

THE PREOPERATIVE PERIOD

 *A*SSESSMENT DATA BASE

1. Physical examination based on an assessment of auditory status (Appendix I) may reveal reports of:
   - diminished hearing with otosclerosis.
   - vertigo attacks, which can be accompanied by nausea and sometimes vomiting, tinnitus, a feeling of fullness in the ear, and progressive hearing loss.
2. See Preoperative and Postoperative Care (page 738).

THE POSTOPERATIVE PERIOD

 *A*SSESSMENT DATA BASE

1. On receiving the patient:
   - Inspect the ear dressing.
   - Assess for pain and nausea.
   - Assess hearing acuity.
   - Inquire about dizziness, light-headedness, or unusual sounds in the ear.
2. See Preoperative and Postoperative Care (page 738).

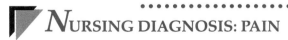

*N*URSING DIAGNOSIS: PAIN

RELATED TO FACTORS: Ear surgery

DEFINING CHARACTERISTICS: Verbalizes discomfort, frowning, moaning, guarding painful site

PATIENT OUTCOME (collaborative): Demonstrates relief from discomfort

EVALUATION CRITERIA: Denies pain, relaxed facial expression, absence of moaning

INTERVENTIONS	RATIONALE
1. Maintain bedrest as ordered with the head of the bed slightly elevated. Instruct the patient to avoid lying on the operative side if a transmastoid approach is used.	Elevation promotes drainage thereby reducing swelling. Lying on the operative side places undue stress on the incision.
2. Administer prescribed analgesic prn and evaluate effectiveness. Consult physician if pain persists or worsens.	Analgesics block the pain pathway. Mild pain is expected. Pain unrelieved by analgesia can indicate infection or bleeding.
3. Administer prescribed antiemetic prn and evaluate its effectiveness.	Vomiting increases pressure within the eustachian tube, which increases discomfort in the ear.

NURSING DIAGNOSIS: HIGH RISK FOR INFECTION

RELATED TO FACTORS: Disruption of tissue secondary to ear surgery

DEFINING CHARACTERISTICS: Returns from surgery with dressing in ear, may show elevation of temperature and WBC

PATIENT OUTCOME (collaborative): Demonstrates no signs of infection

EVALUATION CRITERIA: Temperature below 99°F, absence of purulent ear discharge and pain, WBC between 5,000–10,000/mm^3

INTERVENTIONS	RATIONALE
1. Monitor q4h: • temperature • hearing acuity • ear for drainage • level of comfort	To detect early signs of infection.
2. Consult physician if fever, persistent headache, increased ear pain, or excess drainage from the ear occurs. Culture purulent drainage. Administer antibiotics as prescribed and evaluate effectiveness.	These findings indicate infection. Minimal drainage is expected for the first 24 hours. Antibiotic therapy helps resolve the infective organism identified by the culture.

INTERVENTIONS	RATIONALE
3. Change the ear wick as ordered using universal precautions and aseptic technique (thorough hand-washing before and after patient care, wearing gloves when contact with the blood or body fluid is likely to occur).	Prevents cross-contamination and risk of spread of bacteria.

NURSING DIAGNOSIS: HIGH RISK FOR INJURY

RELATED TO FACTORS: Disturbances in equilibrium secondary to ear surgery

DEFINING CHARACTERISTICS: Reports feeling light-headed or dizzy, sways when standing or walking

PATIENT OUTCOME: Demonstrates no evidence of physical injury

EVALUATION CRITERIA: Reports no falls, absence of bruising on legs

INTERVENTIONS	RATIONALE
1. Keep bed in lowest position, call bell at the bedside, and siderails up. Instruct the patient to signal for assistance before getting out of bed if dizzy or light-headed. Advise the patient to avoid sudden head movements.	To prevent falls.
2. Place the patient on "Falls Precautions" as defined by facility protocol.	To ensure all persons coming into contact with the patient take appropriate actions to ensure patient safety.
3. If Ménière's disease exists, administer meclizine HCL (Antivert) as prescribed and evaluate effectiveness. Instruct the patient to lie or sit and to avoid sudden head movements during episodes of vertigo.	Antivert is the drug of choice for Ménière's disease. It acts by blocking the conduction of impulses along the vestibular portion of the 8th cranial nerve, thus relieving nausea and vomiting associated with the disease. Sudden head movements intensify dizziness.

NURSING DIAGNOSIS: ALTERATIONS IN SENSORY PERCEPTION

RELATED TO FACTORS: Diminished hearing secondary to ear surgery

DEFINING CHARACTERISTICS: Verbalizes diminished hearing, turns head when listening, continually asks for statements to be repeated

PATIENT OUTCOME: Demonstrates absence of sense of isolation

EVALUATION CRITERIA: Denies feeling isolated, reports needs have been adequately met, shows less frustration with communication

INTERVENTIONS	RATIONALE
1. Flag the Kardex and intercom system to indicate "Hearing Impairment." Go directly to the patient's room to address the patient instead of using the intercom system. Also, post a sign above the patient's bed.	All persons coming into contact with the patient should be aware of the hearing deficit. Devising measures to ensure the patient can communicate needs help prevent feelings of isolation.
2. Face the patient when talking. Speak slowly and clearly.	Some patients may be able to lip-read.
3. Keep a pad and pencil at the bedside to write messages if needed.	To facilitate communication.
4. If the patient has a hearing aid for the nonoperative ear, ensure it is in place and turned on. Change the battery if a continuous ringing or buzzing occurs.	Diminished hearing is expected in the operative ear. Hearing is unaffected in the nonoperative ear. A constant noise from a hearing aid indicates a weak battery.

NURSING DIAGNOSIS: HIGH RISK FOR IMPAIRED HOME MAINTENANCE MANAGEMENT

RELATED TO FACTORS: Knowledge deficit about self-care activities on discharge

DEFINING CHARACTERISTICS: Verbalizes lack of understanding, requests information, may report history of noncompliance

PATIENT OUTCOME: Demonstrates willingness to comply with self-care measures for ear on discharge

EVALUATION CRITERIA: Verbalizes understanding of home care instructions, correctly performs required self-care skills, verbalizes satisfaction with home care plans

INTERVENTIONS	RATIONALE
1. Provide written instructions for follow-up care and visits.	Verbal instructions may be easily forgotten.
2. Teach proper care of the ear: • Sneeze or cough with mouth open for one week after surgery. • Avoid blowing the nose for one week to prevent blockage of the eustachian tube. If patient must blow nose, blow one side at a time gently with mouth open. • Avoid airplane flights for one week after surgery. • For sensation of ear pressure, hold nose, close mouth, and swallow to equalize pressure. • Wear noise deafeners for loud noise environment. • Wear the ear wick and change daily and prn. Wash hands before changing the ear wick to prevent infection. • Avoid swimming and shampooing the hair until approved by the physician. Wear a shower cap and cover the ears when taking a shower. Explain that water in the ear provides a good culture medium for bacteria. • Contact physician if bleeding or signs of infection occur: fever, increased ear pain, persistent headache, increased drainage on ear wick. Antibiotic therapy is required to resolve infections.	Discharge teaching is important to ensure a safe recovery and patient compliance.
3. Ensure the patient has: • sufficient supply of ear wicks. Teach and have the patient practice changing the ear wick. • prescription for pain medication if needed.	To ensure a safe and comfortable recovery.

BIBLIOGRAPHY

Alberti, P.W., Ginsberg, I.A., and Goode, R.L. (1988). Managing adult hearing loss. **Patient Care, 22,** 54–58, 63, 67, 70, 73, 76.

Blair, K.A. (1990). Aging: Physiological aspects and clinical implications. **Nurse Practitioner, 15,** 14–16, 18, 23, 26–28.

Maniglia, A.J. (1989). Implantable hearing devices. **The Otolaryngologic Clinics of North America, 22,** 175–199.

Martinelli, A.M. (1991). Glaucoma: Classifications, treatment options, patient care. **Association of Operating Room Nurses, 54,** 743–756.

C

CHAPTER NINE
Problems of the Liver, Biliary, and Pancreatic Systems

Pancreatitis

Pancreatitis refers to inflammation of the pancreas. It can be acute or chronic. The exact mechanism causing the inflammatory reaction is unclear but is believed to be autodigestion (Moorhouse et al, 1988). It is characterized by excess production of proteolytic enzymes that begin to digest pancreatic tissue causing edema, necrosis, and hemorrhage.

The major complications associated with pancreatitis are pseudocyst and abscess formation. These abnormal cavities can ultimately rupture and lead to peritonitis. Pseudocyst can resolve spontaneously; however, surgery is usually required to drain these abnormal cavities to prevent peritonitis (Moorhouse et al, 1988).

The mean LOS for a DRG classification of pancreatitis is 6.1 days (Lorenz, 1991).

General Medical Management

- NPO during acute phase
- Analgesics
- Pancreatic enzymes

Integrative Care Plans

- Pain
- Immobility
- IV therapy
- Shock
- Preoperative and postoperative care (if surgery is planned)

Discharge Considerations

- Follow-up care
- Medications for home use
- Measures to prevent recurrence

ASSESSMENT DATA BASE

1. History or presence of causative factors:
   - chronic alcoholism and biliary disease (primarily gallstones) (most common causes of acute pancreatitis)
   - endoscopic procedure
   - hyperlipidemia
   - hypercalcemia
   - certain drugs
   - organ transplantation
   - peptic ulcer disease

2. Physical examination based on a general survey (Appendix F) may reveal:
   a. Most significant findings:
      - persistent, severe epigastric pain that may radiate to chest and back. Pain is accompanied by nausea, vomiting, and abdominal tenderness. Usually, the pain is lessened by leaning forward or assuming a knee-chest position.
      - hypoactive bowel sounds
      - fever
      - symptoms of hypovolemic shock (page 769)
      - a palpable abdominal mass usually appears about 5–10 days after disease onset
      - steatorrhea (undigested fats in the stool) caused by decreased secretion of lipase and bile in duodenum
   b. Other less common manifestations:
      - jaundice
      - xanthomas
      - subcutaneous nodules
      - umbilical (Cullen's sign) or flank (Turner's sign) hemorrhagic discoloration of the skin
      - tetany

3. Diagnostic studies:
   - Elevated serum amylase, serum lipase, and urine amylase establish the diagnoses. Amylase and lipase are produced by the pancreas and cleared by the kidney. The degree of serum amylase or lipase elevation does not reflect the severity of pancreatitis.
   - Ultrasound and CT scan of the pancreas are useful in detecting complications.

   Additional laboratory studies include liver function studies, serum electrolytes, serum calcium, serum glucose, ABG, CBC, serum lipids, and stools for blood and fat.

4. Assess patient's emotional response and understanding of condition and treatment program.

NURSING DIAGNOSIS: PAIN

RELATED TO FACTORS: Pancreatitis

DEFINING CHARACTERISTICS: Verbalizes discomfort, moaning, frowning, guarding painful site

PATIENT OUTCOME (collaborative): Demonstrates relief from discomfort

EVALUATION CRITERIA: Fewer reports of pain, relaxed facial expression, absence of moaning

INTERVENTIONS	RATIONALE
1. Maintain bedrest in a semi-Fowler's position with knee of bed slightly gatched. Keep NPO.	To facilitate breathing and to relieve tension on abdominal muscles. Food in the duodenum activates release of pancreatic enzymes that increases pain.
2. Administer prescribed narcotic analgesic prn and evaluate effectiveness. Avoid giving morphine sulfate if pancreatitis occurred secondary to biliary tract disease; suggest meperidine HCl (Demerol) instead.	Analgesics block the pain pathway. Narcotics are needed to control severe pain. Morphine sulfate causes spasms of the sphincter of Oddi, which can intensify pain if pancreatitis occurred secondary to biliary tract disease.
3. Insert an N/G tube as ordered and irrigate prn with normal saline. While the tube is in place, keep the patient NPO and provide oral care q2h.	An N/G tube helps control nausea and vomiting by maintaining gastric decompression thereby reducing pancreatic activity. Oral care helps lubricate the oral cavity thus preventing drying, which can occur when patient is NPO for several hours.
4. Administer antacids such as cimetidine (Tagamet) and ranitidine (Zantac) as prescribed and evaluate effectiveness.	These agents reduce gastric secretion thereby reducing stimulation of the pancreas.
5. Administer sedatives or tranquilizers as prescribed and evaluate effectiveness.	To promote rest thereby reducing pancreatic activity.
6. Consult physician if pain persists or worsens.	This can indicate abcess formation and a need for further diagnostic evaluation.

NURSING DIAGNOSIS: HIGH RISK FOR INFECTION

RELATED TO FACTORS: Pancreatitis

DEFINING CHARACTERISTICS: Fever, WBC greater than 10,000/mm^3

PATIENT OUTCOME (collaborative): Demonstrates no manifestations of infection

EVALUATION CRITERIA: Temperature within normal limits, WBC between 5,000–10,000/mm^3

INTERVENTIONS	RATIONALE

1. Monitor:
  • temperature q4h
  • results of CBC reports, particularly WBC
	To identify indications of progress toward or deviations from expected outcome.

2. Administer prescribed antibiotics and evaluate effectiveness. Adhere always to universal precautions (good handwashing technique, wearing gloves when contact with blood or body fluid is likely to occur).	Usually, fever is associated with abcess formation. The inflamed pancreas is susceptible to bacterial growth. Caregivers are the most common source of nosocomial infections. Universal precations help prevent cross-contamination, and also protect the caregiver as well as the patient.

NURSING DIAGNOSIS: ALTERATIONS IN FLUID VOLUME: DEFICIT

RELATED TO FACTORS: Decreased oral intake secondary to nausea and vomiting, gastric suctioning, third spacing, hemorrage

DEFINING CHARACTERISTICS: Serum sodium below normal value, reports thirst, dry ashy skin, voiding concentrated urine, blood pressure below baseline value, daily weight loss, poor skin turgor

PATIENT OUTCOME (collaborative): Demonstrates adequate fluid volume

EVALUATION CRITERIA: Stable vital signs, good skin turgor, strong peripheral pulses, good capillary refill, urinary output above 30mL/hr

INTERVENTIONS	RATIONALE
1. Monitor: • results of electrolyte studies • intake and output q8h or qh if symptoms of shock are present • vital signs q2h or q4h if stable • general status (Appendix F) q8h	To identify indications of progress toward or deviations from expected outcome.
2. Administer prescribed electrolyte supplements and evaluate effectiveness.	Calcium gluconate may be required to correct hypocalcemia that occurs when large amounts of calcium are lost through the stool caused by increased calcium binding calcium with free fats in the small intestine.
3. Initiate and maintain prescribed IV therapy that can include lactated Ringer's solution or plasma volume expanders. Perform appropriate actions to prevent and correct complications of IV therapy (page 764).	To replace lost fluids and correct hypovolemic shock. Bleeding and a fluid shift from intravascular spaces to interstitial spaces cause hypovolemia. Cardiac output falls, and symptoms of hypovolemic shock appear.
4. Insert a Foley catheter as ordered for an accurate assessment of renal output. Notify physician if urinary output falls below 30 mL/hr or 240 mL/8 hr.	A drop in urinary output occurs with hypovolemic shock. This finding also indicates inadequate fluid replacement therapy.
5. See Fluid and Biochemical Imbalance (page 773) for additional interventions per imbalance.	

• •

NURSING DIAGNOSIS: ALTERATION IN NUTRITION: LESS THAN BODY REQUIREMENTS

RELATED TO FACTORS: Decreased food intake secondary to nausea and vomiting, prescribed dietary restrictions

DEFINING CHARACTERISTICS: Weight loss, reports anorexia, consumes less than 30% of meals, verbalizes gastric discomfort, poor muscle tone

PATIENT OUTCOME (collaborative): Demonstrates improved nutritional status

EVALUATION CRITERIA: No further weight loss, consumes increased percentage of meals, denies gastric discomfort

• •

INTERVENTIONS	RATIONALE
1. Monitor: • weight daily • amount of food consumed during each meal • results of serum chemistry studies • abdominal status (Appendix B) q8h • blood glucose studies	To identify indications of progress toward or deviations from expected outcome.
2. Keep NPO until nausea and vomiting subside. Administer antiemetic prn and evaluate effectiveness. Administer TPN (page 220) as prescribed.	To control nausea and vomiting. TPN solutions provide all the essential amino acids, vitamins, and provide carbohydrates.
3. Notify physician if sluggish or absent bowel sounds or abdominal distention accompanied by nausea and vomiting occur. Insert an N/G tube to low intermittent suction as ordered. Irrigate tube with normal saline prn to maintain patency.	These findings indicate paralytic ileus. Gastric decompression allows the pancreas to rest.
4. If blood glucose is above normal value, administer regular insulin as ordered.	Transient hyperglycemia can occur as a result of beta cell damage and pancreatic necrosis.
5. When oral feedings are allowed, administer prescribed pancreatic supplements such as pancrelipase (Cotazym, VioKase) pancreatin, or bile salts. Provide a bland, low-fat, high-protein diet as ordered.	Pancreatic supplements aid in digestion of fats, proteins, and carbohydrates. Expect an increase in food intake and passage of normal stools after taking these supplements. Spices and fats stimulate pancreatic activity. Fats need lipase and bile to be completely digested. Protein aids in tissue repair. The pancreas produces and secretes lipase and protease, all important for digestion in the small intestine.

INTERVENTIONS	RATIONALE
1. See Nursing Diagnosis: Anxiety (page 262).	

. . . .

NURSING DIAGNOSIS: HIGH RISK FOR IMPAIRED HOME MAINTENANCE MANAGEMENT

RELATED TO FACTORS: Knowledge deficit about self-care on discharge

DEFINING CHARACTERISTICS: Verbalizes lack of understanding, requests information, may report history of noncompliance

PATIENT OUTCOME: Demonstrates willingness to comply with self-care activities on discharge

EVALUATION CRITERIA: Verbalizes understanding of home care instructions, verbalizes satisfaction with home care plans

. . . .

INTERVENTIONS	RATIONALE
1. Inform the patient that prescribed pancreatic supplements must be taken until pancreatic enzyme values return to normal.	Patients are more cooperative with the treatment plan if they understand how the treatments help correct their illness.
2. Provide a written appointment for a follow-up visit and written home care instructions, including name, dosage, purpose, schedule, and reportable side effects of medications prescribed for home use.	Verbal instructions may be easily forgotten.
3. Advise the patient to seek medical attention if symptoms recur and to refrain from alcohol consumption. Refer patient to an alcoholic support group if alcohol consumption is a problem.	One episode of pancreatitis does not confer immunity against repeat episodes. Excessive alcohol intake is well documented as a major contributing factor in pancreatitis.

H epatitis

Hepatitis refers to an acute inflammation of the liver. It can be caused by bacteria or toxic injury, but viral hepatitis is seen most often (Alter et al, 1990).

The primary types of viral hepatitis are (Hollinger, 1991):

1. Hepatitis A:
   - transmitted by oral-anal practices, contaminated food, water, and shellfish
   - incubation period about 2–6 weeks, which is the most contagious period
   - prophylaxis: immune globulin before and after exposure provides passive immunity for 2–3 months

2. Hepatitis B:
   - transmitted by blood and blood products through contaminated transfusions and broken skin and mucous membranes via contaminated needles, sexual intercourse, tattooing, direct contact with an open wound, or through handling of infected equipment and supplies
   - incubation period about 6 weeks to 6 months.
   - person is considered contagious as long as surface antigen appears. A carrier state or chronic hepatitis B virus (HBV) exists when the surface antigen remains detectable after six months.
   - prophylaxis: HBV vaccine before exposure provides active immunity. To maintain immunity, the vaccine must be repeated after one month, six months, and seven years. Administering hepatitis B immuneglobulin (HBIG) provides passive immunity to unvaccinated persons exposed to the virus.

3. Hepatitis C:
   - transmitted by same route as HBV
   - incubation period about 2 weeks to 6 months
   - prophylaxis: Immune globulin before and after exposure provides passive immunity for 2–3 months
   - believed to be responsible for posttransfusion hepatitis.

Delta hepatitis, another variant form of viral hepatitis B, is often seen in IV drug users (Hollinger, 1991). It carries a high mortality rate. For delta hepatitis virus to remain viable, hepatitis B virus also must be present. This variant form of viral hepatitis is transmitted in the same manner as hepatitis B and has similar characteristics (Alter et al, 1990). Thus, the prophylaxis used for hepatitis B is also effective against both hepatitis C and delta hepatitis.

Complete recovery of liver function occurs with type A hepatitis. Chronic (active/persistent) hepatitis is a major sequalae of type B. Chronic active hepatitis is characterized by progressive liver damage in which case the prognosis for recovery is poor.

With chronic persistent hepatitis, the patient is clinically asymptomatic except for persistent elevation of serum transaminase levels. No liver damage occurs, and the prognosis for recovery is good.

Usually, hospitalization is not required for treatment, except in severe cases when supportive IV therapy is needed. The mean LOS for a DRG classification of hepatitis B is 6.7 days (Lorenz, 1991).

General prophylaxis against hepatitis B is recommended for:

- persons traveling to high endemic areas
- all healthcare workers exposed to blood
- all patients who have hemophilia or any sickle cell disease
- infants of mothers who are antigen-positive
- patients receiving hemodialysis
- homosexually active males

Contacts of infected persons also must receive prophylaxis. For patients with hepatitis A, contacts receive immune globulin G (Gamastan, Gammar, or Immuglobin). Contacts of patients with hepatitis B receive hepatitis B vaccine (Heptavax-B). Heptavax-B vaccine is derived from plasma. Because of the increased incidence of AIDS, a yeast-derived vaccine (Recombivax-HB) may be used as primary prophylaxis instead of the plasma-derived agent. These vaccines provide short-term immunity (less than four months). The vaccine is given in a series of three intramuscular injections, with the second dose one month after the initial injection and the third dose six months after the initial injection.

General Medical Management

There are no specific medications for treating viral hepatitis. As a general measure against nosocomial infections, healthcare workers should always follow blood and body fluid precautions when providing any patient care.

Integrative Care Plans

- Loss if chronic hepatitis occurs
- IV therapy

Discharge Considerations

- Follow-up care
- Measures to prevent cross-contamination
- Signs and symptoms of exacerbation

ASSESSMENT DATA BASE

1. Inquire about source of exposure.

2. Inquire about contacts.

3. Assess for clinical manifestations. The manifestations are the same for each type of viral hepatitis; however, with hepatitis A the onset of symptoms is more abrupt. Symptoms occur in three phases:

    • preicteric phase (period in which infectivity is greatest)—nausea, vomiting, diarrhea, constipation, weight loss, malaise, headache, low-grade fever, joint aches, skin rash

    • icteric phase—jaundice (most prominent finding), dark smoky urine (caused by increased levels of bilirubin), hepatomegaly with tenderness, lymph node enlargement, pruritus (result of accumulation of bile salts in the skin); symptoms of the preicteric phase subside as these symptoms emerge

    • posticteric phase—previous symptoms subside but fatigue continues; four months needed for complete recovery

4. Assess feelings about condition and understanding of diagnostic studies and treatment plan.

5. Diagnostic studies:

    • For hepatitis A — presence of antihepatitis A antibodies (immunoglobulin M) in serum

    • For hepatitis B — presence of surface antigen (HBSAg) in serum; carrier state is diagnosed by the presence of hepatitis B core antibodies in serum

    • Liver function studies such as serum and urine bilirubin, alkaline phosphatase, aspartate aminotransferase (AST), alanine aminotransferase (ALT), are elevated, reflecting injury to the liver

    • Biopsy of the liver (if hepatitis persists for more than six months) to differentiate between chronic active and persistent active.

    There is no specific test for hepatitis C, non-A, non-B, and delta hepatitis because they have no detectable antigen and antigenic subtypes.

    A diagnosis of non-A or non-B hepatitis is established if the serology tests are negative for hepatitis A and B and nonviral causes (alcohol abuse, medications, heart failure, bacteria) cannot be confirmed.

• •

NURSING DIAGNOSIS: ACTIVITY INTOLERANCE

RELATED TO FACTORS: Inadequate nutritional intake secondary to hepatitis, general malaise, depression, imposed activity restriction

DEFINING CHARACTERISTICS: Reports fatigue and weakness when performing ADL, experiences tachycardia and tachypnea in response to activity

PATIENT OUTCOME (collaborative): Demonstrates improved tolerance to activities

EVALUATION CRITERIA: Denies fatigue with exertion, absence of tachycardia and tachypnea when performing ADL

• •

INTERVENTIONS	RATIONALE

1. Monitor:
  • results of clotting studies (PT and PTT) and serum liver enzymes
  • weight qod
  • results of liver function studies
  • general status (Appendix F) q8h
  • amount of food consumed with each meal
	To identify indications of progress toward or deviations from expected outcome.

2. Encourage rest. Assist with ADL as needed. Allow progressive activity as the serum liver enzyme levels decrease.	Excess physical activity increases metabolic rate that places strain on an already poorly functioning liver.
3. Consult physician if any prescribed medication is contraindicated for patients with liver dysfunction.	Such drugs should be avoided as long as liver enzymes are elevated. A damaged liver cannot perform its normal function of metabolizing drugs.
4. Administer prescribed nutritional supplements such as multiple vitamin supplements or vitamin K injections.	Vitamins are essential for tissue repair. Vitamin K, which is normally stored by the liver, is essential for normal clotting. Bleeding predisposes patient to anemia, which causes fatigue.
5. Provide a high-carbohydrate, low-fat diet. Refer the patient to a dietitian for assistance with meal planning. If food intake is less than 30%, suggest a supplemental feeding such as Ensure or Sustacal. Explain the purpose of dietary modifications. Emphasize there is no specific diet to alter the course of the disease. Diet modifications ensure an adequate intake of calories to meet the energy needs of the body and to reduce protein catabolism.	Carbohydrates exert a protein-sparing effect. Dietary proteins can be increased if serum ammonia level is not elevated. Bile salts, produced by the liver, are needed for fat digestion. A dietitian is a nutritional specialist who can assist the patient in planning a menu to meet nutritional needs in view of current illness.

NURSING DIAGNOSIS: HIGH RISK FOR IMPAIRED SKIN INTEGRITY

RELATED TO FACTORS: Itching secondary to bile salt accumulation in the tissues

DEFINING CHARACTERISTICS: Verbalizes discomfort, scratch marks on skin

PATIENT OUTCOME (collaborative): Demonstrates relief from discomfort

EVALUATION CRITERIA: Denies joint discomfort with movement, no scratches on skin, reports feeling comfortable

INTERVENTIONS	RATIONALE
1. Initiate comfort measures: • cool shower or bath • backrub • warm liquids • low-energy diversional activities (reading, watching TV, board games) • cold cloth to forehead for headache • eggcrate mattress • quiet environment	These measures promote rest. Rest reduces the body's energy needs thus reducing the strain on the liver.
2. Administer prescribed antipyretic and evaluate effectiveness.	To resolve fever. Fever is associated with increased warmth and sweating as the fever resolves. Warmth coupled with moisture increases itching.
3. Keep linen and clothing dry.	Wet clothing from sweating is a source of discomfort.
4. Encourage visits from family and friends.	Isolation can cause boredom that triggers depression and heightens discomfort.
5. Initiate measures to relieve pruitus: • take cool shower or bath • use baking soda or cornstarch in water • avoid alkaline soaps	A cool temperature restricts vasodilation thus reducing the escape of bile salts to the skin surface. Baking soda and cornstarch help neutralize acids on the skin surface. Alkaline soaps have a drying effect, which increases itching. Caladryl lotion contains

INTERVENTIONS	RATIONALE
• apply Caladryl lotion • wear loose fitting clothing • keep room temperature cool	an antihistimine, Benadryl, which also counteracts skin surface acids and supresses sensory nerve ends that trigger itching sensation.
6. Keep patient's nails cut short. Instruct the patient to use knuckles to rub skin or use fingertips to press on the skin if a desire to scratch is great.	To reduce the risk of breaking the skin when scratching.

NURSING DIAGNOSIS: HIGH RISK FOR FLUID VOLUME DEFICIT

RELATED TO FACTORS: Diarrhea and vomiting secondary to hepatitis

DEFINING CHARACTERISTICS: Poor skin turgor, dry ashy skin, voiding concentrated urine, serum sodium above normal value, blood pressure below baseline value, reports thirst

PATIENT OUTCOME (collaborative): Demonstrates adequate fluid status

EVALUATION CRITERIA: Serum sodium within normal range, moist mucous membranes, urinary output greater than 30mL/hr, fewer reports of thirst, good skin tugor, brisk capillary refill, serum sodium within normal range

INTERVENTIONS	RATIONALE
1. See Fluid and Biochemical Imbalance (page 773).	
2. Administer prescribed antidiarrheal prn and evaluate effectiveness.	To control diarrhea. Uncontrolled, diarrhea can cause further fluid and electrolyte deficit.

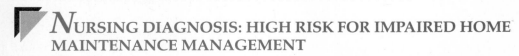

NURSING DIAGNOSIS: HIGH RISK FOR IMPAIRED HOME MAINTENANCE MANAGEMENT

RELATED TO FACTORS: Knowledge deficit about condition and self-care on discharge

DEFINING CHARACTERISTICS: Verbalizes lack of understanding, noncompliance with isolation procedures, requests information

PATIENT OUTCOME: Demonstrates willingness to comply with home care plan

EVALUATION CRITERIA: Adheres to isolation precautions, verbalizes understanding of illness and treatment plan, identifies names of at-risk contacts, verbalizes satisfaction with home care plan

• •

INTERVENTIONS	RATIONALE
1. Provide information about hepatitis: how it is transmitted, how it can be prevented. Reassure the patient with hepatitis A that the disease is self-limiting and that jaundice eventually subsides as liver function returns to normal. Explain the purpose of prescribed medication. Let the patient know there are no specific drugs to cure hepatitis because it is caused by a virus. Time is the best curative approach. Explain that urine is dark or smoky until liver function returns to normal.	Health teaching enhances patient compliance with the treatment program.
2. Initiate blood and body fluid precautions or universal precautions for all types of hepatitis. Explain rationale for protective care procedures. Emphasize the importance of handwashing. Explain purpose of isolation precautions to visitors.	The hepatitis virus can be transmitted by the oral-fecal route, blood, and body fluid.
3. Encourage the patient to report previous direct contacts. Explain that prophylaxis is required for sexual and immediate contacts.	To prevent the spread of hepatitis.
4. Notify infection control nurse of the patient's admission.	Community-acquired infections must be monitored and appropriate steps taken to prevent nosocomial infections.

INTERVENTIONS	RATIONALE
5. Provide a written appointment for a follow-up visit and self-care. Explain the importance of follow-up testing and what it entails: within three months follow-up testing for hepatitis B surface antigen is done. If no surface antigen is found, the patient is no longer infectious. If surface antigen is still present, the patient is considered a carrier and needs to be retested in three months. Contacts of carriers should receive the hepatitis B vaccine.	Verbal instructions may be easily forgotten. A knowledge of what to expect helps promote compliance.
6. Instruct the patient to seek medical attention if symptoms of hepatitis recur or persist.	One episode does not confer immunity against repeat episodes.
7. Instruct the patient to avoid intake of alcohol if excess alcohol intake is a problem. Refer the patient to a community alcoholic support group.	Alcohol is detoxified by the liver. A diseased liver cannot detoxify substances. A support system is essential to successful recovery from alcoholism.

Diabetes Mellitus

Diabetes mellitus (DM) is a chronic incurable but controllable metabolic disorder characterized by hyperglycemia subsequent to an insulin deficiency or inadequate insulin utilization.

There are two types of diabetes: type I and type II. Type I DM, also called insulin-dependent diabetes mellitus (IDDM), begins abruptly and before the age of 30. It is believed linked to either a viral attack, an autoimmune response in which the body triggers destruction of pancreatic beta cells, or an HLA histocompatibility antigen-antibody response (Guthrie & Guthrie, 1991).

Type II DM, also called non–insulin-dependent diabetes mellitus (NIDDM), occurs most often in adulthood, especially in obese individuals. Contributing etiological factors are heredity, diminished islet cell sensitivity to glucose, delayed insulin secretion due to beta cell dysfunction, or increased resistance to insulin due to a decreased insulin-receptor density (Guthrie & Guthrie, 1991).

The major acute complications associated with DM are diabetic ketoacidosis (DKA), hyperglycemic hyperosmolar nonketotic syndrome (HHNKS), and hypoglycemia. The major long-term complications associated with DM are macrovascular disease, microvascular disease, and neuropathy. Ketoacidosis is more prevalent among type I diabetics because no insulin is produced, whereas type II DM diabetics produce some insulin but not enough to maintain normal blood glucose levels. Microvascular disease and neuropathy occur more readily among type II DM diabetics because of the difficulty in determining hyperglycemia onset. The best means of preventing these complications is through glycemic control.

DKA is an acute potentially life-threatening metabolic disorder that occurs as a result of a prolonged insulin deficiency. It is characterized by extreme hyperglycemia (greater than 300 mg/dL). DKA is manifested as an exaggerated pathophysiological state of DM (Guthrie & Guthrie, 1991). The patient appears severely ill and requires emergency intervention to reduce the blood glucose level and correct the severe acidosis, electrolyte, and fluid inbalances. Factors precipitating ketoacidosis include:

- drugs (steroids, diuretics, alcohol, immunosuppressive agents)
- decreased fluid intake
- failure to take insulin as prescribed
- severe emotional stress

- failure to follow dietary modifications
- underlying disease (renal and cardiovascular disorders)
- severe illness (infection, surgery, trauma)
- TPN (total parenteral nutrition) therapy

DKA usually occurs in type I diabetics. Because type I diabetics produce no endogenous insulin, the onset of manifestations is abrupt. Physical and laboratory examination reveal:

- severely elevated blood glucose, which may range from 200–800 mg/dL
- ketonuria
- normal osmolality but in some cases slightly increased
- elevated BUN
- decreased pH and bicarbonate level
- decreased, normal, or increased serum sodium and potassium
- rapid, deep respirations (Kussmaul breathing)
- acetone breath
- polyuria and polydipsia
- dehydration (low BP, rapid pulse, weakness, warm dry skin, decreased level of consciousness, elevated temperature)

These changes occur when glucose uptake is impaired because of an insulin deficiency. To counteract this deficit, secretion of glucagon, epinephrine, cortisol, and growth hormone increases. In response to these hormones, glycogenolysis, gluconeogenesis, lipolysis, and ketogenesis increase. Ketones accumulate as a result of increased lipolysis and ketogenesis, giving rise to the acetone breath and large amounts of urinary ketones. The by-products of protein conversion to glucose give rise to the elevated BUN. The acidic by-products of both fat and protein conversion to glucose cause metabolic acidosis, reflected by a decreased pH and bicarbonate level. The respiratory rate increases in an attempt to blow off the excess carbon dioxide, which is formed as the body attempts an acid-base equilibrium. Glycosuria occurs that causes osmotic diuresis, polydipsia, and dehydration.

Treatment includes:

- hospitalization
- IV therapy to correct dehydration and electrolyte imbalances, particularly potassium; two infusions are started, normal saline and D5W
- insulin to facilitate the transport of glucose across the cell wall and return blood glucose level to a normal range
- potassium chloride added to the IV infusion after the blood glucose decreases to an acceptable level to prevent extracellular hypokalemia, which may occur when hydrogen ions leave the cell making room for glucose and potassium

HHNKS is a potentially life-threatening metabolic crisis that usually affects type II diabetics. In these patients, ketones are absent in the blood and urine because type II diabetics produce some endogenous insulin so the acidic by-products of fat metabolism do not accumulate in the bloodstream. Also, because some insulin is produced by the pancreas, the onset of manifestations is gradual. Factors that may precipitate HHNKS are the same as those for DKA with the exception of failure to take prescribed oral hypoglycemic agent.

Physical and laboratory examination reveal:

- extremely elevated blood glucose ranging from 600–2000 mg/dL
- normal pH and bicarbonate level
- normal respirations with no acetone breath
- polyuria, polydipsia
- severe dehydration characterized by elevated temperature, decreased BP, extreme thirst
- increased serum osmolality
- extremely elevated BUN
- decreased, normal, or increased serum sodium and potassium
- decreased level of consciousness

The basis for these manifestations and treatment is the same as that for DKA.

Hypoglycemia refers to a blood glucose below 60 mg/dL. It can occur when too much insulin or oral hypoglycemic agent is taken or when medications are taken but one does not eat.

Physical examination during a hypoglycemic episode reveals:

- autonomic responses:
  — sweating
  — palpitations
  — tremors
  — nervousness
  — pallor
  — hunger
- neuroglycopenic responses:
  — light-headedness
  — headache
  — confusion
  — irritability
  — difficulty concentrating
  — impaired judgment
  — weakness and seizures
  — coma in severe cases

Treatment includes intake of carbohydrates that act rapidly.

Macrovascular Disease is due to atherosclerosis (Guthrie & Guthrie, 1991). It primarily affects large and medium blood vessels. In the presence of an insulin deficiency, fats are converted to glucose for energy. Alterations in the synthesis and catabolism of fats result in elevated levels of VLDL (very low-density lipoproteins) and LDL (low-density lipoproteins). Vascular occlusion from atherosclerosis can cause coronary artery disease, peripheral vascular disease, and cerebral vascular disease.

Microvascular Disease primarily affects the small blood vessels and is caused by capillary basement membrane thickening from chronically elevated blood glucose levels. This causes diabetic retinopathy, neuropathy, and nephropathy.

Neuropathy is believed to be caused by impairment of nerve conduction velocity subsequent to a high glucose concentration and microvascular disease (Guthrie & Guthrie, 1991). Sensory motor neuropathy contributes to leg and foot ulcers and infection. Autonomic neuropathy contributes to a neurogenic bladder, impotence, constipation alternating with diarrhea, diminished sweating, gastroparesis, and orthostatic hypotension.

Hospitalization usually is not required for treatment of DM unless a complication develops. The mean LOS for a DRG classification of DM with complications is 5.8 days (Lorenz, 1991).

General Medical Management

* For type I DM:
  — insulin (because no endogenous insulin is produced)
* For type II DM:
  — dietary modification, exercise, and oral hypoglycemic agents

Integrative Care Plans

* Loss

Discharge Considerations

* Follow-up care
* Dietary modifications
* Planned exercise program
* Signs and symptoms of hypoglycemia with intervention
* Management of insulin therapy
* Community support agencies
* Blood glucose monitoring

 # ASSESSMENT DATA BASE

1. History or presence of risk factors:
   * family history of the disease
   * obesity
   * history of chronic pancreatitis
   * history of births over nine pounds
   * history of glucosuria during stress (pregnancy, surgery, trauma, infection, illness) or drug therapy (glucocorticosteroids, thiazide diuretics, oral contraceptives)

2. Assess for manifestations of DM:
   * polyuria (result of osmotic diuresis when renal threshold of glucose reabsorption is reached and excess glucose escapes through the kidney)

- polydipsia (caused by dehydration from polyuria)
- polyphagia (caused by increased energy expenditure from altered synthesis of proteins and fats)
- weight loss (result of increased protein and fat catabolism)

    Additional symptoms common to type II DM include:

- vulvular pruritus, fatigue, visual disturbances, irritability, and muscle cramps. These findings reflect electrolyte disturbances and development of atherosclerotic complications.

3. Diagnostic studies:

- Glucose tolerance test (GTT) is prolonged (greater than 200 mg/dL). Usually, this test is recommended for patients who demonstrate elevated blood glucose levels under stressful conditions.
- Fasting blood sugar (FBS) is normal or above normal.
- Glycosylated hemoglobin assay is above normal range. This test measures the percentage of glucose attached to hemoglobin. Glucose remains attached to hemoglobin for the life of the RBC. Normal range is 5–7%.
- Urinalysis is positive for glucose and ketones. In response to intracellular deficiency of glucose, proteins and fats are converted to glucose (gluconeogenesis) for energy. During this conversion process, free fatty acids are broken into ketone bodies by the liver. Ketosis develops as reflected by ketonuria. Glucosuria reflects that the renal threshold of glucose reabsorption is reached. Ketonuria signals ketoacidosis.
- Serum cholesterol and triglyceride levels can be elevated indicating inadequate glycemic control and increased propensity for development of atherosclerosis.

    A diagnosis of DM is made when the FBS is above 140 mg/dL for two or more occasions, and patient exhibits symptoms of DM (polyuria, polydipsia, polyphagia, weight loss, ketonuria, and fatigue). Also, a diagnosis can be established when the GTT sample for the 2-hour period and another period (30 minutes, 60 minutes, or 90 minutes) exceeds 200 mg/dL.

4. Assess the patient's understanding of condition, treatment, diagnostic studies, and self-care measures to prevent complications.
5. Assess the patient's feelings about the condition.

NURSING DIAGNOSIS: HIGH RISK FOR IMPAIRED HOME MAINTENANCE MANAGEMENT

RELATED TO FACTORS: Knowledge deficit about condition and therapeutic management, lack of adequate support system

DEFINING CHARACTERISTICS: Verbalizes lack of understanding, may report history of non-compliance, may verbalize lack of available support system

PATIENT OUTCOME (collaborative): Demonstrates willingness to comply with prescribed home management plan

EVALUATION CRITERIA: Verbalizes understanding of condition and treatment plan, performs health maintenance skills correctly, verbalizes understanding of relation between condition and treatments, verbalizes satisfaction with home maintenance plan

• •

INTERVENTIONS	RATIONALE
1. Teach the patient about DM, prescribed treatments for DM, and other aspects of care outlined on the patient teaching guide (Table 9–1). Evaluate effectiveness of teaching.	The more patients know about their condition, the more likely they are to comply with prescribed treatments.
2. Refer the patient to a diabetic self-care class, if provided by the facility, or a community agency or organization.	Because DM is a chronic lifelong disorder, continual support is essential in helping the person adapt to the lifestyle changes imposed by the therapeutic plan for self-maintenance, which may include blood glucose monitoring, fingerstick procedure, and possibly self-administration of insulin.
3. Refer the patient to the local chapter of the American Diabetic Association.	This organization provides written information about diabetes.
4. Keep patient informed about blood glucose results. Explain significance of the results in relation to the therapy.	To encourage patient involvement in assuming responsibility for self-care.
5. Refer the patient to a dietitian for instructions on meal planning for the prescribed diet. Emphasize the need to restrict alcohol intake because it has many calories and inhibits the release of insulin from the pancreas. If diabinese is used, tell the patient that an Antabuse-like reaction (headache, facial flushing) occurs if alcohol is taken.	A dietitian is a nutritional specialist who can assist the patient in planning meals using the diabetic exchange list to meet specific nutritional needs.

INTERVENTIONS	RATIONALE
6. Provide specific instructions for managing insulin therapy if insulin is required at home. Instructions should include: • Avoid giving cold insulin. Allow refrigerated insulin to warm at room temperature for one hour before taking. • Check expiration date on the insulin and discard vial if outdated. • Take prescribed dose of insulin at least 30 minutes before meals so peak action is reached with postprandial hyperglycemia. • Rotate subcutaneous injection sites. • Eat three meals daily. Eat a light snack to coincide with insulin peaks to prevent hypoglycemia. • Monitor blood glucose level daily and when a hypoglycemic reaction is suspected.	To minimize hypoglycemic episodes and prevent lipodystrophy, the two most common complications associated with long-term insulin therapy.
7. Teach proper foot care. Instructions should include: • Inspect all surfaces of feet and between toes daily. Bathe feet with mild soap and warm water. Dry feet thoroughly. Use a mild foot powder between toes and in the shoes if perspiration is a problem. • Lubricate feet with a light moisturizer if dry. • Change socks daily. Wear white cotton socks. • Trim toenails straight across so nail is even with toe. Seek a podiatrist to manage ingrown toenails, calluses, or corns. Do not use potent medicines to remove corns, calluses, or ingrown toe nails.	To maintain skin integrity and reduce the risk of amputation.

INTERVENTIONS	RATIONALE
• Seek medical treatment for signs of skin breakdown. • Avoid using a heating pad or hot water bottle on feet if cold; wear extra socks instead. • Do not go barefoot. • Wear well-fitted shoes that are not tight.	
8. Assist in planning a regular exercise program that can be easily incorporated into the daily routine. Explain benefits of exercise.	For reasons unclear, exercise facilitates cellular uptake of glucose thus lowering the blood glucose level. Also, it facilitates weight loss and reduces the risk of atherosclerosis.
9. Teach the patient manifestations of hypoglycemia and appropriate actions to restore adequate blood glucose levels: • During sleep — nightmares, restlessness, and diaphoresis • When awake — hunger, nausea, sweating, tremors, irritability, headache, diplopia, tachycardia, nervousness, light-headedness, confusion, numbness of lips and tongue If hypoglycemia occurs: • Assess blood glucose level. • Consume a source of refined sugar (orange juice, candy, jelly). Follow with a long-acting carbohydrate (bread, milk, crackers). • Recheck blood glucose level in 15 minutes. If symptoms persist, repeat snack and recheck blood glucose.	Hypoglycemia is a common manageable problem associated with insulin therapy and oral hypoglycemics. Left untreated, convulsions, coma, and death can occur.

INTERVENTIONS	RATIONALE
10. Explain basis for hypoglycemic symptoms: results from stimulation of the sympathetic nervous system in response to a decreased blood glucose because glucose is the main energy source for the brain.	The more patients understand their condition and can anticipate potential problems, the more likely they are to comply with the therapeutic program.
11. Inform the patient that if hypoglycemia occurs, note the symptoms and the order in which they occur.	For rapid recognition and intervention in the future. The patient experiences the same symptoms in the same order with each hypoglycemic episode.
12. Teach the patient about factors known to cause hypoglycemia: inadequate food intake, unexpected exercise, excess insulin. Emphasize the importance of eating three nutritious meals daily.	To minimize the risk of hypoglycemic episodes.
13. Advise the patient to always carry candy.	For rapid treatment of hypoglycemia when needed.
14. Advise the patient to purchase and wear a Medic Alert bracelet.	To alert emergency personnel to condition if an emergency occurs.

· ·

◤NURSING DIAGNOSIS: HIGH RISK FOR DISTURBANCE IN SELF-CONCEPT.

RELATED TO FACTORS: Actual and perceived losses associated with chronic condition

DEFINING CHARACTERISTICS: May report depression, may verbalize low self-esteem, may report history of noncompliance

PATIENT OUTCOME: Demonstrates progress toward acceptance of self in current situation

EVALUATION CRITERIA: Verbalizes realistic plans, seeks additional information about condition, verbalizes positive statements about self

· ·

INTERVENTIONS	RATIONALE
1. See Loss (page 733).	

Cirrhosis of the Liver

Hepatic cirrhosis is a chronic progressive disease characterized by diffuse inflammation and fibrosis of the liver. Scar tissue replaces normal liver parenchymal cells as the liver attempts to regenerate necrotic cells. Because blood cannot flow freely through a cirrhotic liver, it backs up in splanchnic veins (portal vein, pyloric vein, coronary vein, esophageal vein, and mesenteric vein) ultimately causing engorgement, vascular hemostasis, and hypoxia of organs supplied by these vessels. Moreover, the damaged liver cannot perform its normal metabolic functions such as protein, fat, and carbohydrate metabolism, drug metabolism, synthesis of bile, storage of vitamins, and synthesis of clotting factors.

The major complications of hepatic cirrhosis are:

- hepatic encephalopathy caused by elevated blood ammonia levels
- ascites caused by extravasation of serous fluid into peritoneal cavity caused by increased portal hypertension, increased renal reabsorption of sodium, and decreased serum albumin
- portal hypertension caused by obstruction of portal circulation from continual destruction of liver tissue
- hepatorenal syndrome caused by dehydration or infection
- endocrine disturbances caused by depressed secretion of gonadotropins

The mean LOS for a DRG classification of cirrhosis of the liver is 7.2 days (Lorenz, 1991).

General Medical Management

- Low-protein, low-fat, high-carbohydrate diet
- For ascites:
  — sodium restricted diet
  — diuretics
  — abdominal paracentesis or surgery (peritoneovenous shunt)
- For bleeding esophageal varices secondary to portal hypertension:
  — blood transfusions
  — iced saline lavage

— IV infusion of vasopressin or propranolol

— endoscopic sclerosis or surgery (portocaval or splenorenal shunt)

• For hepatorenal syndrome:

— fluid replacement if caused by dehydration

• For endocrine imbalances:

— no specific treatment

• For hepatic encephalopathy:

— lactulose (Cephulac) or neomycin sulfate

— liver transplant

Integrative Care Plans

• Loss

• Immobility

• Fluid and biochemical imbalances

Discharge Considerations

• Follow-up care

• Medications for home use

• Signs and symptoms requiring medical attention

*A*SSESSMENT DATA BASE

1. History or presence of risk factors:

   • alcoholism

   • viral hepatitis

   • chronic obstruction of the common bile duct and infection (cholangitis)

   • chronic severe right-sided heart failure associated with cor pulmonale

2. Physical examination based on a general survey (Appendix F) may reveal:

   • Early findings:

     — GI disturbances: nausea, anorexia, flatulence, dyspepsia, vomiting, changes in bowel habits (caused by altered nutrient metabolism)

     — right upper quadrant abdominal pain (caused by liver enlargement)

     — enlarged, palpable liver. (In the late stage of the disease, increased formation of scar tissue causes contraction of liver tissue hence shrinkage of the liver)

     — low-grade fever (caused by reduced production of antibodies)

- Later findings:
  — ascites: manifested by weight gain and abdominal distention, accompanied by dehydrated appearance in severe cases (dry skin and mucous membranes, muscle wasting, weakness, low urinary output)
  — portal hypertension: evidenced by GI bleeding from esophageal varices
  — hepatorenal syndrome: manifested by progressive renal failure (rising BUN and serum creatinine, decreasing urinary output)
  — endocrine imbalances manifested by:
    a. hypogonadism (atrophy of the breast, decreased libido, alterations in menstrual periods, gynecomastia in males, testicular atrophy with impotence)
    b. spider angiomas
    c. palmar erythema (can be result of estrogen excess)
  — hepatic encephalopathy manifested by neuropsychiatric alterations such as apathy, hyperreflexia, sleep disturbances, confusion, drowsiness, fetor hepaticus, asterixis, disorientation, and ultimately coma and death.
- Additional findings:
  — fatigue (result of anemia secondary to disturbances in nutrient metabolism)
  — peripheral edema (result of sodium retention and decreased albumin)
  — bleeding tendencies (caused by impaired synthesis of clotting factors and thrombocytopenia secondary to bone marrow depression) evidenced by epistaxis, easy bruising, gingival bleeding, heavy menstrual bleeding
  — jaundice (result of impaired bilirubin metabolism)

3. Diagnostic studies:
   a. Liver function studies are abnormal:
      - elevated serum bilirubin (caused by impaired bilirubin metabolism)
      - elevated blood ammmonia level (result of impaired protein metabolism)
      - decreased serum albumin (caused by impaired protein metabolism)
      - elevated serum alkaline phosphatase, ALT, and AST (result of liver tissue destruction)
      - prolonged PT (result of impaired synthesis of prothrombin and clotting factors)
   b. Liver biopsy can confirm diagnosis if serum studies and radiologic studies are inconclusive.
   c. Ultrasound, CT scan, or MRI is done to assess liver size, degree of obstruction, and hepatic blood flow.
   d. Serum electrolytes reveal hypokalemia, alkalosis, and hyponatremia (caused by increased secretion of aldosterone in response to extracellular fluid volume deficit secondary to ascites).
   e. CBC reveals decreased RBC, hemoglobin, hematocrit, platelets, and WBC (result of bone marrow depression secondary to renal failure and impaired nutrient metabolism).
   f. Urinalysis reveals bilirubinuria.

4. Assess the patient's understanding of condition, treatments, and diagnostic studies.

5. Assess the patient's feelings about condition and impact on lifestyle.

> ### ◢ NURSING DIAGNOSIS: ACTIVITY INTOLERANCE
>
> **RELATED TO FACTORS:** Alteration in nutrition, fatigue, weight loss
>
> **DEFINING CHARACTERISTICS:** Verbalizes fatigue with activity, observation of tachypnea with exertion
>
> **PATIENT OUTCOME:** Demonstrates improved tolerance to activities
>
> **EVALUATION CRITERIA:** Performs ADL without reporting fatigue, dyspnea, or tachycardia

INTERVENTIONS	RATIONALE
1. Monitor: • vital signs q8h if stable, otherwise q4h • general status (Appendix F) q8h	To evaluate effectiveness of therapy.
2. Provide assistance with ADL as needed.	To conserve energy. As end-stage liver disease approaches, the patient is increasingly debilitated.
3. Plan activities to allow frequent rest periods.	Rest reduces metabolic demands of the liver.
4. Maintain a semi-Fowler's position if ascites is present.	To facilitate breathing and to reduce discomfort.
5. If on bedrest, initiate measures to prevent complications of impaired physical mobility (see Immobility, page 725).	
6. Provide oxygen via nasal cannula if dyspnea persists and ABG reveal hypoxia.	To increase arterial oxygen tension to combat hypoxia.
7. Administer prescribed antipyretic and antibiotic.	To resolve fever. Metabolism is increased with fever that causes unnecessary energy expenditure.

••••••••••••••••••••••••••••••

NURSING DIAGNOSIS: ALTERATIONS IN NUTRITION: LESS THAN BODY REQUIREMENTS

RELATED TO FACTORS: GI disturbances, faulty absorption, metabolism, and storage of nutrients

DEFINING CHARACTERISTICS: Weight loss, reports anorexia, muscle wasting, vomiting

PATIENT OUTCOME (collaborative): Demonstrates improved nutritional status

EVALUATION CRITERIA: Increased intake of food, stable weight, no further increase in edema or ascites, serum albumin and ammonia levels remain stable

••••••••••••••••••••••••••••••

INTERVENTIONS	RATIONALE
1. Monitor: • weight daily • vital signs q4h • results of liver function studies and serum electrolyte reports • extent of ascites: measure and record abdominal girth daily • amount of food consumed during each meal	To identify indications of progress toward or deviations from expected outcomes.
2. Provide a high-carbohydrate, low-fat, low-protein, low-sodium diet if serum ammonia level is elevated or edema and ascites are present. If food intake is less than 30%, consult the dietitian about appropriate nutritional supplements such as Ensure or Sustacal.	Ammonia is a by-product of protein metabolism. Sodium is restricted to control ascites and edema because of its natural osmotic action. A high protein intake can be followed if the serum ammonia level is within normal range. A dietitian is a nutritional specialist who can evaluate the patient's nutritional status and plan meals to meet the relate nutritional needs relative to the illness.
3. Provide six small meals instead of three large meals.	Small, frequent meals are often better tolerated than three large meals because there is less distention of the stomach. Nausea can be triggered by stomach distention.
4. Instruct the patient to avoid intake of alcohol. Explain that the damaged liver cannot break down alcohol. Refer the patient to Alcoholics Anonymous (AA) if there is a history of alcoholism.	Alcohol is the most common cause of cirrhosis of the liver. AA is a community-based support group composed of recovering alcoholics.

INTERVENTIONS	RATIONALE
5. Provide oral hygiene before meals.	To enhance appetite.
6. Administer prescribed antiemetic 30 minutes before meals if nausea is present.	Foods are better tolerated when nausea is absent.
7. Initiate prescribed IV therapy if patient cannot tolerate oral feedings. Perform appropriate actions to prevent and correct complications of IV therapy (page 764).	IV therapy is required to prevent dehydration if the patient cannot tolerate oral feedings.
8. Administer prescribed medications that can include diuretics, antidiarrheal agents, stool evacuants, and Cephulac. Evaluate effectiveness of each prescribed agent. Tell the patient that Cephulac causes diarrhea. If diarrhea starts, inform the physician because diarrhea signals a need to reduce the dosage. Consult physician if ascites persist or worsen.	Diuretics rid the body of excess fluid and control ascites. Antidiarrheal agents control diarrhea. Persistent diarrhea can cause a fluid and biochemical imbalance. Persistent constipation can cause bloated feelings and further contribute to anorexia. Cephulac reduces the serum ammonia level by trapping it in the intestine where it is expelled. A paracentesis may be required to relieve discomfort arising from severe ascites.

• •

 # NURSING DIAGNOSIS: HIGH RISK FOR ALTERATIONS IN SKIN INTEGRITY.

RELATED TO FACTORS: Impaired physical mobility

DEFINING CHARACTERISTICS: Reddened areas on bony prominences, scratches on the body, taut dry skin in areas of edema ascites

PATIENT OUTCOME: Skin integrity remains intact

EVALUATION CRITERIA: Absence of scratches on the skin, absence of reddened areas over bony prominences

• •

INTERVENTIONS	RATIONALE
1. Instruct the patient to bathe with a mild hypoallergenic soap (such as Lowilla or Neutrogena). Apply an emollient lotion over the entire body after bathing.	Dry irritated skin is more susceptible to breakdown. Hypoallergenic soaps do not dry the skin.
2. While on bedrest, implement measures to prevent complications of immobility (page 725).	Ascites and edema increase the risk of skin breakdown.
3. Keep nails trimmed. If pruritus occurs, apply Calamine or Caladryl lotion to the skin prn. Provide cool or warm baths. Avoid hot baths because heat increases itching. Keep the patient cool to prevent sweating.	Scratching dry edematous skin increases the risk of skin breakdown.

NURSING DIAGNOSIS: ALTERATIONS IN FLUID VOLUME: EXCESS

RELATED TO FACTORS: Decreased oral intake, abnormal fluid retention, fluid shift from intravascular space to extravascular space and abdominal cavity

DEFINING CHARACTERISTICS: Bleeds easily, dry mucous membranes, poor skin turgor, hyperatremia, voiding concentrated urine

PATIENT OUTCOME (collaborative): Demonstrates improved fluid status

EVALUATION CRITERIA: Absence of bleeding, serum sodium within normal limits, denies thirst, less concentrated urine with output above 50 mL/hr, abdominal girth shows no further enlargement

INTERVENTIONS	RATIONALE
1. Monitor: • intake and output q8h • results of coagulation studies (PT, PTT)	To identify indications of progress toward or deviations from expected outcome.

INTERVENTIONS	RATIONALE
• urine, stool, and emesis for evidence of bleeding by Hematest® prn (dark urine, black tarry stools, or coffee-ground emesis) • measure abdominal girth q8h	
2. Consult physician of the following: • ecchymotic areas on the skin • prolonged bleeding after parenteral injection • bleeding gums • positive Hematest® of urine, stool, or emesis • PT or PTT above the normal range Administer vitamin K as ordered. Implement bleeding precautions (see Table 6-1).	These findings indicate bleeding. Vitamin K promotes clotting. Bleeding precautions are safety measures to prevent further bleeding.
3. Use a soft bristle toothbrush for brushing teeth.	To prevent disrupting gum tissue.
4. Use a small gauge needle for intramuscular (IM) injections. Apply pressure to injection sites for at least 2–3 minutes.	To ensure clot formation.
5. Avoid giving narcotics and sedatives if altered mental status exists.	These drugs further depress consciousness and are poorly metabolized by a diseased liver. Special care is required to ensure safety and to meet the physiological needs of the unconscious patient.
6. Protect patient from injury. Keep siderails up if the patient demonstrates impaired mentation or altered levels of consciousness.	As the disease progresses to encephalopathy, disorientation, confusion, and varying degrees of consciousness occur. Siderails protect the patient from falls.
7. See Fluid and Biochemical Imbalances (page 773) specific for dehydration and metabolic acidosis.	

• •

◣ NURSING DIAGNOSIS: HIGH RISK FOR ALTERATIONS IN HOME MAINTENANCE MANAGEMENT

RELATED TO FACTORS: Knowledge deficit about condition and treatment plan; difficulty accepting a chronic, incurable condition; lack of adequate support system

DEFINING CHARACTERISTICS: Verbalizes lack of understanding, may report history of noncompliance, may report depression

PATIENT OUTCOME (collaborative): Demonstrates willingness to comply with home care measures on discharge

EVALUATION CRITERIA: Verbalizes understanding of illness and treatments, reports satisfaction with discharge plans

• •

INTERVENTIONS	RATIONALE
1. Explain prescribed diagnostic studies: • purpose • preparation required before test • nursing care to expect after test • if discomfort is expected	Anxiety interferes with learning. A knowledge of what to expect helps lessen anxiety.
2. Teach the patient about the nature of the illness and purpose of prescribed treatments. Emphasize the following points: • There is no cure. • Medical treatment is aimed at controlling complications. • Rate of disease progression can be slowed by following prescribed therapy.	The more patients know about their condition, the more likely they are to accept it. Persons who understand their disease have more reasonable expectations, are more compliant with the treatment plan, and assume greater responsibility for their therapy.
3. Assist patient or significant other in identifying home care needs. Refer to social services or discharge planning department to arrange for home care assistance as needed.	Compliance is enhanced with thorough discharge planning and teaching. Social services or discharge planners are specialists who can coordinate available community resources to meet the patient's home care needs.

▶ NURSING DIAGNOSIS: HIGH RISK FOR INEFFECTIVE INDIVIDUAL COPING

RELATED TO FACTORS: Chronic incurable illness

DEFINING CHARACTERISTICS: Verbalizes depression and inability to cope with condition

PATIENT OUTCOME: Demonstrates progress toward acceptance of condition

EVALUATION CRITERIA: Verbalizes acceptance of self in current situation, reports realistic plans, verbalizes positive statements about self

INTERVENTIONS	RATIONALE
1. Suggest loose clothing that does not emphasize a distended abdomen and light color fabrics that do not accentuate jaundice.	Finding the right style and color of clothing to complement body size and skin tone is a trial-and-error process. Looking attractive helps improve self-esteem.
2. See Loss (page 733).	

Cholecystitis

Cholecystitis refers to acute inflammation of the gallbladder. It usually develops in association with cholelithiasis (gallstones). Gallstones irritate the lining of the gallbladder. They may become impacted in the cystic duct causing obstruction and inflammation of the gallbladder wall, predisposing to infection.

The gallbladder is located below the right lobe of the liver. Its primary function is the concentration and storage of bile produced by the liver. Bile is needed to emulsify fats. The gallbladder contracts and releases bile into the duodenum when fatty foods enter the intestine.

Gallbladder disease is acute or chronic. The acute form is characterized by severe pain of sudden onset. Chronic disease is characterized by milder symptoms (dull ache, dyspepsia, belching, bloating, flatulence) of shorter duration than symptoms with acute disease (Evans & Harvey, 1991).

Gallstones precipitate most often because of excess concentration of cholesterol in the bile. No specific diet can prevent gallstone formation or prevent small stones from becoming larger. The major complications associated with cholelithiasis are empyema and gallbladder perforation with peritonitis (Evans & Harvey, 1991).

Acute cholecystitis is most often treated with surgical removal of the gallbladder (cholecystectomy) either via the traditional abdomenal approach involving an incision on the right side of the abdomen just below the rib cage or via laparoscopy.

With endoscopic cholecystectomy (laparoscopic laser cholecystectomy) recovery is easier and faster with few complications. The mean LOS is 2–3 days, with patients generally returning to work in 2–4 days. With this procedure, four small punctures are made in the abdomen: one slightly above the umbilicus, two beneath the rib cage (right midclavicular line and right axillary line), and a fourth to the right of the midsection. A laparoscope attached to a microscopic camera is inserted through the puncture above the umbilicus, and grasping forceps are inserted through each puncture below the rib cage. The dissection laser is inserted through the fourth puncture. The surgeon then retracts, dissects, and removes the gallbladder using a closed-circuit monitor to see the abdominal cavity. The procedure takes about 90 minutes. Postoperative pain is minimal. Some patients experience mild shoulder pain for one week after, which may be due to irritation of the diaphragm from stretching the abdomen during the procedure.

With the traditional approach, a T-tube is placed into the common bile duct and brought out through the abdominal wall via a small stab incision if stones are found in the common bile duct. It then is connected to a sterile collection receptacle to allow gravity to drain bile. The T-tube maintains common bile duct patency until swelling subsides. Complications that can occur with a T-tube include biliary obstruction or peritonitis if bile leaks into the peritoneal cavity. About one week after cholecystectomy, a T-tube cholangiogram is performed. If the common bile duct is patent, the physician removes the tube; if not, the patient is discharged with the tube in place for later removal. Before removal, the physician may clamp the tube to assess common bile duct patency.

Both surgical approaches are performed under general anesthesia. Preoperative preparation is the same as any patient undergoing surgery. Supportive therapy is initiated to stabilize the patient in preparation for surgery, which usually includes IV therapy, narcotic analgesia, restricting oral intake, insertion of an N/G tube for gastric decompression to reduce stimulation of the gallbladder and pancreas, and insertion of a Foley catheter.

Postoperatively, the patient returns to the medical/surgical unit with :

- IV infusion
- abdominal dressing
- wound drainage device (with the traditional approach)
- nasogastric (N/G) tube
- possibly a T-tube if stones were found in the common bile duct
- Foley catheter

The mean LOS for a DRG classification of cholecystectomy (traditional approach) is 14.0 days (Lorenz, 1991). No special diet must be followed after cholecystectomy. Some patients can experience postcholecystectomy syndrome characterized by recurrence of symptoms such as:

- dyspepsia and intolerance to certain foods, symptoms believed due to causes unrelated to the gallbladder
- diarrhea (possibly caused by excess secretion of bile salts)
- biliary pain (possibly caused by spasms of the sphincter of Oddi)

Integrative Care Plans

- Preoperative and postoperative care
- IV therapy
- Pain

Discharge Considerations

- Follow-up care
- Activity limitations
- Signs and symptoms of wound infection
- Wound care
- Care of T-tube

THE PREOPERATIVE PERIOD

 # ASSESSMENT DATA BASE

1. History or presence of risk factors:
   - diabetes mellitus
   - sickle cell anemia
   - pancreatitis
   - cirrhosis of the liver
   - obesity
   - chronic use of oral contraceptives
   - cancer of the gallbladder

2. Physical examination based on an abdominal assessment (Appendix B) may reveal:
   - biliary colic that can be accompanied by nausea and vomiting. This is the most signifi-cant finding. Biliary colic is severe pain episodic in nature and intense during acute attack.It is characterized by a sudden onset of severe epigastric or right upper quadrant pain, which often radiates to the back. The intensity of the pain peaks within one hour or less and remains persistent for several hours. The pain is caused by contraction of the gallbladder against a stone lodged in the gallbladder neck or cystic duct. The pain sub-sides when the stone falls into the gallbladder or passes into the intestine.
   - fever
   - positive Murphy's sign (sharp localized pain occurring when the gallbladder is palpated and patient is instructed to inhale deeply)
   - jaundice (if stone obstructs common bile duct)

3. Diagnostic studies:
   - Serum amylase and lipase are markedly elevated if the stone obstructs the pancreatic duct at the sphincter of Oddi.
   - Serum bilirubin is elevated if the common bile duct is obstructed.
   - Ultrasound is the initial screening test for detecting stones in the gallbladder but cannot assess the patency of the common bile duct. Ultrasound must be followed by radionu-clide scanning to confirm diagnosis.
   - Cholescintigraphy confirms a diagnosis of acute cholecystitis and gallstones revealed by ultrasound and assesses patency of the common bile duct.
   - Oral cholecystogram is done if ultrasound capabilities are not available. This study provides diagnostic data about gallbladder contraction, duct patency, and composition of the stone.
   - CBC reveals leukocytosis.
   - Endoscopic retrograde cholangiopancreatography (ERCP) is useful for assessing chole-docholithiasis (stones in the common bile duct). Stones found the common bile duct by ERCP are removed at the time of the procedure.

4. Assess the patient's understanding of the condition, treatment, and diagnostic studies.

◣ NURSING DIAGNOSIS: PAIN

RELATED TO FACTORS: Acute cholecystitis

DEFINING CHARACTERISTICS: Verbalizes discomfort, frowning, guarding painful site, moaning

PATIENT OUTCOME: Demonstrates relief from discomfort

EVALUATION CRITERIA: Reports less intense pain, relaxed facial expression, absence of moaning

INTERVENTIONS	RATIONALE
1. Maintain bedrest and assist with assuming a position of comfort.	Rest reduces gastric and pancreatic stimulation.
2. Keep in a semi-Fowler's position.	To facilitate breathing.
3. Insert a N/G tube and connect to intermittent suction as ordered. Irrigate the tube prn with normal saline. Keep NPO. Provide oral care q4h while NPO. Allow to moisten mouth q2h with a wet cloth.	N/G suctioning prevents gastric distention. Gastric distention triggers nausea and vomiting. Normal saline is an isotonic solution that does not cause fluid and electrolyte loss. Keeping the oral mucosa moist promotes comfort.
4. Prepare the patient for surgery as ordered. See Preoperative and Postoperative Care (page 738).	Routine preoperative preparation helps ensure the patient is physiologically ready for surgery thus minimizing the risk of postoperative complications.
5. Administer prescribed narcotic analgesic prn and evaluate effectiveness.	Narcotic analgesia is required for severe pain.

THE POSTOPERATIVE PERIOD

 ## ASSESSMENT DATA BASE

1. See Preoperative and Postoperative Care (page 738).

NURSING DIAGNOSIS: HIGH RISK FOR IMPAIRED TISSUE INTEGRITY

RELATED TO FACTORS: Presence of a T-tube secondary to cholecystectomy

DEFINING CHARACTERISTICS: Observation of T-tube in place connected to collection receptacle

PATIENT OUTCOME: Tissue integrity remains intact

EVALUATION CRITERIA: Absence of manifestations of leakage of bile from T-tube, continued T-tube patency

INTERVENTIONS	RATIONALE
1. Monitor color and amount of drainage from the T-tube q4h. Notify physician if output continually exceeds 500 mL daily.	Normally, T-tube output during the first 24 hours after insertion ranges from 300–500 mL. Afterward, output decreases daily to less than 150 mL/day. Persistent excessive output signals obstruction.
2. Take no action if drainage from the T-tube gradually decreases, stools are brown, and jaundice subsides.	These findings indicate a return of common bile duct patency.
3. Notify physician immediately if drainage from the T-tube suddenly stops and the patient complains of severe abdominal pain. Check for kinks and blood clots in the tubing.	This can indicate leakage of bile into the peritoneal cavity.
4. Ensure the tubing from the T-tube is securely taped to the patient. Remind the patient to avoid lying on the tubing or on the collection receptacle.	To prevent accidental dislodgment.
5. Keep the collection receptacle in a dependent position.	To aid gravitational flow of bile.
6. If the T-tube has been clamped in preparation for removal, unclamp the tubing immediately and notify physician if abdominal pain, nausea, or feeling of fullness occur.	The findings signal obstruction.

INTERVENTIONS	RATIONALE
7. If discharged home with a T-tube: a. Teach and have the patient practice: • emptying the collection receptacle using aseptic technique. Stress the importance of hand-washing before emptying receptacle. • dressing change. b. Instruct the patient to contact the physician if fever, redness, swelling, and drainage around the tube, increased jaundice, abdominal distention, brown urine, clay stools, nausea, or vomiting occur.	To ensure safe management of the device at home. The risk of bile duct obstruction remains as long as the T-tube is in place.
8. Tell the patient that some discomfort can continue for several weeks. Advise the patient to avoid foods that cause discomfort if dyspepsia occurs. Instruct the patient to notify physician if diarrhea or biliary pain recurs.	These findings suggest postcholecystectomy syndrome. Cholestyramine (Questran) can be prescribed to control diarrhea. For biliary pain, an endoscopic sphincterotomy may be done or nitrates and calcium channel blockers can be prescribed to control spasms.
9. See Preoperative and Postoperative Care (page 738) for the remainder of this plan of care.	

TABLE 9–1. Patient-Centered Teaching Guide for Diabetes Mellitus

Diagnosis: On completion of teaching about diabetes mellitus, the patient can:

1. Define diabetes mellitus.

2. Verbalize the type of diabetes (type I or II) per diagnosis and the primary reason for the elevated blood glucose.

3. Verbalize signs and symptoms of diabetes mellitus.

4. Explain how diabetes mellitus develops.

Medications: On completion of teaching about prescribed medications, the patient should be able to:

1. Explain action and side effects of medication prescribed to control blood glucose (insulin or oral hypoglycemic agents).

2. Verbalize signs and symptoms of hypoglycemia.

3. Verbalize what to do if hypoglycemia occurs.

If insulin prescribed:

4. Demonstrate how to self-administer insulin.

5. Explain reason for rotating injection sites.

6. Identify subcutaneous injection sites.

7. Name places in the community where insulin syringes, insulin, and glucose monitoring equipment can be purchased.

8. Demonstrate how to record rotation of injection sites on a chart.

9. Explain how to store opened vial of insulin and unopened vial of insulin.

10. Verbalize when to discard vial of insulin.

11. State factors that can alter insulin needs (fever, illness, alcohol intake, pregnancy, emotional stress, exercise, inadequate food intake).

12. Demonstrate how to use a blood glucose monitoring device.

13. Demonstrate how to perform a fingerstick using an automatic lancet device.

Diet: On completion of diet teaching, the patient can:

1. Explain the purpose of calorie restriction.

2. State how many calories are allowed on prescribed diet.

3. Explain how to use the diabetic exchange list in planning meals for the prescribed diet.

Lifestyle Changes: On completion of teaching about lifestyle changes, the patient can:

1. Name local community resources that provide information about diabetes mellitus and support groups.

2. Explain the importance of skin care and how to care for feet.

3. Explain reason for Medic Alert identification (bracelet or necklace) and where to obtain identification.

4. Explain mechanism for financing medications and glucose monitoring equipment.

5. Explain importance of an annual ophthalmology examination.

BIBLIOGRAPHY

Alter, M.J., Hadler, S.C., Judson, F.N., Manes, A., Alexander, W.J., Hu, P.Y., & Miller, J.K. (1990). Risk factors for acute non-A, non-B hepatitis in the United States and association with hepatitis C virus infection. **Journal of the American Medical Association, 264,** 2231–2235.

Christensen, M.H., et al (1991). How to care for a diabetic foot. **American Journal of Nursing, 91,** 50–57.

Evans, J.C., & Harvey, C.B. (1991). Gallstone disease: Clinical review. **Physician Assistant, 15,** 14–16, 23–24, 26–29.

Guthrie, D.W., & Guthrie, R.A. (1991). **Nursing Management Of Diabetes Mellitus,** New York: Springer Publishing Co.

Haicken, R.N. (1991). Laser Laparoscopic Cholecystectomy in the Ambulatory Setting. **Journal of Post Anesthesia Nurse, 6,** 33–39.

Hollinger, F.B. (1991). Viral hepatitis: Antibodies and antigens furnish many answers. **Consultant, 31,** 33—36, 41–42.

Lorenz, E.W. (1991). **St. Anthony's DRG Working Guidebook.** Alexandria: St. Anthony's Publishing Company.

Moorhouse, M.F., et al (1988). Patient care guidelines: Acute pancreatitis. **Journal of Emergency Nursing, 14,** 387-391.

Rhoads, J. (1990). Cirrhosis of the liver. **Emergency Medical Service, 19,** 44, 46–47.

Skyler, J.S. (1991). Strategies in diabetes mellitus: Start of a new era. **Postgraduate Medicine, 89,** 45–46, 49, 53.

Smith, A. (1991). When your pancreas self-destructs. **American Journal of Nursing, 91,** 38–48.

C

HAPTER TEN
Problems of the Endocrine System

*T*ranssphenoidal Hypophysectomy

Transsphenoidal hypophysectomy is a procedure that involves removing a pituitary adenoma through a horizontal incision beneath the upper lip. An opening is then created through the nasal cavity and the sphenoidal sinus to expose the sella turcia to access and remove the tumor while leaving the pituitary gland intact. To ensure destruction of any remaining tumor cells, the cavity is usually packed with Gelfoam soaked in alcohol. Sometimes adipose tissue and muscle are taken from the thigh to pack the cavity when structural defects exist in the sella diaphragm (Chipps, 1992).

Preoperatively, the patient undergoes diagnostic evaluation to determine the location of the tumor. Diagnostic evaluation includes radioimmunoassays, 24-hour urine studies, and computed tomography (CT) scan and/or magnetic resonance imaging (MRI). A culture of nasopharyngeal secretions may be done to rule out sinus infection, which increases the risk of postoperative infection.

Postoperatively, the patient returns to the ICU with:

- IV infusion for fluid replacement
- nasal packing, usually Vaseline gauze with an antibiotic ointment, that is removed within 24– 48 hours
- soft nasal airway
- pressure dressing applied under the nose like a moustache

The pituitary gland (also called hypophysis) consists of an anterior lobe and a posterior lobe. Each lobe secretes specific hormones that control glandular secretions of other body organs, for example, thyroid gland, gonads, adrenal cortex, breast, skin, kidneys, and uterus. Removal of a pituitary gland lobe predisposes a patient to conditions reflecting hypofunctioning of the lobe. The patient requires lifetime replacement of hormones normally supplied by target organs of the lobe removed.

Potential postoperative complications are (Chipps, 1992):

a. diabetes insipidus — caused by edema from manipulation of the gland. It is a transient problem characterized by a decrease in secretion of antidiuretic hormone (ADH), which is normally secreted by the posterior pituitary gland

b. meningitis — occurs by bacterial contamination during or after surgery. If the CSF leaks, then bacteria can migrate into the cranial vault and infect the meninges

c. visual disturbances (diplopia, ptosis, or strabismus) - caused by damage to cranial nerves III, IV, V, VI, the optic chiasm, or optic nerves

d. sinusitis — caused by preoperative nasal infection or improper instrumentation during surgery.

The mean LOS for a DRG classification of transsphenodial hypophysectomy is 9.5 days (Lorenz, 1991)

Integrative Care Plans

- Hypothyroidism
- Fluid and biochemical imbalance
- IV therapy
- Preoperative and postoperative care

Discharge Considerations

- Follow-up care
- Medications to continue at home
- Signs and symptoms of pituitary deficit

THE PREOPERATIVE PERIOD

 # ASSESSMENT DATA BASE

1. Physical examination based on a general survey (Appendix F), visual status (Appendix H), and neurological status (Appendix J) may reveal:
   - headache, somnolence (caused by enlargement of the tumor)
   - visual disturbances that can include diplopia, vision loss in a portion of the visual field (resulting from compression of the optic chiasma as the tumor grows)

   Additional manifestations depend on which lobe (anterior or posterior) of the pituitary is affected. The clinical findings can be:

a. Hyperfunctioning:
   — acromegaly in adults (characterized by enlarged hands, feet, and thickened facial features)
   — Cushing's disease (truncal obesity, moonface, thin skin, striae, bruising easily)
   — hyperthyroidism (page 581)
   — gonadotropin imbalance (menstrual irregularities, galactorrhea)
   — increased skin pigmentation

or

b. Hypofunctioning:
  — Addison's disease (weakness, anorexia, weight loss, hypertension, intolerance to stress)
  — hypothyroidism (page 574)
  — dwarfism in children
  — gonadotropin deficits (amenorrhea, impotence, decrease libido, infertility)
  — decreased skin pigmentation

2. Assess the patient's feelings and concerns about surgical outcomes and impact on lifestyle.

3. See Preoperative and Postoperative Care (page 738).

THE POSTOPERATIVE PERIOD

 # ASSESSMENT DATA BASE

1. Perform a neurological assessment (Appendix J), a routine postoperative assessment (Appendix L), and an assessment of visual status (Appendix H).

NURSING DIAGNOSIS: PAIN

RELATED TO FACTORS: Headaches secondary to transsphenoidal hypophysectomy
DEFINING CHARACTERISTICS: Verbalizes headache, moaning, guarding painful site, frowning
PATIENT OUTCOME (collaborative): Demonstrates relief from discomfort
EVALUATION CRITERIA: Denies pain, relaxed facial expression, absence of moaning

INTERVENTIONS	RATIONALE
1. Administer prescribed analgesic prn and evaluate effectiveness.	Mild to moderate headache is expected. Analgesics block the pain pathway.
2. If headache persists, palpate sinuses for tenderness. Consult physician if headache persists or worsens or is accompanied by increased sinus tenderness and low-grade fever.	Although mild to moderate headache is expected, severe headache can indicate intracranial air, which is confirmed by skull x rays or sinusitis if accompanied by low-grade fever.
3. Keep head of bed elevated 30 degrees.	To facilitate breathing and to reduce swelling and pressure on the sella turcica.

INTERVENTIONS	RATIONALE
4. Provide diet as prescribed, usually a clear liquid diet with progression to a dental soft diet if no nausea is experienced. Tell the patient that sense of taste and smell are diminished until the nasal packing is removed and swelling subsides.	Chewing tough, hard foods can be uncomfortable.
5. Allow the patient to rinse mouth with a solution of half strength hydrogen peroxide and cool water q2h. Provide a moisturizer to lips prn.	Hydrogen peroxide helps reduce transient bacteria in the mouth thereby reducing the risk of bacterial invasion of the operative side and meningitis. A moisturizer keeps lips from cracking.
6. Maintain bedside air humidification or administer supplemental oxygen via face mask as ordered. Remove nasal packing as ordered.	To prevent drying of the oral mucosa. Because of the nasal packing, the patient must breathe through the mouth. Supplemental oxygen provides more oxygen to the tissue thereby helping relieve some discomfort.

NURSING DIAGNOSIS: HIGH RISK FOR COMPLICATIONS

RELATED TO FACTORS: Intracranial swelling and incidental injury or manipulation of the pituitary gland

DEFINING CHARACTERISTICS: May show manifestations of diabetes insipidus, sinusitis, meningitis, visual deficits

PATIENT OUTCOME (collaborative): Demonstrates absence of complications

EVALUATION CRITERIA: Absence of manifestations of fluid and electrolyte imbalance, absence of infection, vision remains intact, LOS does not exceed established DRG

- radioiodine therapy
- overdose of antithyroid drugs

2. Inquire about alterations in sexual function:
   - decreased libido
   - impotence, infertility
   - menstrual abnormalities (amenorrhea or prolonged menstrual bleeding)

3. Physical examination based on a general assessment (Appendix F) may reveal:
   - skin or nail changes (dry, coarse skin and thick, brittle nails)
   - hair loss
   - cardiovascular changes (bradycardia)
   - GI changes (anorexia, constipation, weight gain)
   - neurological changes (initially somnolence and irritability progressing to apathy and lethargy, extreme fatigue, slow speech, memory deficits, slow clumsy movements, hyporeflexia of tendon reflexes)
   - metabolic changes (intolerance to cold)
   - general appearance (puffy facial appearance, thickening of tissue on hands and feet, enlarged tongue)

4. Diagnostic studies:
   - Serum T3 and T4 levels are below normal range.
   - CBC reveals anemia (RBC, hemoglobin, and hematocrit below normal levels).

5. Assess the patient's feelings and concerns about condition and impact on lifestyle.

6. Assess understanding of condition and treatments.

NURSING DIAGNOSIS: HIGH RISK FOR CONSTIPATION

RELATED TO FACTORS: Decreased peristalsis, decreased activity level

DEFINING CHARACTERISTICS: Reports passage of hard stool, verbalizes decreased activity level, reports feeling of pressure in rectum, reports straining at stool

PATIENT OUTCOME (collaborative): Demonstrates relief from constipation

EVALUATION CRITERIA: Reports passage of soft formed stool, denies excess straining with defecation, reports bowel movement at least every three days

INTERVENTIONS	RATIONALE
1. Instruct the patient to: • drink at least 2–3 liters of fluid daily • increase intake of high-fiber foods (raw fruits, vegetables, whole grain breads and cereals, prune juice) • use a bulk-forming stool softener such as Metamucil if dietary modifications are ineffective • use a laxative if no bowel movement occurs in three days • contact physician if constipation persists	These measures help soften the stool. Persistent constipation can signal a need for further evaluation to determine if the medication dosage should be increased.
2. Review all other medications prescribed for the patient to determine their potential for causing constipation.	Many medications can cause constipation. Persons with hypothyroidism have a low tolerance for drugs because of reduced metabolism.

 NURSING DIAGNOSIS: ALTERATION IN NUTRITION: MORE THAN BODY REQUIREMENTS

RELATED TO FACTORS: Decreased metabolism secondary to hypothyroidism

DEFINING CHARACTERISTICS: Reports continual weight gain, reports cold sensitivity, laboratory values consistent with anemia, reports anorexia

PATIENT OUTCOME (collaborative): Demonstrates improved nutritional status

EVALUATION CRITERIA: Decreased weight, reports increased intake of food, CBC values within normal range, denies cold sensitivity

INTERVENTIONS	RATIONALE
1. Monitor: • CBC reports, especially RBC, hemoglobin, and hematocrit • percentage of food consumed with each meal • weight weekly	To evaluate effectiveness of therapy.

INTERVENTIONS	RATIONALE
2. Refer the patient to a dietitian for instructions in preparing a low-fat, low-sodium diet. Explain rationale for dietary modifications.	A dietitian is nutritional specialist who can assist the patient in planning meals to meet nutritional needs in relation to current illness. These dietary modifications help prevent weight gain. Sodium contributes to weight gain by causing water retention.
3. Keep the room warm. Encourage the patient to wear extra clothing. Let the patient know that cold intolerance subsides after thyroid hormone medication begins taking effect, usually in 2–3 weeks.	To prevent heat loss. With hypothyroidism, heat production is less because of decreased metabolism.
4. Encourage the patient to engage in a regular exercise program. Suggest walking, swimming, bicycling, or low-level exercise class. Emphasize that exercises should be done at least three times a week.	Exercise promotes energy expenditure thus weight loss.

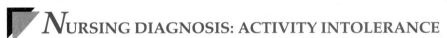

NURSING DIAGNOSIS: ACTIVITY INTOLERANCE

RELATED TO FACTORS: Decreased metabolism secondary to hypothyroidism, anemia

DEFINING CHARACTERISTICS: Verbalizes extreme fatigue, reports slowing of speech and thought processes, reports sedentary lifestyle

PATIENT OUTCOME: Demonstrates improved activity tolerance

EVALUATION CRITERIA: Fewer reports of fatigue with ADL, CBC reveals absence of anemia

INTERVENTIONS	RATIONALE
1. Monitor: • results of CBC reports, especially RBC, hemoglobin, and hematocrit • results of serum T_3 and T_4 levels	To evaluate effectiveness of therapy.

INTERVENTIONS	RATIONALE
2. Encourage intake of foods high in iron, such as organ meats, especially liver.	Iron is essential to erythrocyte synthesis thus resolution of anemia. Anemia contributes to fatigue.
3. Encourage activities to tolerance. Advise the patient to rest at intervals during the day. Explain that as the thyroid replacement hormone begins to take effect, fatigue will resolve.	With hypothyroidism, a decreased metabolic rate causes decreased energy production, hence fatigue. Rest helps conserve energy. Frustration is less likely to occur when the patient feels a sense of accomplishment with an activity.
4. Avoid bombarding the patient with data that require complex decisions. Increase decision-making tasks as mentation improves.	Decision making can be a source of stress and anxiety.

◣ NURSING DIAGNOSIS: HIGH RISK FOR IMPAIRED HOME MAINTENANCE MANAGEMENT

RELATED TO FACTORS: Knowledge deficit about condition and treatment plan, difficulty coping with a chronic condition

DEFINING CHARACTERISTICS: Verbalizes lack of understanding, requests information, verbalizes depression or embarrassment about physical appearance and altered sexual functioning

PATIENT OUTCOME: Demonstrates willingness to comply with self-care measures for home maintenance

EVALUATION CRITERIA: Verbalizes understanding of condition and therapy, verbalizes positive statements about self, verbalizes satisfaction with therapeutic plan

INTERVENTIONS	RATIONALE
1. Allow the patient to express feelings about condition and the need for lifetime hormone replacement therapy. If sexual dysfunction occurs, let the patient know that it may return to normal with adequate thyroid hormone replacement. Also, puffiness will lessen but may not completely disappear.	Expressing feelings helps promote coping. Knowing expected outcomes of treatments helps lessen anxiety and promotes compliance.

INTERVENTIONS	RATIONALE
2. Instruct the patient to seek medical attention if the following occur: • symptoms of hypothyroidism persist • chest pain, skin eruptions, pulse rate over 100 beats per minutes at rest, palpitations, increased nervousness, headache	Persistent symptoms of hypothyroidism indicate medication underdosage thus a need to increase dosage. Overdosage indicates a need to decrease dosage and is reflected by the latter symptoms.
3. Provide information about the nature of the condition and pre-scribed drugs, including name, dosage, schedule, purpose, and reportable side effects. Emphasize the importance of taking medica-tion as prescribed. Remind the patient that lifetime replacement therapy is required because thyroid hormones are essential for life. Caution the patient against expect-ing immediate improvements since it normally takes about 2–3 weeks before improvements are noticeable.	The more patients know about their condi-tion, the more likely they are to have rea-sonable expectations and to comply with prescribed treatments.
4. Encourage the patient to keep fol-low-up appointments. Explain that a low dose of the thyroid hormone is given initially and gradually increased over several weeks until symptoms begin to subside. Tell the patient the dose at which a euthy-roid state is attained becomes the maintenance dose.	To allow physician to monitor effectiveness of drug therapy to determine if a euthyroid state has been reached.
5. Provide written self-care instruc-tions and written appointments for follow-up care. Evaluate patient's understanding of home care instructions.	Verbal instructions may be easily forgotten. Evaluation is important to ensure that learning has occurred.

Thyroidectomy

A **thyroidectomy** can involve partial (subtotal) or complete removal of the thyroid gland as treatment for hyperthyroidism, a condition characterized by oversecretion of thyroid hormones (T_3 and T_4). The abnormal tissue is removed through a horizontal neck incision under general anesthesia.

Preoperatively, measures are taken to reduce the risk of postoperative hemorrhage and thyroid storm. Generally, this involves administering antithyroid drugs and saturated solution potassium iodine (SSKI) if goiter (hypertrophy of thyroid gland) is present. Additional preoperative preparation is the same as for any surgical patient.

Postoperatively, the patient returns to the medical/surgical unit with a neck dressing and an IV infusion. The mean LOS for a DRG classification of thyroidectomy is 2.8 days (Lorenz, 1991).

The major complications associated with thyroidectomy are hemorrhage, injury to the recurrent laryngeal nerve, airway obstruction caused by edema of the glottis, and hypocalcemia (if the parathyroid gland was inadvertently injured or removed during surgery).

Following a subtotal thyroidectomy, it is not unusual for the patient to experience mild hypothyroidism. However, thyroid hormone replacement therapy usually is not required since the remaining thyroid tissue hypertrophies, eventually recovering normal function. Lifetime hormone replacement therapy is required following a total thyroidectomy.

Integrative Care Plans

• Preoperative and postoperative care

Discharge Considerations

• Follow-up care
• Medications to continue at home
• Signs and symptoms requiring medical attention
• Wound care

THE PREOPERATIVE PERIOD

 # Assessment data base

1. History or presence of causative factors:
   - hyperthyroidism unresponsive to antithyroid drugs
   - carcinoma of the thyroid
   - large goiter causing swallowing problems

2. Physical examination based on a general survey (Appendix F) may reveal:
   - skin changes (warm, moist skin, palmar erythema)
   - cardiovascular changes (tachycardia, bounding pulse, tachypnea)
   - GI changes (increased appetite, diarrhea, weight loss)
   - neurological changes (insomnia, irritability, agitation, tremors, restlessness, difficulty focusing eyes, hyperreflexia of tendon reflexes)
   - metabolic changes (intolerance to heat, elevated temperature)
   - exophthalmos

3. Inspect the neck for evidence of a goiter evidenced by swelling in the neck area. If goiter is present, inquire about long-term use of medications and goitrogenic foods:
   - foods (turnips, rutabagas, soybeans, cabbage)
   - medicines (lithium, sulfonylureas, thiocarbanides)
   - use of iodine-free salt

4. See Preoperative and Postoperative Care (page 738).

Nursing diagnosis: anxiety

RELATED TO FACTORS: Knowledge deficit about preoperative and postoperative events, fear of some aspect of surgery

DEFINING CHARACTERISTICS: Verbalizes lack of understanding, requests information, reports feeling nervous or anxious, tense body posture

PATIENT OUTCOME: Demonstrates relief from anxiety

EVALUATION CRITERIA: Fewer reports of feeling nervous, verbalizes understanding of preoperative and postoperative events, relaxed body posture

INTERVENTIONS	RATIONALE
1. See Preoperative and Postoperative Care (page 738).	
2. Inform the patient that some hoarseness and swallowing discomfort can be experienced after surgery but will gradually resolve as swelling subsides in about 3–5 days. If exophthalmos is present, ensure the patient understands that a thyroidectomy does not correct the eye problem but helps prevent further enlargement of eye tissue.	A knowledge of what to expect helps lessen anxiety.
3. Teach and have the patient practice how to support the neck to avoid tension on the incision when getting out of bed or coughing. Instruct the patient to place both hands behind the neck for support of the neck.	Practicing postoperative activities helps ensure a less complicated postoperative course.
4. Administer prescribed antithyroid medications and SSKI and evaluate effectiveness. Notify physician if serum T_3 and T_4 levels remain above normal range and goiter size (if present) remains unchanged.	Antithyroid drugs achieve a euthyroid state; SSKI reduces the size and vascularity of the thyroid gland if goiter is present. These measures help reduce the risk of postoperative hemorrhage.

THE POSTOPERATIVE PERIOD

 # A SSESSMENT DATA BASE

1. On receiving the patient,
   - Perform a routine postoperative assessment (Appendix L).
   - Assess voice quality and difficulty swallowing.
   - Assess status of neck dressing by looking at the sides and feeling the back of the neck.

NURSING DIAGNOSIS: PAIN

RELATED TO FACTORS: Thyroidectomy

DEFINING CHARACTERISTICS: Verbalizes discomfort, frowning, moaning, guarding painful site

PATIENT OUTCOME (collaborative): Demonstrates relief from discomfort

EVALUATION CRITERIA: Denies pain, absence of moaning, relaxed facial expression

INTERVENTIONS	RATIONALE
1. Administer prescribed narcotic analgesic prn and evaluate effectiveness.	Narcotic analgesia is necessary with severe pain to block the pain pathway.
2. Remind the patient to follow measures to prevent strain on the incision: • support the neck when moving in bed and when getting out of bed • avoid hyperextension and acute flexion of the neck	Strain on the suture line is a source of discomfort.

NURSING DIAGNOSIS: HIGH RISK FOR COMPLICATIONS

RELATED TO FACTORS: Thyroidectomy, edema in and around incision, accidental removal of parathyroids, hemorrhage, damage to laryngeal nerve

DEFINING CHARACTERISTICS: May show early manifestations of hemorrhage, airway obstruction, laryngeal nerve damage, wound infection, hypocalcemia

PATIENT OUTCOME (collaborative): Demonstrates no further tissue injury

EVALUATION CRITERIA: Absence of manifestations of excess bleeding, hypocalcemia, laryngeal nerve damage, airway obstruction, thyroid hormone imbalance, and infection; discharged home within allotted DRG time frame

INTERVENTIONS	RATIONALE
Hemorrhage:	
1. Monitor: • BP, pulse, and respiration q2h x 4 hours, then q4h if stable • status of dressing: inspect and feel behind the neck q2h x 24 hours, then q8h thereafter	To detect early signs of hemorrhage.
2. Notify physician if bright red drainage on the dressing or falling BP accompanied by rising pulse and respiratory rate occur.	These findings indicate excess bleeding and a need for prompt medical attention.
3. Place call bell at bedside. Instruct the patient to signal if a choking or pressure sensation at the incision site is felt. If these symptoms occur, loosen the dressing, obtain vital signs, inspect the site, keep the patient in a semi-Fowler's position, and notify physician immediately.	These findings can indicate bleeding and a need for prompt medical attention.
Airway Obstruction:	
1. Monitor respirations q2h x 24 hours.	To detect early signs of airway obstruction.
2. Notify physician if complaints of difficulty breathing, irregular respirations, or choking sensations occur.	These findings signal tracheal compression, which can be caused by excess swelling but usually by bleeding. Prompt medical attention is required to prevent respiratory arrest.
3. Maintain a semi-Fowler's position with a pillow behind the head for support. Apply ice collar to neck.	An erect position allows fuller lung expansion and helps reduce swelling. Cold promotes vasoconstriction and prevents swelling.
4. Encourage use of the incentive spirometer q2h to stimulate deep breathing.	Deep breathing keeps the alveoli open to prevent atelectasis.

INTERVENTIONS	RATIONALE
5. Ensure that tracheostomy set, oxygen, and suction equipment are readily available on the unit.	For use if tracheal compression occurs.
Wound Infection:	
1. Change dressing as prescribed using sterile technique.	To guard against introducing bacteria.
2. Notify physician if redness, increased tenderness or drainage from the wound, or fever occur. Obtain a wound specimen for culture to identify the infective organism. Administer antibiotics as ordered.	These findings indicate wound infection and a need for antibiotic therapy.
Laryngeal Nerve Damage:	
1. Instruct the patient to refrain as much as possible from talking.	To reduce strain on the vocal cords.
2. Report increasing hoarseness and weakness of the voice.	Such changes reflect laryngeal nerve damage for which there is no cure.
Hypocalcemia:	
1. Monitor serum calcium reports.	A change in serum calcium level occurs before overt manifestations of a calcium imbalance.
2. Notify physician if complaints of numbness, tingling of lips, fingers, or toes, muscle twitching, or serum calcium level below normal range occur. Check for a positive Chvostek's sign (facial twitching when face is tapped just below the temple) and a positive Trousseau's sign (carpopedal spasms of hand when arm circulation is temporarily restricted with a tourniquet).	These findings indicate hypocalcemia and a need for replacement with calcium salts such as calcium gluconate or calcium chloride. The parathyroid gland may have been injured or inadvertently removed during surgery.

INTERVENTIONS	RATIONALE
Thyroid Hormone Imbalance:	
1. Monitor serum T_3 and T_4 levels.	To detect early indications of thyroid hormone imbalance.
2. Administer thyroid replacement hormones as ordered.	Thyroid hormones are essential for normal metabolic functions.

NURSING DIAGNOSIS: HIGH RISK FOR IMPAIRED HOME MAINTENANCE MANAGEMENT

RELATED TO FACTORS: Knowledge deficit about self-care on discharge

DEFINING CHARACTERISTICS: Verbalizes lack of understanding, requests information

PATIENT OUTCOME: Demonstrates willingness to comply with home maintenance plan

EVALUATION CRITERIA: Verbalizes understanding of discharge instructions, performs exercises correctly, verbalizes satisfaction with home care plan

INTERVENTIONS	RATIONALE
1. Provide instructions for neck exercises: flexion, extension, and rotation exercises. Instruct the patient to begin exercises after sutures are removed, usually within seven days.	These exercises help prevent contracture of neck muscles.
2. Instruct the patient to inspect the neck sutures daily using a mirror. Contact physician if signs of wound infection occur: redness, increased tenderness, drainage, fever.	Antibiotic therapy is required to resolve infections.

INTERVENTIONS	RATIONALE
3. If a total thyroidectomy was performed, provide information about prescribed thyroid hormone replacement medication. Remind the patient that the medication must be taken for a lifetime. Emphasize that the source of thyroid hormone was removed with thyroidectomy and that thyroid hormone is essential for life. Allow the patient to express feelings about having to take medication for a lifetime. Instruct the patient to report symptoms of hypothyroidism (page 574) or recurring symptoms of hyperthyroidism.	Understanding the relation between condition and therapy helps foster patient compliance. Periodic dosage adjustment may be required, especially with prolonged exposure to conditions associated with increased metabolism (fever, chronic inflammatory conditions).
4. Provide written instructions for self-care activities, follow-up appointments, and prescribed medications, including name, dosage, purpose, schedule, and reportable side effects. Evaluate understanding of instructions.	Verbal instructions may be easily forgotten.
5. If exophthalmos is present, advise the patient to continue wearing sunglasses with exposure to the sun.	To protect the delicate eye tissue.
6. See Preoperative and Postoperative Care (page 738).	

Adrenalectomy

Removal of the adrenal gland (adrenalectomy) is done through an abdominal incision. Preoperative preparation is the same for any patient undergoing surgery.

Postoperatively, the patient is kept in the ICU for a few days. Major problems encountered are hypertension, hypotension, and cardiac arrhythmias. For this reason, hemodynamic monitoring is often required, including an arterial catheter, pulmonary artery catheter, and ECG. Hypotension can be life threatening and requires aggressive treatment with fluid volume replacement and vasopressors. The mean LOS for a DRG classification of adrenalectomy is 9.5 days (Lorenz, 1991).

Removal of the adrenal gland predisposes a patient to adrenocortiosteroid deficiency (Addison's disease). If bilateral adrenalectomy is done, cortisol therapy is started preoperatively and continued postoperatively for a lifetime.

Integrative Care Plans

- Hypertension if pheochromocytoma is present
- Preoperative and postoperative care

Discharge Considerations

- Follow-up care
- Wound care
- Signs and symptoms of wound infection
- Medications for home use
- Activity limitations

THE PREOPERATIVE PERIOD

 # ASSESSMENT DATA BASE

1. History or presence of causative factors:
   - pheochromocytoma (rare benign catecholamine-producing tumor of the adrenal medulla).
   - carcinoma of the prostate or breast (done as palliative treatment for these estrogen-dependent cancers)
2. Physical examination based on a general assessment (Appendix F) may reveal hypertension if caused by pheochromocytoma.
3. Diagnostic studies for pheochromocytoma:
   - CT scan and renal ultrasound reveal a mass.
   - 24-hour urine for excretion of catecholamines confirms the diagnosis.
4. See Preoperative and Postoperative Care (page 738).

THE POSTOPERATIVE PERIOD

See integrative care plans Preoperative and Postoperative Care. In addition, discharge teaching should include recognition of manifestations of glucocoticosteroid deficiency (Addison's disease) and special instructions about self-administration of cortisol.

BIBLIOGRAPHY

Chipps, E. (1992). Transsphenoidal surgery for pituitary tumors. **Critical Care Nurse, 12,** 30–39.

DeGroog, L.J. (1989). **Endocrinology.** 2nd ed., Philadelphia: W.B. Saunders Company.

Hershman, J.M. (1989). Getting the most from thyroid tests. **Patient Care, 23,** 86–90, 99–101, 105–106.

Isley, W.L. (1990). Thyroid disorders. **Critical Care Nurse, 13,** 39–49.

Lorenz, E.W. (1991). **St. Anthony's DRG Working Guidebook.** Alexandria: St. Anthony's Publishing Company.

Reasner, C.A. (1990). Adrenal disorders. **Critical Care Nurse, 13,** 67–73.

Yeomans, A.C. (1990). Assessment and management of hypothyroidism, **Nurse Practitioner, 15,** 8, 11–12, 14.

Yucha, C., & Blakeman, N. (1991). Pheochromocytoma. **Cancer Nursing, 14,** 136–140.

C

HAPTER ELEVEN
Problems of the Nervous System

Vertebral Column Surgery

Laminectomies and spinal fusion are the most common vertebral column surgeries performed on adults. They are done for decompression of the spinal cord or peripheral nerves, repair of unstable vertebrae, and spinal vascular anomalies.

Laminectomy involves removal of fragments of a herniated intervertebral disc through an incision made over the affected vertebrae. To prevent adhesions, small pieces of subcutaneous fatty tissue are placed over the excised dura mater.

With spinal fusion, fragments of bone taken from the patient's iliac crest are used to graft adjacent vertebrae together to eliminate vertebral instability.

Preoperative preparation is the same for any patient undergoing surgery.

Postoperatively, the patient returns to the medical/surgical unit with:

- small dressing over the vertebral incision. (Following a spinal fusion, the patient has two dressing sites: the back and iliac crest from which the bone was taken).

- IV infusion

- Foley catheter (most often with spinal fusion).

Ambulation often begins the first postoperative day following a laminectomy; the second or third postoperative day following a spinal fusion. The patient with a spinal fusion must wear a back brace before getting out of bed.

The patient is kept flat in bed but can be log-rolled in a side-lying position. Meals are taken with assistance in a side-lying position. After ambulation is allowed, the head of the bed may be raised about 30–40 degrees for meals.

When out of bed, sitting and standing are restricted because such activities place too much stress on the back. A spinal fusion is often more painful than a laminectomy because the patient has two surgical sites (back incision and iliac crest incision).

The average recuperation time following a laminectomy is about 4–6 weeks and about three months following a spinal fusion.

Constipation can be a problem due to self-imposed decreased physical activity and chronic use of pain medication and muscle relaxants. It is not uncommon to find depression with chronic back pain. Often the pain has resulted in loss of work and impairment in performance of role functions in the home environment.

The major postoperative complications are urinary retention, wound infection, and disruption of the bone graft (following spinal fusion) (Feingold, 1991).

The mean LOS for a DRG classification of vertebral column surgery is 9.9 days (Lorenz, 1991).

Integrative Care Plans

- Immobility
- Loss
- Pain
- Preoperative and postoperative care

Discharge Considerations

- Follow-up care
- Activity limitations
- Application of back brace if spinal fusion performed
- Signs and symptoms requiring medical attention
- Wound care

THE PREOPERATIVE PERIOD

 # ASSESSMENT DATA BASE

1. History or presence of causative factors:
   - chronic back pain that can be accompanied by paresthesia. Foot-drop and loss of ankle reflex with lumbar involvement can be present.

2. Assess motor and sensory functioning of the lower extremities:
   - Have the patient wiggle toes and feet.
   - Palpate and mark pedal pulses.
   - Check color and temperature of the feet.
   - Assess capillary refill.
   - Assess sensation to light touch and temperature.

3. Assess pain:
   - What makes pain worse?
   - What relieves pain?
   - Is pain localized or does pain radiate?
   - Is pain constant or intermittent?
   - What does pain feel like (burning, aching, stabbing)?

4. Assess for problems with bowel and bladder elimination.

5. Diagnostic studies:
   - CT and MRI scan show structural abnormality and bulging of the disc.
   - Myelogram confirms diagnosis of herniated nucleus pulposus (HNP).
   - Bone scan can be done to assess for degenerative changes.

6. See Preoperative and Postoperative Care (page 738).

NURSING DIAGNOSIS: PAIN

RELATED TO FACTORS: Herniated nucleus pulposus, unstable vertebrae

DEFINING CHARACTERISTICS: Verbalizes discomfort, frowning, moaning, tense body posture

PATIENT OUTCOME (collaborative): Demonstrates less discomfort

EVALUATION CRITERIA: Fewer reports of back pain, less moaning, relaxed facial expression

INTERVENTIONS	RATIONALE
1. Assist the patient to assume a position of comfort such as supine with knees slightly flexed.	To relieve stress on the back muscles.
2. Apply heat pack or ice pack to back as ordered.	Heat relaxes muscles. Cold helps reduce inflammation and desensitizes nerve endings.
3. Administer prescribed muscle relaxant, analgesic, and anti-inflammatory agent and evaluate effectiveness.	These agents act systemically to produce generalized relaxation and to reduce inflammation. Analgesics block the pain pathway.
4. Prepare the patient for surgery as ordered. Have the patient practice: a. log-rolling from side-to-side. b. getting out of bed from the side-lying position: Have the patient move close to the edge of the bed while supine, roll to a side-lying position, and then use arms to push self to a sitting position as legs are brought to a dangling position. c. coughing and deep breathing.	Practicing these activities ensures a smoother postoperative recovery.

THE POSTOPERATIVE PERIOD

 ASSESSMENT DATA BASE

1. On receiving the patient:
   - perform a routine postoperative assessment (Appendix L)
   - assess motor and sensory function in both lower extremities
   - assess urge to void, if a Foley catheter is not in place; palpate and inspect the suprapubic region for distention

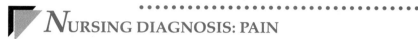

NURSING DIAGNOSIS: PAIN

RELATED TO FACTORS: Laminectomy, spinal fusion
DEFINING CHARACTERISTICS: Verbalizes discomfort, frowning, moaning, rigid body posture
PATIENT OUTCOME (collaborative): Demonstrates relief from pain
EVALUATION CRITERIA: Denies pain, relaxed facial expression, absence of moaning

INTERVENTIONS	RATIONALE
1. Assist in assuming a comfortable side-lying or back-lying position. Place pillows between legs and securely behind back while in the side-lying position. Ensure proper body alignment while in the side-lying or back-lying position. Gatch knee of bed slightly while in the back-lying position. Avoid turning the patient to the iliac crest donor side (with spinal fusion).	Slight flexion of the knees while supine helps relieve tension on back muscles. A pillow between legs when in a lateral position keeps hips abducted thus relieving tension on back muscles. Repositioning helps relieve pressure on dependent body parts.
2. Log-roll from side-to-side. Place a draw sheet on the bed to make turning easier. Always get assistance when repositioning or getting the patient out of bed.	Twisting increases tissue damage at the operative site and pain.
3. See Pain (page 700).	

NURSING DIAGNOSIS: HIGH RISK FOR COMPLICATIONS

RELATED TO FACTORS: Laminectomy, spinal fusion

DEFINING CHARACTERISTICS: Demonstrates early manifestations of wound infection, urinary retention, pseudarthrosis (with spinal fusion)

PATIENT OUTCOME (collaborative): Demonstrates absence of complications

EVALUATION CRITERIA: Absence of manifestations of wound infection, adequate urinary output, and absence of neurovascular deficits, discharged within LOS for DRG

INTERVENTIONS	RATIONALE
Wound Infection:	
1. See Preoperative and Postoperative Care (page 738).	
Urinary Retention:	
1. Monitor fluid intake and output q8h.	These parameters are a valuable indicator of the amount of body fluid that needs to be replaced when losses exceed gains. Also, provides reliable data about the status of the urinary system. Normally, fluid intake should approximate urinary output.
2. Notify physician of suprapubic distention with complaints of the inability to void despite the urge, or if frequently voiding small amounts. Catheterize as ordered.	A full bladder places stress on the back, increasing discomfort.
3. If a Foley catheter is in place, ensure no kinks are in the tubing. After removal, provide fluids to ensure the patient voids. Note time and amount of first voiding. Inquire about problems with voiding, such as burning or difficulty initiating the flow. Obtain a specimen for culture and sensitivity tests. Administer prescribed antibiotic and evaluate effectiveness (normal urinalysis, denies voiding discomfort).	The bladder is kept in a deflated position while the Foley catheter is in place. Bladder tone can be reestablished by providing fluids. Burning with voiding can indicate a urinary infection. Antibiotic therapy is required to resolve an infection. Appropriate antibiotic therapy is ensured with a urine culture and sensitivity test.

INTERVENTIONS	RATIONALE
Pseudoarthrosis:	
1. Monitor neurovascular status of lower extremities q2h x 24 hours, then q4h if stable.	Neurovascular deficits can occur if severe swelling or bleeding occur at the operative site and compress the spinal cord.
2. Use a log-rolling technique when positioning the patient side-to-side, placement on a bedpan, or changing bed linen. Instruct the patient to keep the back straight. Apply a draw sheet to the bed for use when turning the patient.	Maintains normal vertebral column alignment. A draw sheet makes turning easier.
3. Apply a back brace **before** getting the patient with a spinal fusion out of bed.	Keeping the back straight helps maintain alignment of the vertebrae, reducing the risk of graft dislocation.
4. Avoid prolonged sitting and standing in one position. When sitting is allowed, place patient in a semi-Fowler's position for meals; otherwise, keep patient flat when in bed. Instruct patient to keep moving when out of bed.	To reduce stress on the vertebrae.
5. Avoid having the patient use the trapeze bar to move self in bed.	To prevent excess strain on the back.
6. Refer to physical therapist for instructions on muscle-strengthening exercises.	A physical therapist is a specialist who can plan an exercise program to complement the patient's current condition.

• •

NURSING DIAGNOSIS: HIGH RISK FOR IMPAIRED HOME MAINTENANCE MANAGEMENT

RELATED TO FACTORS: Knowledge deficit about self-care activities on discharge, lack of adequate support system

DEFINING CHARACTERISTICS: Verbalizes lack of understanding, requests information, observation of inappropriate posture, may report need for assistance with some ADL but lives alone

PATIENT OUTCOME (collaborative): Demonstrates willingness to comply with self-care measures for home maintenance

EVALUATION CRITERIA: Verbalizes understanding of instructions, performs required skills correctly, verbalizes satisfaction with discharge plans to meet home care needs

• •

INTERVENTIONS	RATIONALE
1. Provide home care instructions and evaluate understanding. Instructions should include: • Follow exercise protocol to strengthen abdominal, back, and leg muscles. Explain that strong abdominal muscles help support the back. • Avoid prolonged sitting and standing. Walk at intervals. Sit in a semireclining position to relieve stress on the back. • Avoid bending, twisting, and lifting. When lifting is permitted, maintain good body mechanics for lifting objects: bend knees and hips while keeping the back straight to lift an object. Explain that extra weight places added stress on the vertebrae. • Abstain from sexual intercourse until approved by physician to avoid placing undue stress on the back. • Wear comfortable shoes that keep the body balanced so undue tension is not placed on back muscles. • Keep appointments for follow-up evaluations because x rays are required to assess healing.	Discharge teaching makes a smoother transition from facility to home. It is a safety measure that helps the patient or significant other know what to do to maintain or improve health.

INTERVENTIONS	RATIONALE
2. Ensure the patient has a prescription for an analgesic for use at home prn.	Some back discomfort still will be experienced.
3. Provide home care instructions and appointment for follow-up visit in writing.	Verbal instructions may be easily forgotten.
4. For spinal fusion, advise the patient to wear the back brace until discontinued by physician. Have the patient practice applying the brace before discharge. Remind the patient to apply the back brace **before** getting out of bed. Tell the patient that the back brace must be worn for about three months until the graft has healed, determined by an x ray.	Return demonstrations are essential for evaluating teaching and assessing an individual's level of independence with a required skill.
5. Evaluate need for assistance with ADL and adequacy of support system at home. Initiate a referral to the social services or discharge planning department if patient expresses a need for assistance with ADL.	Social service personnel or discharge planners are liaisons that ensure patients' rehabilitative needs are met on discharge.

Guillain-Barré Syndrome

Guillain-Barré syndrome is a progressive and acute demyelinating inflammatory neuritis (also called polyneuropathy) that affects the peripheral nervous system. The etiology is unknown. However, it is believed to involve an autoimmune reaction to a viral infection such as cytomegalovirus, Epstein-Barr virus, or Campylobacter jejuni. The major pathological finding is patchy demyelination of peripheral nerves (Morgan, 1991).

The symptoms of Guillain-Barré syndrome usually appear within 1–7 weeks after a viral infection. Accordingly, the influenza vaccine is not a risk factor in the disease (Morgan, 1991).

Guillain-Barré syndrome is characterized by progressive paralysis, which occurs in an ascending pattern. Motor and sensory losses occur symmetrically, starting in the feet and legs. The disease severity and progression rate are variable: the disease can advance rapidly within 24 hours ultimately paralyzing respiratory muscles, or develop slowly over weeks. It can affect only the lower extremities or travel up the body, ultimately involving the thorax and face.

Often within 2–3 weeks of the onset of neurological symptoms, clinical deterioration reaches a peak. The patient slowly shows signs of recovery. Return of normal motor and sensory function commonly occurs in a descending pattern. Most patients recover within 4-6 months; however, some patients need one year for recovery (Morgan, 1991).

Because of the possibility of rapid progression to respiratory failure, patients with Guillain-Barré syndrome are initially cared for in an ICU. Prognosis for recovery is poor for persons who (Morgan, 1991):

- are elderly
- experience rapid progression of symptoms
- require mechanical ventilation
- have electrophysiologic studies showing severe nerve impairment

During the acute phase, patients express fear and anxiety over the possibility of permanent paralysis. Anger and depression can be expressed during the peak and recovery phases of the illness.

The mean LOS for a DRG classification of Guillain-Barré syndrome is 6.7 days (Lorenz, 1991).

General Medical Management

There is no specific treatment to halt the process. Treatment is symptomatic and can include:
- mechanical ventilation for respiratory failure
- chest physiotherapy and endotracheal suctioning if ability to cough is lost and secretions begin to pool in the lungs
- insertion of a nasogastric tube for tube feedings if patient cannot swallow
- analgesics to control pain during the recovery period
- physical therapy to restore muscle strength, initiated when patient shows signs of recovery
- plasmapheresis (therapeutic plasma exchanges)
- beta-blockers to control hypertension
- continuous ECG monitoring
- IV therapy to increase fluid volume and correct hypotension

Integrative Care Plans

- Immobility
- Mechanical ventilation if respiratory paralysis occurs

Discharge Considerations

- Follow-up care

 # ASSESSMENT DATA BASE

1. Inquire about a recent exposure to a viral infection or recent flulike symptoms (most common antecedent infection), diarrhea, surgery, blood transfusion, vaccination, or unusual illness within the past few weeks.

2. Physical examination based on a rapid neurological assessment (Appendix J) may reveal:
   - paresthesia, progressive weakness, and pain beginning in both feet and legs; ultimately paralysis occurs

     As these neurological deficits progress upward, additional manifestations begin to emerge:

   - low back pain
   - tachycardia with episodic bouts of bradycardia
   - hypertension with varying periods of orthostatic hypotension
   - muscle cramps, light-headedness, facial weakness
   - respiratory failure with paralysis of the diaphragm

3. Diagnostic studies:

  • Lumbar puncture analyses reveals elevated CSF protein and a low white cell count.
  • Electrophysiologic studies reveal a slowing of nerve conduction velocity, indicating demyelination.
  • Stool culture is done to assess for **Campylobacter jejuni** if diarrhea is present.

4. Assess the patient's feelings and concerns about illness.

5. Assess the patient's understanding of condition, treatment, and diagnostic studies.

NURSING DIAGNOSIS: HIGH RISK FOR IMPAIRED GAS EXCHANGE

RELATED TO FACTORS: Paralysis of the diaphragm secondary to Guillain-Barré syndrome

DEFINING CHARACTERISTICS: Reports increasing difficulty breathing, abnormal pulmonary function studies, observation of shallow respirations

PATIENT OUTCOME (collaborative): Demonstrates adequate gas exchange

EVALUATION CRITERIA: Denies dyspnea, arterial blood gases (ABG) within normal limits, respiratory rate between 12–24 per minute, normal skin color

INTERVENTIONS	RATIONALE

1. Monitor:
  • vital signs q2h initially, then q4h when stable
  • respiratory status (Appendix A) q8h
  • results of ABG reports
	These parameters provide objective data for evaluating the effectiveness of therapy.

2. Notify physician if respiratory rate less than 12 per minute, diminished breath sounds or PO_2 less than 85–90 mm Hg occur.	These findings signal eminent respiratory failure. Mechanical ventilation is required to support breathing until recovery begins.
3. Perform nasotracheal suctioning prn if patient cannot clear secretions.	Suctioning helps clear the airway of secretions.
4. Encourage use of an incentive spirometer q2h.	To promote deep breathing and expansion of the alveoli.

INTERVENTIONS	RATIONALE
5. As respirations become increasingly difficult, maintain a semi-Fowler's position.	An erect position allows fuller lung expansion.
6. Administer prescribed analgesia prn and evaluate effectiveness. Assist the patient in assuming a position of comfort.	Individuals normally restrict breathing when in pain. Analgesics block the pain pathways. Changing positions relieves pressure and prevents joint stiffness.

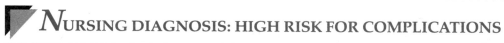

NURSING DIAGNOSIS: HIGH RISK FOR COMPLICATIONS

RELATED TO FACTORS: See Immobility (page 725).

INTERVENTIONS	RATIONALE
1. See Immobility (page 725).	
2. Refer to the physical therapy department for muscle strengthening exercises as ordered.	A physical therapist is a specialist who can plan and provide an exercise program in relation to the patient's current condition.
3. Monitor ability to perform activities of daily living (ADL). Assist as needed. Allow the patient to do as much as possible for self.	Self-care promotes a sense of control and independence. Performing ADL also provides active exercise to help maintain joint flexibility and muscle strength.
4. Check for soiling frequently if incontinent of stool and urine. Provide perineal care prn. Apply a disposable brief as needed.	Dry and clean skin is less susceptible to breakdown.
5. Keep call bell always within the patient's reach. Arrange for a call bell system that the patient can trigger depending on voluntary control present (for example, chin activated if patient can only move head).	Being able to communicate needs prn helps reduce frustration and fosters a sense of control.

▶ NURSING DIAGNOSIS: ANXIETY

RELATED TO FACTORS: Knowledge deficit about condition, treatments, and threat of permanent paralysis (see Anxiety, page 262)

▶ NURSING DIAGNOSIS: HIGH RISK FOR ALTERATION IN NUTRITION: LESS THAN BODY REQUIREMENTS

RELATED TO FACTORS: Dysphagia secondary to Guillain-Barré syndrome

DEFINING CHARACTERISTICS: Reports increasing difficulty with swallowing, observation of excessive coughing with oral feedings, weekly weight loss

PATIENT OUTCOME (collaborative): Nutritional status maintained

EVALUATION CRITERIA: No further weight loss

INTERVENTIONS	RATIONALE
1. Monitor: • amount of food consumed at each meal • weight weekly	To evaluate effectiveness of therapy.
2. Provide supplemental feedings if dietary intake is less than 30%. Refer to dietitian for assistance with meal planning.	An adequate intake of nutrients, especially proteins, vitamins, and minerals, is essential for tissue repair. The dietitian is a nutritional specialist who can evaluate the patient's nutritional status and plan meals to ensure adequate nutrition.
3. If swallowing difficulty occurs, insert a feeding tube as ordered.	Giving oral feedings when dysphagia is present can cause aspiration.

Spinal Cord Injury

Injury to the spinal cord can be a contussion, compression, concussion, laceration, partial transection, or complete transection. The injury can involve the cervical, thoracic, lumbar, or sacral vertebrae. With spinal cord injury, movement and sensation below the level of injury are affected.

The patient displays a variety of emotional reactions (anger, depression, withdrawal) in response to the immediate losses incurred and the uncertainty of the extent of residual effects of the injury. Having to readjust one's lifestyle to accommodate permanent physical impairments and alterations in bodily functioning is frightening and frustrating. These emotional reactions represent the normal grief process in response to loss.

The mean LOS for a DRG classification of spinal cord injury is 7.1 days (Lorenz, 1991).

A major complication associated with spinal cord lesions above the sixth thoracic vertebrae is autonomic dysreflexia. This syndrome represents a life-threatening emergency. If not corrected promptly, it can cause a stroke. It represents an overstimulation of the sympathetic system to a mild stimulus. The most common cause of this syndrome is visceral distention (distended bladder, fecal impaction, and pain). The patient can continue to experience this syndrome throughout life.

General Medical Management

- Measures to immobilize and maintain alignment of the vertebrae:
  — cervical collar, sandbags, or IV bags to stabilize the neck, and a backboard when transporting the patient
  — skeletal traction for cervical fractures, which involves applying Crutchfield, Vinke, or Gardner-Wells tongs to the skull
  — bedrest and application of a halo brace for simple stable cervical fractures
  — surgery (laminectomy, spinal fusion, or Harrington rod insertion) for decompression of the spine if x rays indicate an unstable spine
- Measures to reduce spinal cord swelling using IV glucocorticosteroids.

ASSESSMENT DATA BASE

1. Physical examination based on a rapid neurological assessment (Appendix J) may reveal motor and sensory deficits below the level of injury:

   • spinal shock characterized by flaccid paralysis or areflexia (loss of all reflexes below the site of injury). This is often a temporary event lasting from several days to six months. However, with complete cord transection, spastic or hyperreflexic muscle movements occur later as edema subsides. These involuntary movements often indicate spinal shock is ending. Medications such as baclofen, valium, or dantrolene can reduce spasticity.

   • pain

   • altered bladder function:

   — neurogenic bladder (autonomic bladder) is characterized by uncontrollable and spontaneous voiding of small quantities at frequent intervals. This type of incontinent voiding pattern represents an upper motor neuron lesion. The reflex arc remains intact but inhibiting mechanisms are lost. Minor stimulation such as stroking the abdomen, thigh, or genitalia can trigger voiding.

   — atonic bladder is characterized by urinary retention with no awareness of the need to void. The bladder overdistends, and constant dribbling occurs. This type of bladder dysfunction represents lower motor neuron involvement. The reflex arc is lost and impulses no longer reach the brain.

   • impaired sexual functioning. In men, impotence, decreased sensation, and ejaculation difficulties often occur. These findings occur most often with spinal cord damage in the sacral area. Sexual functioning is more likely to remain intact with injuries occurring above the sacral area although sexual satisfaction can be diminished. Sexual functioning in females usually remains unaffected.

   • altered bowel functioning, including incontinence and constipation

2. Assess the patient's feelings and concerns about condition.

3. Diagnostic studies.

   • X rays of the vertebrae reveal the type and site of the fracture.

NURSING DIAGNOSIS: HIGH RISK FOR INFECTION

RELATED TO FACTORS: Bladder dysfunction secondary to spinal cord injury
DEFINING CHARACTERISTICS: May experience urinary retention, incontinence
PATIENT OUTCOME: Demonstrates no urinary tract infection
EVALUATION CRITERIA: Passage of clear urine without foul smell, normal urinalysis

INTERVENTIONS	RATIONALE
1. Monitor intake and output q8h.	To assess bladder function and to evaluate fluid needs.
2. Apply disposable briefs for incontinent females. Use an external catheter or disposable brief for incontinent males. Keep skin clean and dry.	Achieving continence helps improve self-esteem. In addition, clean dry skin is less susceptible to breakdown.
3. Notify physician of suprapubic distention or constant dribbling (which indicates overflow incontinence). Insert a Foley catheter as ordered, or perform intermittent catheterization as ordered.	These findings indicate urinary retention. A catheter is used to drain the bladder. A full bladder provides a good culture medium. Intermittent catheterization is often preferred treatment for persistent urinary retention because UTI is more likely to occur with an indwelling bladder catheter.
4. Provide at least 1–2 liters of fluid daily.	To keep the kidneys flushed.

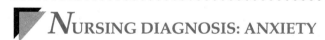

NURSING DIAGNOSIS: ANXIETY

RELATED TO FACTORS: Fear of threat of permanent paralysis, knowledge deficit about treatment plan

DEFINING CHARACTERISTICS: Verbalizes nervousness, fear, anger, depression, frustration, and lack of understanding about outcome and treatment plan

PATIENT OUTCOME (collaborative): Demonstrates relief from anxiety

EVALUATION CRITERIA: Fewer reports of feeling nervous and afraid, verbalizes understanding of possible outcomes and treatment plans

INTERVENTIONS	RATIONALE
1. See Anxiety (page 262).	

INTERVENTIONS	RATIONALE
2. If cord injury does not involve transection, remind the patient that the extent of residual motor and sensory impairment is best determined after tissue swelling has subsided. Explain that when spinal cord injury occurs, edema forms, which further contributes to more compression of the cord.	A knowledge of what to expect helps lessen anxiety.
3. Refer the patient for psychological counseling if impairment of motor, sensory, and sexual functioning will be permanent.	Patients who experience permanent loss of some aspect of body functioning will grieve that loss. The greater the significance of the loss to the individual, the longer and more intense the grief reaction is likely to be. These persons often need professional help to cope with permanent loss arising from an acute situation.
4. If cord injury has resulted in impotence, encourage the patient to discuss the possibility of a penile implant with the physician. Let the patient know that there are other ways of expressing sexuality such as touching, talking, and kissing.	A knowledge of alternatives available to amend a loss helps lessen the threat of altered body image.
5. Offer praise for accomplishments made in learning how to regain independence.	Positive reinforcement helps motivate one to learn.
6. Initiate rehabilitative therapy by making a referral to occupational therapy and physical therapy.	Early rehabilitation helps promote a sense of hope. An occupational therapist can assess the patient's rehabilitation potential and design a rehabilitation program that focuses on developing usable skills in view of physical limitations. The physical therapist is an exercise specialist who can assess the patient's potential for mobility and design an exercise program to regain mobility, to improve muscle strength and tone, or both.

INTERVENTIONS	RATIONALE
7. Consult social services for assistance in arranging rehabilitation services for the patient after discharge.	Social services can link the patient with the appropriate community services so all the patient's rehabilitative needs are met. Also, they can also assist with financing rehabilitative services.

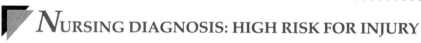

NURSING DIAGNOSIS: HIGH RISK FOR INJURY

RELATED TO FACTORS: Vertebral fracture

DEFINING CHARACTERISTICS: X rays confirm an unstable fracture, neuromuscular deficits below the site of injury, verbalizes pain with movement

PATIENT OUTCOME (collaborative): Demonstrates no further injury

EVALUATION CRITERIA: No further motor and sensory impairment

INTERVENTIONS	RATIONALE
1. Monitor: • neurovascular status of the extremities (Appendix D) below the level of injury q2h x 48 hours, then q4h thereafter • vital signs q2h x 24 hours, then q4h if stable.	To evaluate effectiveness of therapy.
2. Notify physician immediately if the following occur: • further neurological deficits • sudden changes in respiratory rate and pattern	Further neurological deficits can indicate further cord compression and the need for immediate surgery. Patients with cervical injuries are at great risk of respiratory impairment.
3. Maintain traction and/or bedrest as prescribed.	Traction helps maintain vertebral alignment. A supine position reduces stress on the spine.
4. Perform measures to prevent autonomic dysreflexia: • Ensure passage of a soft bowel movement at least every three days. Give a stool softener as	Pain, constipation, and a distended bladder can trigger autonomic dysreflexia.

INTERVENTIONS

prescribed, especially if there is
a history of constipation. Provide
a fluid intake of 1–2 liters daily,
unless contraindicated. Give a
laxative if no bowel movement
occurs in three days or if stools
are hard and lumpy. Provide
foods high in fiber such as raw
fruits and vegetables, prune juice,
bran cereals, and whole wheat
breads.
- Keep indwelling urinary catheter
  patent.
- Administer prescribed pain medication as needed.

5. Take action immediately if manifestations of autonomic dysreflexia
   occur: "gooseflesh," nasal congestion, slow pulse rate, extremely
   high systolic pressure. If these
   symptoms occur:
   - Place the patient in an upright
     position immediately to lower
     blood pressure.
   - Search for and remove the stimu-
     lus (kink in the catheter tubing
     causing bladder distention, pain,
     something causing pressure on
     the skin, fecal impaction).
   - Monitor BP every 15 minutes until
     stable. Notify physician if unable
     to locate the stimulus. Administer
     prescribed ganglionic blocking
     agent (Hyperstat or Apresoline)
     to relieve hypertension.

6. Administer prescribed gluco-
   corticosteroid. Ensure the patient
   receives medication such as
   cimetidine (Tagamet) or ranitidine
   (Zantac) to control gastric acidity
   while on steroid therapy.

RATIONALE

An erect position reduces venous return
thus lowering blood pressure. Unrelieved,
hypertension can cause a stroke.

Steroids help reduce spinal cord edema
and are also ulcerogenic.

INTERVENTIONS	RATIONALE
7. Place the patient with paralysis on a Roto Rest bed if available.	This special bed allows repositioning without movement of the vertebrae.
8. If a regular bed is used, place a backboard beneath the mattress to prevent sagging of the mattress. Place an eggcrate or air pressure mattress on the bed to guard against skin breakdown.	Pressure areas can develop easily when the patient has lost sensory and motor functions of a body part.
9. Ensure proper wearing and application of the prescribed brace.	A brace helps maintain vertebral alignment.
10. If a standard bed is used, avoid turning the patient until ordered by the physician. When turning the patient on a standard bed, ensure a draw sheet is on the bed. Instruct the patient to keep the spine straight when turning. Use a log-roll technique when turning side-to-side. Ensure the body is properly aligned using pillows to provide support as needed. Always get extra help when turning a patient.	Log-rolling keeps the spine straight. A draw sheet makes positioning easier. Additional assistance provides a safeguard to make turning easier for the patient and the caregiver.
11. Administer prescribed analgesic sparingly prn and evaluate its effectiveness. Avoid overmedication.	Heavy use of analgesics can mask symptoms, making it difficult to detect further neurological deficits.
12. Reposition q2h.	To relieve pressure on dependent bony areas.

. . . .

◤NURSING DIAGNOSIS: HIGH RISK FOR IMPAIRED HOME MAINTENANCE MANAGEMENT

RELATED TO FACTORS: Knowledge deficit about continual rehabilitative measures on discharge, lack of adequate resources at home to perform rehabilitative plan, lack of sufficient finances, paralysis

DEFINING CHARACTERISTICS: Verbalizes lack of understanding about rehabilitative plans, reports lives alone, may report financial distress in meeting continuing care needs

PATIENT OUTCOME (collaborative): Demonstrates willingness to comply with rehabilitative plan

EVALUATION CRITERIA: Performs prescribed exercises correctly, verbalizes understanding of how to manage physiological impairments on discharge, verbalizes satisfaction with rehabilitative plans

• •

INTERVENTIONS	RATIONALE
1. Evaluate significant other's ability to manage the patient at home. Consult a social service representative to make arrangements for home care assistance or placement in an extended care facility or rehabilitation facility if there is no assistance at home.	Social service representatives are specialists in arranging and coordinating community resources to meet continuing care needs of patients.
2. If the patient is cared for at home, teach the patient and significant others how to manage physiological impairments as the need arises. **For Bladder Dysfunctions, Teach:** 1. Intermittent catheterization using a clean technique if urinary retention exists. Provide a written schedule of times. Instruct to catheterize q6h; however, if output is greater than 350 mL, change catheterization schedule to q4h. Explain the urge to void is normally felt when bladder capacity reaches 350 mL. 2. Recognition of urinary tract infection. Instruct to notify physician if urine is foul smelling and cloudy. Encourage daily fluid intake of at least 2-3 liters to keep the kidneys flushed. As prevention against UTI, encourage daily intake of cranberry juice to keep the urine acid. Explain that an alkaline urine predisposes to UTI.	Discharge planning involves identifying and using the patient's existing support systems and providing new support systems as the need arises. When significant others assume responsibility as the patient's primary caregiver, discharge planning also entails providing support for them. Discharge teaching helps promote continual recovery.

INTERVENTIONS	RATIONALE
For Autonomic Dysreflexia, Teach: 1. Prevention, recognition, and treatment. **For Paralysis of Extremities, Teach:** 1. Range-of-motion (ROM) exercises as planned by physical therapy department and how often to perform them. 2. Prevention of skin breakdown. 3. Correct application of back or neck brace if one is required. Stress the importance of inspecting the skin beneath the brace for signs of irritation. Encourage the patient to wear a T-shirt beneath the brace to minimize skin irritation. **For Bowel Dysfunction, Teach:** 1. Measures to ensure passage of a soft stool. 2. Measures to relieve constipation. **General:** 1. Provide information about local resources to obtain needed medical supplies such as wheelchair and catheterization equipment.	

Craniotomy

A **craniotomy** is a surgical opening of the skull. Preoperative preparation is the same for any patient undergoing surgery. Usually when the hair is shaved, it is placed in a bag and returned to the patient. Many patients fear disability from a craniotomy.

Postoperatively, the patient can be kept in the ICU for several days until stable and is connected to an ECG monitor to provide continuous monitoring of cardiac status. The patient returns to the ICU with:

- IV infusion
- arterial line for obtaining blood samples for arterial blood gases (ABG) analysis and to provide constant monitoring of BP
- triple or double lumen central venous catheter
- endotracheal tube for connection to a mechanical ventilator
- possibly, a ventriculostomy catheter for monitoring intracranial pressure (ICP) if very high before surgery
- Foley catheter to monitor output
- dressing around the head

Bedrest is maintained until stable. If ABG are stable and the gag and swallowing reflex return, the respiratory therapist, physician, or nurse removes the endotracheal tube.

A craniotomy predisposes the patient to:

- increased ICP caused by cerebral edema
- injury to cranial nerves
- seizures caused by cortical disturbances
- infection (meningitis)

The mean LOS for a DRG classification of craniotomy is 12.2 days (Lorenz, 1991).

Integrative Care Plans

- Preoperative and postoperative care
- Epilepsy
- Immobility

Discharge Considerations

- Follow-up care
- Rehabilitative measures to continue at home
- Medications for home use

THE PREOPERATIVE PERIOD

 # ASSESSMENT DATA BASE

1. History or presence of conditions associated with the need for a craniotomy
   - intracranial lesions (tumor, abscess, bleeding, aneurysm)
   - hydrocephalus
   - skull fracture
   - congenital arteriovenous malfunction

2. Physical examination based on a rapid neurological assessment (Appendix J) and a general survey (Appendix F) to establish baseline values.

3. If the patient is conscious, assess feelings and concerns about the surgery.

4. See Preoperative and Postoperative Care (page 738).

NURSING DIAGNOSIS: ANXIETY

RELATED TO FACTORS: Knowledge deficit about preoperative and postoperative events, fear of possible permanent loss of body function

DEFINING CHARACTERISTICS: Reports feeling nervous, anxious, or afraid; verbalizes lack of understanding

PATIENT OUTCOME: Demonstrates relief from anxiety

EVALUATION CRITERIA: Verbalizes understanding of preoperative and postoperative events, reports feeling less nervous

INTERVENTIONS	RATIONALE
1. Allow the patient and significant others to express feelings and concerns. Provide clear explanations to questions. Refer specific questions about the surgery to the neurosurgeon. Explain that chances of disability depend on the quantity of brain tissue damaged by the primary lesion or injury and the amount of tissue removed.	Expressing feelings helps lessen anxiety.
2. Ask the patient if the hair shaved from the scalp should be saved. Flag the chart with the patient's request. Suggest wearing a wig or decorative headscarf until the hair grows back.	Hair can hold a cultural significance. Baldness, in most situations, alters body image and is associated with feelings of lowered self-esteem. An important nursing role when medical intervention causes altered body image is to assist the patient in reestablishing self-esteem.
3. Have the patient practice turning and deep breathing. Inform the patient that coughing should be avoided since it causes a transient increase in ICP.	Preoperative teaching and practice help promote a smoother recovery from surgery.
4. See Preoperative and Postoperative Care (page 738).	

THE POSTOPERATIVE PERIOD

 # ASSESSMENT DATA BASE

1. Perform a routine postoperative assessment (Appendix L) and a rapid neurological assessment (Appendix J).

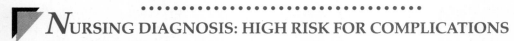

NURSING DIAGNOSIS: HIGH RISK FOR COMPLICATIONS

RELATED TO FACTORS: Craniotomy

DEFINING CHARACTERISTICS: May show early manifestations of increasing ICP, seizures, and infection

PATIENT OUTCOME (collaborative): Demonstrates no further neurological deficits

EVALUATION CRITERIA: Absence of manifestations of increasing ICP, seizures, and infection; discharged within LOS for DRG

● ●

INTERVENTIONS	RATIONALE
Increasing ICP:	
1. Monitor: • neurological status (Appendix J) q2h x 48 hours, q4h once stable • intake and output q2h x 48 hours, then q8h if urinary output is above 240 mL/8-hours • specific gravity of urine q4h and prn, especially if urine is pale and volume is significantly greater than fluid intake	To evaluate effectiveness of therapy.
2. Keep head of bed elevated 30–40 degrees. A small pillow may be placed beneath the head.	To prevent increasing ICP.
3. Notify physician of manifestations of ICP and intervene as ordered (Table 11–1).	Prompt intervention is required to relieve pressure. Respiratory arrest can occur if elevated ICP is untreated.
4. Administer glucocorticosteroids as prescribed.	To reduce ICP by inducing diuresis.
5. Perform measures to guard against increasing ICP: a. Remind the patient to avoid coughing. b. Administer prescribed stool softener and evaluate effectiveness. c. Administer prescribed antiemetic if the patient complains of nausea. d. Maintain patency of the N/G tube, if present, to decompress the stomach and reduce the possibility of vomiting.	Coughing, straining with defecation, and vomiting trigger the Valsalva maneuver (holding the breath). The Valsalva maneuver increases intrathoracic pressure that forces a surge of blood to the brain by compressing the central venous network. This venous engorgement increases ICP.

INTERVENTIONS	RATIONALE
6. Notify physician if the urine specific gravity is low, accompanied by excess urinary output in relation to fluid intake.	This finding can indicate diabetes insipidus, reflecting injury to the pituitary gland.
7. Notify physician of changes in neurological status that are different from the baseline values.	The extent of residual neurological deficits is not realized until cerebral edema resolves. Increasing ICP can cause further neurological deficits.
Seizures 1. Administer prescribed anticonvulsant. Monitor results of laboratory studies that measure anticonvulsant level in serum.	To control seizures, anticonvulsants exert a depressant effect on the brain's electrical activity. A therapeutic blood level of each anticonvulsant varies. An established blood level is essential to maintain to guard against seizure activity.
2. Notify physician immediately if a seizure occurs and intervene appropriately (Table 11–2).	Cerebral edema occurring secondary to increased ICP and irritation of the meninges can trigger a seizure.
Infection (meningitis): 1. Monitor: • vital signs qh until stable, then q2h x 48 hours, then q4h • neurological status (Appendix J) q2h x 48 hours, then q4h x 48 hours, then q8h	To evaluate effectiveness of therapy.
2. Notify physician of: • complaints of stiff neck • headache • restlessness • diminished sensorium • fever	These collective findings can suggest meningitis. The physician may perform a spinal tap to confirm the diagnosis. Prompt antibiotic therapy is required to resolve the infection.
3. Administer prescribed antibiotics.	As a prophylaxis against infection.

INTERVENTIONS	RATIONALE
4. Perform prescribed measures to resolve fever (101°F or greater): • antipyretics • increase fluid intake • antibiotics • hypothermia blanket (for persistently high temperatures unresponsive to drug therapy) • sheet used as top covering	Antipyretics readjust the body's thermostat. Blood circulates more rapidly when viscosity is lessened. Circulation increases the body's cooling capacity. Antibiotics resolve infections. Body cooling through evaporation is enhanced by a hypothermia blanket and by removing a heavy top covering.
5. Follow universal precautions (wash hands thoroughly before and after patient contact, wear gloves when contact with blood or body fluid is likely to occur) when providing patient care activities. Use aseptic technique for all wound care procedures.	Surgery temporarily weakens the immune system, making the individual more susceptible to infection. Caregivers are the most common source of nosocomial infections.

NURSING DIAGNOSIS: HIGH RISK FOR IMPAIRED HOME MAINTENANCE MANAGEMENT

RELATED TO FACTORS: Knowledge deficit about self-care management on discharge, lack of adequate support system

DEFINING CHARACTERISTICS: May show residual sensory/motor deficits but lives alone, may verbalize lack of understanding, requests information, significant other may report inability to care for person because of own physical or financial deficits

PATIENT OUTCOME (collaborative): Demonstrates willingness to comply with rehabilitative plan

EVALUATION CRITERIA: Patient or significant other verbalizes understanding of home care instructions, correctly performs prescribed exercises, verbalizes satisfaction with discharge plans

INTERVENTIONS	RATIONALE
1. Involve the patient and significant other in ADL. Start with simple tasks such as holding a washcloth and wiping the face, brushing teeth, and so on. Assist with hygienic care, toileting, feeding, turning, and ambulation until independent.	Self-performance of ADL promotes joint flexibility and helps maintain self-esteem.
2. Evaluate level of comprehension and ability to follow instructions and perform self-care activities. Discuss with the patient and significant others arrangements for continual care after discharge. If the patient continues to have neurological deficits, contact the appropriate service that focuses on rehabilitation for the specific deficit (physical therapy, occupational therapy, speech therapy). Consult social services or discharge planning department to arrange for home care or placement in an extended care or rehabilitation facility depending on the preference of the patient and significant others.	Discharge planning is essential to ensure continuation of care to help the patient regain an optimal level of functioning.

Alzheimer's Disease

Alzheimer's disease is a progressive degenerative disease in which the primary pathological findings are the formation of neuritic plaques around the neurons and a decreased level of acetylcholine in the brain. The primary areas involved are the cerebral cortex, hypocampus, limbic system, and brain stem (Hull, 1991).

The disease primarily affects persons in late adulthood. It has an unknown etiology and is irreversible. There is no specific diagnostic test to establish a diagnosis of Alzheimer's disease. Diagnosis is based on negative diagnostic test findings of other possible causes of deterioration in mental status. If all test results are negative and the patient shows progressive deterioration six months after the tests, a diagnosis of Alzheimer's disease is then established.

As the person's mental status and physical condition become progressively worse, placement in an extended care facility is an alternative when the patient's family can no longer provide care.

The mean LOS for a DRG classification of Alzheimer's disease is 6.9 days (Lorenz, 1991).

General Medical Management

• No specific drug therapy is available

Integrative Care Plans

• Immobility

Discharge Considerations

• Follow-up care
• Safety measures
• Community support services

 ## ASSESSMENT DATA BASE

1. Physical examination based on a neurological assessment (Appendix J) may reveal progressive deterioration of mental and physical status. Significant others generally report

the patient has shown mild memory lapses, loss of interest in surroundings, and short attention span. As the disease progresses, memory loss becomes more pronounced, especially for recent events; however, memory for past events remains intact. Personality begins to deteriorate, and motor deficits such as apraxia become apparent. In the end stage, hand and eye coordination is impaired, bowel and bladder control is lost, the person cannot recognize the family, verbal communication is often incoherent, gait becomes ataxic, and mood swings are prominent. Weight loss occurs as the patient forgets to swallow, becomes increasingly agitated, and resists feeding.

2. Assess significant other's response to the patient's condition and impact on home environment.

• •

NURSING DIAGNOSIS: SELF-CARE DEFICIT

RELATED TO FACTORS: Impaired mental status secondary to Alzheimer's disease
DEFINING CHARACTERISTICS: Observation of inability to perform ADL
PATIENT OUTCOME: Demonstrates no deficits in ADL
EVALUATION CRITERIA: Intact skin, absence of body odor

• •

INTERVENTIONS	RATIONALE
1. Initiate a bowel and bladder training program if incontinent. Keep a record of bowel evacuation pattern for several days. Place patient on the commode when bowel movement is anticipated. Place the patient on the commode every 2–3 hours during the day for voiding.	To reduce incidence of accidental soiling. Normally, individuals defecate every 1–2 days, usually in the mornings about one hour after meals. The bladder capacity of the elderly person normally decreases with aging. Normally, individuals void about 1–2 hours after consuming liquids.
2. Apply disposable briefs if incontinent and change prn.	Disposable briefs prevent soiling of clothing for the incontinent patient.
3. Limit fluid intake before bedtime. Give largest portion of fluids during the day. Reduce intake of caffeinated beverages.	Gauging fluid intake provides a means of bladder control. Caffeine acts as a diuretic.
4. Provide hygienic care. Allow the patient to do self-care with supervision as much as possible.	Self-performance of ADL promotes joint flexibility.

INTERVENTIONS	RATIONALE
5. Involve the patient in a daily exercise program.	Exercise helps promote musculoskeletal tone, peristalsis, circulation, and cardiac muscle tone.

· ·

◢ NURSING DIAGNOSIS: ALTERATION IN NUTRITION: LESS THAN BODY REQUIREMENTS

RELATED TO FACTORS: Deterioration in mental status

DEFINING CHARACTERISTICS: May refuse food, weight loss, holds food in mouth and needs constant reminder to swallow

PATIENT OUTCOME: Demonstrates adequate nutritional status

EVALUATION CRITERIA: No further weight loss, consumes more than 40% of each meal

· ·

INTERVENTIONS	RATIONALE
1. Feed the patient. Change consistency of food as needed to facilitate swallowing. For the patient who forgets to swallow, try pureed foods placed on the back of the tongue and finger foods. Be accepting of the patient eating with fingers and spills.	Pureed foods require no chewing. They mix readily with saliva to become more fluid; therefore, as saliva is swallowed, food is also swallowed. Socially learned skills are often lost. The more simple and natural the task, the easier it is done.
2. Insert a feeding tube for tube feedings as ordered if dietary intake continues to be less than 20% and weight loss continues.	To ensure adequate nutritional intake.
3. Provide snacks between meals.	Extra feedings are needed to meet nutritional needs especially when dietary intake becomes poor.
4. Provide enough time for eating. Do not force food or argue with the patient about eating. Wait until the patient is in a cooperative mood before continuing with the meal.	The use of force with an agitated patient intensifies the agitation.

• •

NURSING DIAGNOSIS: HIGH RISK FOR INJURY

RELATED TO FACTORS: Mental deterioration secondary to Alzheimer's disease

DEFINING CHARACTERISTICS: Observation of confusion, disorientation, loss of memory, ataxic gait, wandering, nocturnal confusion, restlessness

PATIENT OUTCOME: Demonstrates no physical injury

EVALUATION CRITERIA: No bruising noted on skin, no falls reported

• •

INTERVENTIONS	RATIONALE
1. Keep siderails up when sleeping. Check on the patient frequently. Use vest and wrist restraints only if needed to protect patient from self-injury or injury to others. Leave a dim light on at night when nocturnal confusion exists.	To prevent wandering without supervision, especially when mental status deteriorates and gait is unsteady. Often restraints intensify agitation. Confusion may be exacerbated at night as darkness occurs, commonly called sundowner's syndrome.
2. Administer prescribed neuroleptic (antipsychotic) such as haloperidol or thioridazine HCL when patient becomes extremely agitated and uncontrollable. Do not argue with the patient during episodes of suspiciousness and agitation. Approach patient in a calm, confident manner. Reduce environmental stimuli. Determine what precipitates the agitated or paranoid state and try to avoid exposure to these situations if possible.	To prevent self-injury. Neuroleptic agents help control paranoid delusions. Developing a trusting relationship is essential to helping the patient work through paranoid attacks.
3. Maintain a regular schedule for daily activities, especially when demonstrating confusion. Provide daily exercise such as walking. Engage the patient in some routine activity to divert attention from wandering.	Establishing a routine helps diminish the frequency of wandering.

INTERVENTIONS	RATIONALE
4. Avoid rushing the patient. Keep the pace slow. Speak softly, distinctly, and in simple sentences using nonverbal signals such as pointing or touching when the patient demonstrates difficulty in verbally expressing self.	Impaired communication is often a source of frustration that can trigger agitation.

▶ Nursing Diagnosis: Ineffective Family Coping: Compromised

RELATED TO FACTORS: Difficulty dealing with patient's physical and mental deterioration

DEFINING CHARACTERISTICS: Family members verbalize lack of understanding about patient's condition, report frustration and exhaustion in caring for patient at home, report disruption in family network because of patient's chronic condition

PATIENT OUTCOME (collaborative): Significant others demonstrate effective coping

EVALUATION CRITERIA: Verbalizes understanding of the patient's condition, identifies community resources that provide assistance with Alzheimer's patients, reports relief from frustration

INTERVENTIONS	RATIONALE
1. Allow significant others to express feelings about having a family member with Alzheimer's disease. Assist the family in anticipating problems in caring for the patient and in obtaining community resources to resolve those problems.	Caring for an Alzheimer's patient can be exhausting and frustrating. Significant others need support in caring for the patient.
2. Refer significant others to community support groups and agencies that provide care on a short-term basis (adult day care center, respite care facilities).	The primary caregivers will benefit from brief breaks because caring for an Alzheimer's person places tremendous stress on the caregivers.

INTERVENTIONS	RATIONALE
3. Provide significant others with information about the nature of Alzheimer's disease. Refer to local chapter of Alzheimer's Disease Foundation.	This agency provides written information about the disease and sources of financial and social support.
4. If the family cannot provide care at home, refer the family to a social service agency for assistance in planning where to place the person with Alzheimer's disease.	Eventually, the patient may have to be placed in an extended care facility when significant others can no longer provide care.

*M*ultiple Sclerosis

Multiple sclerosis (MS) is a demyelinating disorder of the CNS (central nervous system). The disease attacks the myelin sheath around the axon of nerve fibers in the brain and spinal cord in a scattered pattern (Clark, 1991). Myelin is the white laminated material coating the nerve fiber that is essential for normal nerve conduction.

MS is characterized by periods of remission and exacerbations. During remission, partial remyelination occurs, and the patient appears to improve. Repeated attacks cause inflammation, thickening, and eventual destruction of myelin sheath. Damaged myelin is removed by astrocytes (scavenger cells) leaving behind scar tissue or harden plaques (Clark, 1991). These plaques impede the transmission of normal nerve impulses resulting in irreversible neurological deficits.

The etiology is unknown but is believed linked to viral agents and autoimmune mechanisms (Clark, 1991).

Because symptoms of MS mimic other neurological disorders, diagnosis can take several months as the patient undergoes extensive diagnostic studies to rule out other disorders. Usually, a diagnosis is established by finding at least two or more lesions (each in a different area of the CNS) and remission and exacerbation of two or more neurological symptoms, with remission lasting at least one month (Clark, 1991).

The course of the disease is variable. Although extremely rare, it can stop completely after one or two attacks without residual neurological deficits. In most cases, repeated attacks terminate in permanent motor and sensory deficits. An increase in core body temperature makes the symptoms worse.

The mean LOS for a DRG classification of multiple sclerosis is 6.7 days (Lorenz, 1991).

General Medical Management

- There is no cure for MS and no specific treatment.
- Traditional treatments have included:
  a. steroids to suppress inflammation:
    — adrenocorticotropic hormone (ACTH) given intramuscular (IM)
    — prednisone

b. drugs to suppress the immune system:
  — cyclophosphamide (Cytoxan)
  — Imuran
c. antispasmodics to control spasticity of the extremities;
  — baclofen
d. physical therapy to maintain muscle strength and tone
e. plasmapheresis in some cases (with questionable results)

Integrative Care Plans

• Loss
• Immobility

Discharge Considerations

• Follow-up care
• Rehabilitative program
• Exercises to continue at home
• Signs and symptoms of exacerbation
• Medications to continue at home

ASSESSMENT DATA BASE

1. Physical examination based on a neurological assessment (Appendix J) may reveal:
   • reports of burning or prickling sensation and paresthesia in the extremities
   • gait disturbances
   • visual disturbances due to optic neuritis (diplopia, blurred vision, loss of color vision, unilateral loss of vision, one pupil larger than other)
   • extraocular movement abnormalities: nystagmus or lateral or upward gaze
   • lack of coordination
   • muscle weakness
   • positive Babinski reflex
   • ticlike facial pain
   • bladder and sexual dysfunction (with extensive cord damage)
   • slow, monotonous, or slurred speech
   • exaggerated asymmetrical deep tendon reflexes with spasticity of the lower extremities

2. Diagnostic studies:
   • Spinal tap reveals elevated protein, gamma globulin, and lymphocytes in cerebral spinal fluid (CSF).
   • Electrophoresis studies of CSF may reveal oligoclonal bands of globulins.

- Evoke potentials (visual and auditory) reveal a delayed response in cerebral nerve transmission with a given stimulus (light, touch, or sound).
- CT scan and MRI may show lesions in the white matter of the brain.

3. Assess the patient's feelings and concerns about having a chronic incurable disorder.
4. Assess the patient's understanding of condition, diagnostic studies, and treatments.

NURSING DIAGNOSIS: HIGH RISK FOR INFECTION: URINARY

RELATED TO FACTORS: Altered bladder function secondary to MS

DEFINING CHARACTERISTICS: Observation of urinary retention, incontinence

PATIENT OUTCOME (collaborative): Demonstrates no urinary tract infection

EVALUATION CRITERIA: Denies dysuria, absence of foul-smelling urine, passage of clear amber or yellow urine, normal temperature

INTERVENTIONS	RATIONALE
1. Monitor: • intake and output q8h • vital signs q4h • results of urinalysis reports	To identify indications of progress toward or deviations from expected outcome.
2. Apply disposable briefs on incontinent females. Apply an external catheter or disposable briefs on incontinent males. Change the briefs prn. Remove the external catheter daily to cleanse and inspect the skin of the penis. Do **not** apply an external catheter if the skin of the penis shows signs of irritation.	Disposable briefs help keep clothing dry. Moisture accumulates beneath an external catheter creating a good culture medium for bacterial growth.
3. Notify physician of manifestations of urinary retention: suprapubic distention, constant dribbling (indicating overflow incontinence), frequent voiding of small amounts. Insert a Foley catheter or perform intermittent catheterization, as	Stasis of urine provides a good culture medium for microbes. Catheter care helps reduce the number of transient bacteria around the urinary meatus.

INTERVENTIONS	RATIONALE
ordered, to empty the bladder. Provide catheter care according to facility protocol and procedures for indwelling catheters.	
4. Provide at least 1–2 liters of fluid daily. Encourage daily intake of cranberry juice.	To keep the kidneys flushed and maintain an acid urine. Bacteria cannot thrive in a acid medium.

. . . .

◤ NURSING DIAGNOSIS: DISTURBANCE IN SELF-CONCEPT

RELATED TO FACTORS: Threat of permanent physical disability

DEFINING CHARACTERISTICS: May verbalize low self-esteem, depression, anger, frustration

PATIENT OUTCOME (collaborative): Demonstrates acceptance of self in current situation

EVALUATION CRITERIA: Verbalizes positive statements about self, cooperates with planned rehabilitative activities, verbalizes realistic plans

. . . .

INTERVENTIONS	RATIONALE
1. Allow the patient to express feelings about condition.	Expressing feelings helps promote coping.
2. Refer the patient for psychological counseling, as ordered, if displaying behaviors indicative of mal-adaptation: persistent depression, apathy, lack of involvement in planned activities, verbal statements of depression and inability to handle physical impairment.	Professional help may be required to deal with problems of psychological adaptation.
3. Offer praise for accomplishments made in learning how to regain independence.	Reinforcement enhances learning.

INTERVENTIONS	RATIONALE
4. Allow the patient to do as much as possible for self.	Self-help promotes better self-esteem.
5. Refer patient to occupational therapy and physical therapy.	The occupational therapist can assess the patient's functional level and plan a rehabilitation program that focuses on developing useable skills in view of physical limitations. The physical therapist can assess the patient's musculoskeletal deficits and plan program of muscle-strengthening exercises and teach use of assistive devices for ambulation.
6. Plan ways to foster the patient's independence, for example, using a shower chair for bathing, applying Velcro closings to clothes and shoes instead of buttons or strings, using a hand mit with soap for bathing. Advise to keep the environment cool. Discourage taking hot showers or baths.	Heat worsens symptoms of weakness. Being able to care for oneself helps maintain self-esteem.
7. Administer prescribed anti-inflammatory and/or immunosuppressant drugs. Ensure patient has an antacid prescribed while on steroidal anti-inflammatory agents. Report side effects.	These drugs are not curative but may offer some relief in controlling painful spasms. Steroids are ulcergenic.
8. Apply an overhead trapeze to the bed.	To allow the patient to assist with moving self in and out of bed.

NURSING DIAGNOSIS: INEFFECTIVE FAMILY COPING: COMPROMISED

RELATED TO FACTORS: Difficulty dealing with the patient's physical deterioration, knowledge deficit about condition and treatment plan

DEFINING CHARACTERISTICS: Verbalizes lack of understanding, reports frustration, requests information

PATIENT OUTCOME: Patient and significant others demonstrate effective coping

EVALUATION CRITERIA: Verbalizes understanding of condition, treatment, diagnostic studies, and rehabilitative measures to continue at home; correctly performs required rehabilitative skills; verbalizes realistic plans

• •

INTERVENTIONS	RATIONALE
1. Evaluate significant others ability to manage the patient at home. Consult a social service representative to arrange for home care assistance or placement in an extended care or rehabilitation facility if there is nobody to provide assistance at home. If the patient can be cared for at home, teach the patient and significant others how to manage physiological alterations as the need arises: • bladder dysfunction — intermittent catheterization • muscle strengthening exercises • constipation	Discharge planning involves identifying and using the patient's existing support systems and providing new support systems as the need arises. Discharge teaching helps promote continual rehabilitation.
2. Provide information about: • nature and course of disease • purpose of prescribed treatments • prescribed medications, including name, dosage, schedule, purpose, and reportable side effects • prescribed diagnostic studies, including: — brief description — purpose — preparation required before test — care after test	Health teaching promotes safety in self-care, better compliance with the treatment program, and helps the patient develop realistic expectations.
3. Refer the patient and significant others to the local chapter of the National Multiple Sclerosis Society.	This agency provides information about the condition and availability of other local support services for the patient and family.

INTERVENTIONS	RATIONALE
5. If the person is hospitalized with uncontrolled seizures: • Pad siderails. • Keep siderails up. • Post a "Seizure Precautions" sign above patient's bed. • Make sure suction equipment is readily available if patient has grand mal seizures. • Ensure patient has vascular assess established, either an IV infusion or a heparin lock. • Keep a bite block and oral airway at the bedside.	Safety precautions must be initiated to prevent injury. Vascular access allows for rapid administration of urgent medications.
6. If the patient is admitted with a history of seizure, flag the Kardex with a notice. Ensure the patient has medication ordered for seizure control if on medication before hospitalization.	A consistent blood level of the anticonvulsant is essential for effective seizure control.
7. Administer prescribed anticonvulsant. Notify physician if seizure activity persists or worsens.	This can indicate a need for a change in drug therapy or further diagnostic studies.

• •

 Nursing Diagnosis: HIGH RISK FOR IMPAIRED HOME MAINTENANCE MANAGEMENT

RELATED TO FACTORS: Knowledge deficit about condition and treatment plan, ineffective coping with a chronic condition

DEFINING CHARACTERISTICS: Verbalizes lack of understanding, may report history of noncompliance, may verbalize difficulty coping with chronic condition

PATIENT OUTCOME: Demonstrates willingness to comply with home management therapy

EVALUATION CRITERIA: Verbalizes understanding of condition, treatments, and preventive self-care measures; verbalizes satisfaction with therapeutic plan; verbalizes realistic plans

• •

INTERVENTIONS	RATIONALE
1. Provide information about: • underlying pathological mechanism triggering seizure activity • purpose of prescribed treatments • prescribed medication, including name, dosage, schedule, purpose and reportable side effects • diagnostic studies, including: — brief description — purpose of test — preparation required before test — care after test	Patients are more likely to comply if they understand their condition and how prescribed treatments will help them.
2. Teach the patient self-care management for seizures: • Seek safety and lie down when you sense an impending seizure. • Take medication as prescribed. • Wear a Medic Alert bracelet or necklace. • Avoid intake of alcohol while on anticonvulsant therapy. • Pursue an occupation that allows for safety. Avoid jobs that involve working at heights or being submerged in water. • Follow state laws about driving. Most states require the person to be free of seizures for at least two years before issuance of a driver license.	These instructions are designed to ensure physical safety.

INTERVENTIONS	RATIONALE
3. Teach family members what to do when a seizure occurs (see Table 11–2). Explain that it is not necessary to seek emergency care after each seizure provided the seizure pattern remains the same. Advise to contact the physician if the seizures become more intense or more frequent.	A change in the pattern of the seizures warrants a thorough evaluation: serum level of the anticonvulsant and neurological examination.
4. Allow the patient and family members to express feelings about seizure care. Correct any misconceptions.	Expressing feelings helps facilitate coping and allows the caregiver to identify and correct any misconceptions.

Cerebral Vascular Disorders

Cerebrovascular accident (CVA) refers to a constellation of neurological events that occur when arterial blood flow to or within an area of the brain is disrupted. Atherosclerosis is the most common pathological antecedent in CVA; others include thrombus (blood clot), emboli, or intracranial hemorrhage.

The occlusion can occur in any cerebral arterial network cause temporary cerebral ischemia or an infarction. When infarction occurs, collateral circulation forms to bypass the infarcted area and reestablish cerebral blood flow. In some cases this allows the person to regain some degree of functional recovery. In other cases, the lesion may be so extensive that coma and eventually death may occur.

Based on the type and duration of symptoms, a CVA is classified as:

1. **Transient ischemic attack** (TIA), which is characterized by a focal neurological event of sudden onset that lasts a few minutes or hours, often less than 24 hours. It may resolve spontaneously without residual deficits or it may progress to a complete stroke within months or one year.

2. **Reversible ischemic neurological deficits** (RIND), which are neurological symptoms lasting a few days to a few weeks. Symptoms can resolve spontaneously without residual deficits or can progress to a complete stroke within several months to one year.

3. **Stroke in evolution** (SIE), which is characterized by progressive neurological deficits that are initially hallmarked by hemiparesis, terminating in complete stroke.

4. **Complete stroke** (CS), which is characterized by cerebral infarct. Neurological deficits become fixed and permanent, although with time the person can regain some degree of functional recovery as a result of collateral circulation. A complete recovery does not occur.

The mean LOS for a DRG classification of CVA is 7.2 days (Lorenz, 1991). During the acute phase, the patient is often hospitalized in an ICU because of the threat of respiratory compromise.

General Medical Management

- Pharmacotherapy:
  - — antihypertensive agents
  - — anticoagulants (for stroke caused by thrombus)
  - — corticosteroids to reduce cerebral edema
  - — aminocaproic acid (Amicar) for subarachnoid hemorrhage
- Surgery
  - — endarterectomy (for carotid occlusion caused by atherosclerosis)

Integrative Care Plans

- Loss
- Immobility

Discharge Considerations

- Follow-up care
- Medications to continue at home
- Rehabilitative activities
- Signs and symptoms requiring medical attention

ASSESSMENT DATA BASE

1. Physical examination based on a rapid neurological assessment (Appendix J) and a general survey (Appendix F) may reveal a variety of manifestations depending on the site and extent of the lesion (see Table 11–3). With obstruction of the carotid artery, symptoms occur unilaterally. Also, because motor fibers crossover in the spinothalamic tract, symptoms occur contralateral (on the opposite side) from the site of the lesion, with obstruction of the carotid and cerebral arteries. Symptoms of vertebrobasilar obstruction occur bilaterally.

2. Diagnostic studies:
   - EEG detects disturbances in transmission of electrical impulses in the brain.
   - Brain scan (radionuclide scan) or MRI identifies location of the lesion.
   - Angiography identifies cause and location of lesion.
   - Doppler ultrasound of carotid artery assesses vessel patency.

3. Assess airway patency.

4. Assess patient's and significant other's feelings and concerns about condition.

NURSING DIAGNOSIS: HIGH RISK FOR IMPAIRED VERBAL COMMUNICATION

RELATED TO FACTORS: Aphasia

DEFINING CHARACTERISTICS: May show frustration when attempting to verbally communicate, slurred speech, inappropriate statements

PATIENT OUTCOME (collaborative): Communicates needs with minimal frustration

EVALUATION CRITERIA: Relaxed body posture and facial expression with communications, fewer episodes of agitation

INTERVENTIONS	RATIONALE
1. Initiate appropriate measures to allow the patient to communicate needs based on the type of aphasia (see Table 11–4). Anticipate the patient's needs. Show patience. Avoid rushing the patient. Continue to explain actions even when the patient does not understand.	The ability to verbally communicate is an important aspect in maintaining independence. The frustration and anger commonly demonstrated with aphasia reflect the individual's perception of self as being dependent.
2. Initiate referral to a speech therapist as required.	A speech therapist can assess the patient's language deficit and plan an individualized program of speech rehabilitation.
3. Flag the Kardex and intercom system with "Communication Deficit."	To alert caregivers of the need to go to the patient's room when the call light is signaled.

NURSING DIAGNOSIS: ALTERATION IN NUTRITION: LESS THAN BODY REQUIREMENTS

RELATED TO FACTORS: Dysphagia, inability to feed self caused by paralysis or weakness of upper extremities or altered mentation such as confusion or disorientation

DEFINING CHARACTERISTICS: Drooping of one side of mouth with constant drooling, persistent coughing with oral feedings, difficulty swallowing

PATIENT OUTCOME: Demonstrates no nutritional deficits

EVALUATION CRITERIA: Stable weight

INTERVENTIONS	RATIONALE
1. Weigh weekly.	To evaluate effectiveness of therapy.
2. If dysphagia occurs, place the patient in an erect position and place the food back on the tongue to promote swallowing. Use pureed foods. If aspiration occurs with oral feeding, insert N/G tube and initiate tube feedings as ordered.	Pureed foods are easier to swallow because of their semiliquid state. Tube feedings can meet the patient's nutritional needs.
3. Evaluate ability to feed self. Provide assistance with meals as needed.	To ensure dietary intake until patient can feed self without assistance.

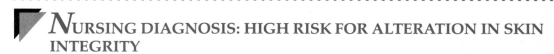

NURSING DIAGNOSIS: HIGH RISK FOR ALTERATION IN SKIN INTEGRITY

RELATED TO FACTORS: Bowel and bladder incontinence, immobility

DEFINING CHARACTERISTICS: Unaware of voiding, observation of soiled bed linen from urine or feces, paralysis of extremities

PATIENT OUTCOME: Skin integrity maintained

EVALUATION CRITERIA: Absence of skin breakdown

INTERVENTIONS	RATIONALE
1. Keep the skin dry and clean. Use disposable briefs for incontinent females. For incontinent males, apply a condom catheter or disposable brief. If a condom catheter is used, remove it daily. Cleanse and inspect the skin of the penis. Reapply a clean condom and connect it to a urinary drainage bag. Avoid applying a condom catheter to irritated skin.	The acid urine increases the risk of skin breakdown. Moisture accumulates beneath a condom catheter, creating a good medium for bacterial growth.
2. See Immobility (page 725).	

•••••••••••••••••••••••••••••••••••

◤ NURSING DIAGNOSIS: HIGH RISK FOR INJURY

RELATED TO FACTORS: Extension of impaired cerebral tissue perfusion

DEFINING CHARACTERISTICS: Diagnostic studies reveal continued intracranial bleeding, shows no improvement in two days

PATIENT OUTCOME (collaborative): Demonstrates no further cerebral tissue impairment

EVALUATION CRITERIA: Absence of further neurological deficits, discharged within LOS for DRG

•••••••••••••••••••••••••••••••••

INTERVENTIONS	RATIONALE
During Acute Phase: 1. Monitor: • results of arterial blood gases (ABG) reports • neurological status (Appendix J) q2h x 48 hours, then q4h • vital signs q2h x 48 hours, then q4h • general status (Appendix F) q8h • ECG tracings frequently • intake and output q8h, or qh if eight-hour urinary output is less than 240 mL	To identify indications of progress toward or deviations from expected outcomes.
2. Notify physician of any changes in neurological status from the baseline findings.	The initial 24 hours are the most critical. Prompt intervention plays a significant role in reducing the risk of permanent motor and sensory deficits.
3. Connect to an ECG monitor for continuous monitoring of cardiac status. Place a strip of the ECG tracing on the chart q8h and prn if an arrhythmia is detected.	Persons with CVA often have other underlying disorders that may have contributed to the CVA (heart disease, hypertension, diabetes, obesity, hyperlipidemia).
4. Insert a Foley catheter as ordered. Provide catheter care twice a day according to facility protocol and procedures.	An indwelling catheter provides accurate monitoring of urinary output. Cleansing the genitalia helps reduce the number transient bacteria, minimizing the risk of urinary tract infection.
5. Administer prescribed antihypertensive and evaluate effectiveness.	Preexisting hypertension is common with CVA. Higher blood pressure cause further ischemia.

INTERVENTIONS	RATIONALE
For Hemorrhagic CVA: 1. Administer aminocaproic acid (Amicar) as ordered. 2. Notify physician if calf pain, sudden chest pain or dyspnea, or falling blood pressure accompanied by rising pulse rate occur. 3. Implement measures to reduce intracranial pressure that include maintaining bedrest in a semi-Fowler's position, reducing environmental stimulation, and administering stool softeners as ordered.	Amicar is an antifibrinolytic that inhibits resolution of the clot by preventing the fibrin breakdown. Thrombosis can occur elsewhere. Increased intracranial pressure increases the risk of further bleeding.
For Thrombotic CVA: 1. Administer anticoagulants and antiplatelet agents as ordered and evaluate effectiveness. 2. Notify physician if PT and PTT exceed upper and lower values. 3. Report signs of bleeding that include epistaxis, hematuria, ecchymosis, petechiae, melena. 4. Prepare to administer protamine sulfate for heparin excess and vitamin K for Coumadin excess.	These agents help prevent further clot formation. Bleeding is the major complication with these agents, which indicates overdosage and a need to reduce dosage. The PT is used to evaluate serum levels of Coumadin, and PTT monitors serum level of heparin.
For CVA Caused by Carotid Occlusion; 1. Prepare for endarterectomy as prescribed.	Carotid occlusion is caused by atherosclerotic plaques that must be surgically removed to reestablish vessel patency.

 NURSING DIAGNOSIS: HIGH RISK FOR INEFFECTIVE AIRWAY CLEARANCE

RELATED TO FACTORS: Depressed level of consciousness

DEFINING CHARACTERISTICS: Constant snoring or gurgling respirations, persistent moist cough

PATIENT OUTCOME: Airway remains patent

EVALUATION CRITERIA: ABG within normal limits, absence of noisy respirations, normal skin color

INTERVENTIONS	RATIONALE
1. Monitor: • results of ABG reports • respiratory status (Appendix A) q4h	To detect early signs of respiratory distress and to evaluate effectiveness of therapy.
2. If comatose and tongue falls back to obstruct the airway, insert an oral airway. Suction prn. Keep patient in a side-lying position.	To maintain a patent airway.
3. Administer supplemental oxygen via nasal cannula as ordered.	To prevent further cerebral ischemia.

NURSING DIAGNOSIS: DISTURBANCE OF SELF-CONCEPT

RELATED TO FACTORS: Grief over perceived and actual loss of function and role responsibilities

DEFINING CHARACTERISTICS: May verbalize low self-esteem, worthlessness, and depression; may refuse to participate in rehabilitative activities; may cry frequently

PATIENT OUTCOME: Demonstrates acceptance of self in current situation

EVALUATION CRITERIA: Acknowledges limitations, participates in planned rehabilitation activities, verbalizes positive statements about self

INTERVENTIONS	RATIONALE
1. See Loss (page 733).	

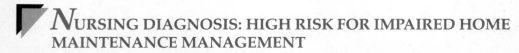

NURSING DIAGNOSIS: HIGH RISK FOR IMPAIRED HOME MAINTENANCE MANAGEMENT

RELATED TO FACTORS: Sensory/motor deficits secondary to CVA, lack of adequate support system, lack of adequate finances

DEFINING CHARACTERISTICS: May report absence of caregiver at home or lack of adequate financial resources, inability to independently perform some ADL caused by residual sensory/motor deficits

PATIENT OUTCOME (collaborative): Patient or significant others demonstrate ability to meet continuing care needs

EVALUATION CRITERIA: Verbalizes satisfaction with discharge plan, verbalizes understanding of home care instructions, identifies community resources that provide needed assistance

INTERVENTIONS	RATIONALE
1. Evaluate the patient's continuing care needs and the ability of significant others to meet those needs at home. Consult social services or discharge planning department or for assistance in coordinating continuing rehabilitation services on discharge.	Rehabilitation for the CVA patient requires a multidisciplinary approach and may include a physical therapist, occupational therapist, speech therapist, nurse, dietitian, and physician. Social service personnel or discharge planners are specialists who coordinate community resources to meet the continuing care needs of patients after discharge.
2. Allow the patient and significant others to express feelings about their lifestyle changes resulting from the person's condition. Refer them to community support groups if available. Explain that it takes several months before the full extent of residual motor and sensory deficits can be determined because collateral circulation is developing, which may allow for some functional recovery.	Significant others need support in caring for the patient with a chronic illness. Expressing feelings helps promote coping.
3. Provide information about prescribed medication to be taken at home, including purpose, action, dosage, schedule, and side effects.	Health teaching is important for ensuring safety with self-medication administration.
4. Provide written instructions for follow-up appointment and home care.	Verbal instructions may be easily forgotten.

Traumatic Brain Injury

Acute head injuries are classified according to (Reimer, 1989):

1. Status of the scalp and skull:
   - closed head injuries
   - open head injuries

2. Trauma to the brain tissue:
   - concussion — characterized by momentary loss of consciousness without damage to brain tissue; some cerebral edema occurs
   - contusions — characterized by bruising of brain tissue that causes some bleeding at the site; bruise may be coup (occurring on same side as blow) or contra coup (occurring on side opposite blow)
   - lacerations — characterized by bleeding into the subarachnoid, epidural, or subdural space

   Bleeding of venous origin causes slow formation of a hematoma because of low pressure; an arterial laceration is characterized by rapid hematoma formation caused by high pressure.

   Major complications associated with head injury are increased intracranial pressure (ICP), hemorrhage, and seizure. The patient with a skull fracture, especially at the base of the basal skull, is at risk for leakage of cerebrospinal fluid (CSF) from the nose (rhinorrhea) or ear (otorrhea). A CSF leakage predisposes to meningitis.

   The mean LOS for a DRG classification of traumatic brain injury associated with stupor and coma is 5.9 days and 2.6 days for concussion (Lorenz, 1991).

General Medical Management

- For concussion with loss of consciousness less than 20 minutes:
  - usually no hospitalization required
  - bedrest
  - acetaminophen for headache

- For contussions, lacerations, or loss of consciousness greater than 20 minutes:
  - — hospitalization in an ICU
  - — bedrest
  - — measures to relieve increased ICP (Table 11-1) and to prevent seizures
  - — craniotomy to evacuate the hematoma, especially when bleeding is of arterial origin
  - — burr holes to evacuate epidural hematomas
- Antibiotics to guard against meningitis if CSF leakage is present and placement of sterile cotton ball loosely over leakage to prevent entry of bacteria

Integrative Care Plans

- Epilepsy
- Craniotomy

Discharge Considerations

- Follow-up care
- Signs and symptoms requiring medical attention
- Medications to continue at home
- Activity limitations

*A*SSESSMENT DATA BASE

1. Obtain a history of the head injury:
   - When did the injury occur?
   - Did the person lose consciousness? If so, how long?

   A contussion is suspected if the person is initially alert following closed head trauma and then shows progressive deterioration in level of consciousness (LOC), ranging from lethargy to comatose. A concussion is suspected if the person reports loss of consciousness less than 20 minutes, shows absence of focal neurological deficits, and a rapid return of consciousness.

2. Perform a rapid neurological assessment (Appendix J).

3. Inspect the head and behind the ear for evidence of bruising or swelling.

4. Examine the ears and nose for evidence of serous or bloody drainage. If present, use diabetic TesTape to assess for the presence of CSF. Drainage testing positive for glucose indicates presence of CSF.

5. Diagnostic studies:
   - Cervical and skull x rays detect location and extent of a fracture.
   - CT scan identifies intracranial hematomas.
   - Lumbar puncture confirms meningitis if the patient shows signs of meningeal irritation (fever, nuchal rigidity, seizures).

6. If alert and oriented, assess patient's response to condition and understanding of condition and treatment plan.

◤ NURSING DIAGNOSIS: HIGH RISK FOR INEFFECTIVE AIRWAY CLEARANCE

RELATED TO FACTORS: Altered level of consciousness

DEFINING CHARACTERISTICS: Abnormal arterial blood gases (ABG), noisy gurgling respirations, ineffective cough

PATIENT OUTCOME: Airway remains patent

EVALUATION CRITERIA: ABG within normal range, clear lung sounds, respiratory rate 12–24 per minute, normal color

INTERVENTIONS	RATIONALE
1. Monitor neurological status (Appendix J) q2–4h. If manifestations of increasing ICP are noted, notify physician immediately and intervene appropriately (see Table 11–1).	Cerebral edema or intracranial bleeding predisposes to increased ICP.
2. Keep NPO while consciousness is depressed.	To prevent aspiration.
3. Notify physician immediately and intervene appropriately if a seizure occurs (see Table 11–2).	Seizure activity increases cerebral metabolism, which results in vasoconstriction thus reducing cerebral blood flow. Cerebral ischemia can occur when cerebral blood flow is inadequate to meet cerebral metabolic requirements.
4. If level of consciousness is depressed and ABG reveal hypoxia (PaO_2 less than 60 mm Hg), administer supplemental oxygen as prescribed. Use pulse oximetry to continually monitor oxygenation.	Hypoxia produces cerebral vascular vasodilation, which contributes to increased ICP.

NURSING DIAGNOSIS: PAIN

RELATED TO FACTORS: Head injury
DEFINING CHARACTERISTICS: Reports headache, moaning, frowning
PATIENT OUTCOME (collaborative): Demonstrates relief from discomfort
EVALUATION CRITERIA: Denies headache, relaxed facial expression, absence of moaning

INTERVENTIONS	RATIONALE
1. Administer prescribed analgesic prn and evaluate effectiveness. Avoid narcotics.	Analgesics block the pain pathway. Narcotic analgesics can mask signs of neurologic changes.
2. Maintain bedrest in a semi-Fowler's position as prescribed.	Bedrest reduces oxygen tissue demands. A head-up position aids venous drainage by gravity thereby reducing the risk of increasing ICP.
3. If headache is unrelieved by analgesia within four hours or worsens, evaluate for additional neurological deficits (Appendix J), then notify physician.	This can indicate expansion of the intracranial lesion.
4. Keep environment quiet and room dark.	Stress accentuates headache and can provoke seizure.

NURSING DIAGNOSIS: HIGH RISK FOR IMPAIRED HOME MAINTENANCE MANAGEMENT

RELATED TO FACTORS: Knowledge deficit about self-care on discharge
DEFINING CHARACTERISTICS: Verbalizes lack of understanding, requests information, may report history of noncompliance
PATIENT OUTCOME: Demonstrates willingness to comply with home care on discharge
EVALUATION CRITERIA: Verbalizes understanding of instructions, reports satisfaction with discharge plan

INTERVENTIONS	RATIONALE
1. Provide discharge instructions that should include: • Headache, tinnitus, dizziness, or malaise may occur for several days. • Acetaminophen can be used to relieve headache. • Notify physician or emergency department if any of the following develop: vomiting, progressive drowsiness, progressive loss of balance, progressive dizziness. • Rest with head elevated on two pillows. Resume activities gradually.	Discharge instructions help ensure a safe recovery. Following a concussion, cerebral edema can worsen and cause progressive deterioration in level of consciousness.
2. Provide written instructions for home care and follow-up visit.	Verbal instructions may be easily forgotten.

TABLE 11–1. Increased Intracranial Pressure

The brain is enclosed in a nonexpandable, protective covering called the skull. Any space-occupying lesion can cause increased intracranial pressure (ICP). These lesions include meningitis, tumor, abcess, aneurysm, hematoma, or an abnormality that prevents cerebrospinal fluid outflow from the ventricles.

INTERVENTIONS	RATIONALE
1. Monitor: • neurological status (Appendix J) q2h. • ICP qh if intracranial monitoring catheter has been inserted	To evaluate effectiveness of therapy.
2. Notify physician if the patient shows manifestations of increasing ICP: • change in level of consciousness (earliest sign), for example, irritability, confusion, restlessness, lethargy • headaches • pupillary changes • projectile vomiting • rising systolic pressure with widening pulse pressure, accompanied by a decreasing pulse rate • alternate breathing pattern such as deep stertorous breathing, Cheyne-Stokes respirations, or cessation of respirations • focal motor and sensory changes (progressive weakness, paresthesia) • abnormal posturing (decorticate rigidity, decerebrate rigidity)	Prompt treatment is required. If not relieved, herniation of the brain through the tentorium cerebelli can occur, which ultimately leads to death from respiratory failure.
3. Administer prescribed drugs to reduce ICP and evaluate effectiveness: • osmotic diuretics (mannitol, urea) • corticosteroids (dexamethasone [Decadron])	These agents help reduce ICP by inducing diuresis. Expect an increased urinary output.

INTERVENTIONS	RATIONALE
4. Maintain a semi-Fowler's position.	To prevent further increase in ICP.
5. Administer prescribed medication to prevent coughing, sneezing, vomiting, and constipation. Have the patient roll on the bedpan instead of lifting hips.	These activities trigger the Valsalva maneuver thus causing a transitory rise in ICP with a return to normal after the activity is aborted.
6. Avoid drugs which depress the level of consciousness or cause pupillary constriction (potent narcotics and barbiturates).	To prevent masking of symptoms.
7. Administer supplemental oxygen as ordered.	To relieve hypoxia. An expanding intracranial lesion, shown by a CT scan, causes pressure on the brain, eventually displacing brain tissue and compromising cerebral circulation. As a result, the PCO_2 increases and the pH and PO_2 decrease. These blood gas changes cause vasodilation and contribute to cerebral edema, which further increases intracranial pressure.
8. Administer phenytoin (Dilantin) as ordered.	To control seizures. Increased intracranial pressure (ICP) predisposes patient to seizures.
9. Prepare for surgery as ordered that may include: craniotomy, burr holes, ventricular shunt, ventriculostomy.	These procedures are performed to relieve increased ICP by removing the lesion or by providing an outlet for cerebral spinal fluid flow if normal outflow channnels are obstructed.

TABLE 11–2. Actions To Take When a Seizure Occurs

1. Note time of onset.

2. Note characteristics of body movements.

3. Note time seizure ends and behaviors after the seizure stops.

4. Protect the person's head from injury by pillowing the head with any soft object or your hands.

5. Do **not** restrain the person.

6. Clear the area of all injurious objects.

7. Do **not** attempt to force the teeth apart if clenched.

8. Do **not** insert your fingers or anything in the mouth during the seizure.

9. Loosen tight clothing.

10. Do **not** leave the person alone.

11. If person is standing, lower to the floor.

12. Note any unusual behaviors before the seizure.

13. When seizure ends, inform the person of the seizure and describe the behavior during the seizure. Allow the person to rest.

TABLE 11–3. Neurological Events Commonly Associated With Impairment of Cerebral Vascular Circulation

Carotid Artery:

- bruits heard over affected carotid (assessed with bell of stethoscope)
- facial numbness on one side
- transient hemiparesis
- aphasia (receptive or expressive)
- complete loss of vision in one eye

Vetebrobasilar Arteries:

- perioral numbness
- diplopia
- dizziness (complaints of whirling sensation)
- ataxia
- dysarthria (slurred speech)
- cranial nerve dysfunction
- altered level of consciousness
- altered breathing pattern
- motor and sensory deficits in one or four extremities
- ptosis

Cerebral Arteries:

- hemiparesis or hemiplegia
- changes in mentation (confusion, irritability)
- aphasia
- visual disturbances: homonymous hemianopsia (blindness in corresponding halves of visual fields of both eyes)
- urinary incontinence
- memory loss
- spatial-perceptual deficits: agnosia (inability to recognize objects by sight, sound, or touch), apraxia (loss of ability to perform learned movements in sequence on command)

TABLE 11–4. Types of Aphasia With Communication Techniques

Receptive Aphasia:

Person cannot understand the spoken or written word but can coherently communicate needs. Communicate with this person by using gestures or demonstration.

Expressive Aphasia:

Person can understand the spoken and written word but cannot appropriately communicate thoughts. Person is aware that own verbal responses are inappropriate and often becomes frustrated and agitated when trying to express thoughts. Communicate with this person by:

- keeping patient responses to "yes" and "no." Instruct the person to nod head as a response.
- using a picture album with photos or drawings of typical things people need (food, water, comb, brush). Have person point to desired object.
- keeping questions simple. Focus on one thought at a time.

Global Aphasia:

Person cannot comprehend and express thoughts and ideas. Verbal statements are incoherent. With these persons, anticipate their needs. Continue to explain actions even though the person does not understand.

BIBLIOGRAPHY

Arnason, B.G. (1988). Could it be Guillain-Barré syndrome? **Patient Care, 22,** 22–26.

Clark, C.(1991). Nursing care for multiple sclerosis. **Orthopedic Nursing, 10,** 21–34.

Dunn, K.L. (1991). Autonomic dysreflexia: A nursing challenge in the care of the patient with spinal cord injury. **Journal of Cardiovascular Nursing, 5,** 57–64.

Feingold, D.J. (1991). Complications of spine surgery. **Orthopedic Nurse, 10,** 39–58.

Gray-Vickrey, P. (1988). Evaluating Alzheimer's patients. **Nursing, 18,** 34–41.

Hart, G.(1990). Strokes causing left vs. right hemiplegia: Different effects and nursing implications. **Geriatric Nursing, 11,** 67–70.

Hull, G.R. (1991). This hospital patient has Alzheimer's. **American Journal of Nursing, 91,** 44–51.

Jastremski, M.S., (1988). What to look for in seizure workups. **Patient Care, 22,** 68–72, 74, 76, 81–83, 86, 88–90, 93.

Kane, D.M. (1991). Practical points in the postoperative management of a craniotomy patient. **Journal of Post Anesthesia Nursing, 6,** 121–124.

Lorenz, E.W. (1992). **St. Anthony's DRG Guidebook,** Alexandria: St. Anthony Publishing Company.

Morgan, S.P. (1991). Guillain-Barré: A passage through paralysis. **American Journal of Nursing, 91,** 70–74.

Reimer, M. (1989). Head-injured patients: How to detect early trouble. **Nursing, 19,** 34-41.

Romeo, J.H. (1988). Spinal cord injury: Nursing the patient toward a new life. **RN, 51,** 31–35.

C

HAPTER TWELVE
Problems of the Reproductive System

Hysterectomy
Prostatectomy
Mastectomy
References

Hysterectomy

Hysterectomy is the surgical removal of the uterus. When the uterus is removed, the cervix also is removed. Depending on the reason for surgery, a hysterectomy may be done vaginally or through an abdominal incision. When the uterus alone is removed, the vaginal approach can be used. The abdominal approach is used when other reproductive structures such as the ovaries (oophorectomy) and fallopian tubes (salpingectomy) must also be removed or when the uterus is unusually large.

A midline or Pfannenstiel's incision may be used for an abdominal hysterectomy. The latter is a horizontal incision made just above the symphysis. It is sometimes called a "bikini cut" because it leaves a less visible scar.

Preoperative preparation is the same for any patient undergoing surgery. Postoperatively, the patient returns to the medical/surgical unit with:

- IV infusion
- Foley catheter
- abdominal dressing
- vaginal wound drainage device
- sanitary pad in place
- antiembolism stockings
- vaginal packing if hemostasis was a problem following vaginal hysterectomy

When the cervix is removed during surgery, a purse-string suture is used to create a vaginal cuff when leaves a small opening at the top of the vaginal for drainage of residual fluid. Within a few weeks, this opening eventually heals and closes.

Some individuals think that after a hysterectomy, the vagina is sealed and that intercourse is not possible.

A hysterectomy does not have a negative effect on sexual performance or sexual gratification. Some women express increased enjoyment of sex after surgery because the fear of pregnancy is no longer a concern and menstruation no longer occurs.

A major side effect from hysterectomy is menopausal symptoms that occur as a result of abrupt hormonal changes. Lifetime hormonal replacement therapy is required to control symptoms associated with menopause.

After a vaginal hysterectomy, vaginal sensation is diminished but returns after several weeks when the site heals.

The mean LOS for a DRG classification of hysterectomy is 4.6 days (Lorenz, 1991). The average recovery time is 10–12 weeks.

Integrative Care Plans

- Preoperative and postoperative care
- Loss

Discharge Considerations

- Follow-up care
- Signs and symptoms of wound infection
- Wound care
- Medications for home use
- Activity limitations

THE PREOPERATIVE PERIOD

 # ASSESSMENT DATA BASE

1. History or presence of factors necessitating surgery:
   - carcinoma of the cervix, ovary, or uterus
   - large uterine myomas (fibroids)
   - severe endometriosis
   - chronic dysfunctional uterine bleeding (postmenopausal bleeding, metrorrhagia)
   - symptomatic uterine prolapse

2. Physical examination based on a general survey (Appendix F) to establish baseline values.

3. Assess the patient's feelings and concerns about the surgery and knowledge of preoperative and postoperative events.

4. See Preoperative and Postoperative Care (page 738) for the remainder of the preoperative plan of care.

THE POSTOPERATIVE PERIOD

 # ASSESSMENT DATA BASE

1. On receiving the patient:
   - perform a routine postoperative assessment (Appendix L)
   - check amount of drainage on the perineal pad

NURSING DIAGNOSIS: HIGH RISK FOR COMPLICATIONS

RELATED TO FACTORS: Hysterectomy

DEFINING CHARACTERISTICS: Verbalizes increased pressure and discomfort in legs with sitting, unusual vaginal bleeding

PATIENT OUTCOME (collaborative): Demonstrates no complications

EVALUATION CRITERIA: Absence of unusual vaginal bleeding, less reports of pelvic congestion

INTERVENTIONS	RATIONALE
Pelvic Congestion:	
1. Monitor: • color and amount of drainage on perineal pad at least q2h x 24 hours, then q8h thereafter. • output from vaginal wound drainage device q8h • vital signs q4h	Early detection of complications with prompt intervention can prevent permanent tissue damage.
2. Instruct the patient to avoid prolonged sitting and standing when allowed out of bed.	Gravity and hip flexion increase venous congestion in the pelvis.
3. Notify physician if the patient is passing clots, the pad is saturated with bright red blood, or a large amount of bright red drainage collects in the wound drainage device within one hour continuously.	This indicates hemorrhage and a need for prompt medical intervention. A small amount of wound drainage, usually less than 50 mL in 24 hours, is expected.
4. If a vaginal packing is in place, do **not** remove it until ordered by physician, usually within 24 hours.	The vaginal packing acts as a hemostat.
5. Keep a supply of sterile perineal pads at the bedside for patient use prn. Teach the patient how to apply the pads. Ensure the patient has a sanitary belt.	The perineal pads absorb drainage. Minimizing contamination of the pad when applied lessens the risk of vaginal infection.

NURSING DIAGNOSIS: HIGH RISK FOR DISTURBANCE IN SELF-CONCEPT

RELATED TO FACTORS: Hormonal changes and perceived losses secondary to hysterectomy

DEFINING CHARACTERISTICS: May verbalize depression and loss of femininity, may cry for unknown reasons, may express concerns about alteration in sexual functioning or loss of reproductive capability

PATIENT OUTCOME: Demonstrates acceptance of self in current situation

EVALUATION CRITERIA: Verbalizes understanding of relation between hormonal changes and emotions, verbalizes ways to cope with perceived and actual losses, verbalizes positive statements about self

INTERVENTIONS	RATIONALE
1. Encourage the patient to continue personal grooming practices that she feels enhance femininity (using makeup, perfume).	Gender grooming practices reinforce one's sexual identity.
2. Explore the possibility of adoption if the patient or significant other express a desire to have children.	Exploring ways to fulfill one's perceived role in view of current circumstances helps promote coping with a loss.
3. Suggest alternative ways to express intimacy during the recovery period such as holding hands, kissing, and massage.	An individual's need for reassurance of love and belonging is heightened with surgery of the reproductive system.
4. Encourage the patient and significant other to express their feelings and concerns about the perceived impact of the surgery on the relationship.	Body image changes affect not only the individual but also immediate loved ones.

NURSING DIAGNOSIS: HIGH RISK FOR IMPAIRED HOME MAINTENANCE MANAGEMENT (SEE PAGE 747)

INTERVENTIONS	RATIONALE
1. Instruct the patient to: • avoid sexual intercourse until approved by physician, usually about six weeks. Explain this time is needed to allow vaginal tissue to heal. • avoid douching and tub baths. Take showers to minimize the risk of vaginal infection. • avoid strenuous activities, prolonged standing and sitting, and driving and lifting for six weeks to prevent pelvic congestion. • notify physician if manifestations of infection occur: fever, odorous vaginal discharge, or increased redness, tenderness, and purulent wound drainage. Explain that antibiotic therapy is required to resolve infection. • consume a well-balanced diet consisting of high-fiber foods. Drink at least eight glasses of fluid daily, especially water to prevent constipation. • consume calcium-rich foods or take calcium supplements with vitamin D to prevent osteoporosis. • resume activities slowly. Rest throughout the day as some fatigue is expected for several weeks. Explain a hysterectomy is major surgery, which places a tremendous physiologic stress on the body.	Thorough discharge instructions ensure a safe recovery.

INTERVENTIONS	RATIONALE
2. If estrogen replacement therapy is prescribed, advise to take in the mornings to correlate with the natural hormonal cycle. Remind the patient to inform physician if menopausal symptoms persist or worsen: hot flashes, pain with intercourse (when allowed).	Estrogen replacement therapy requires adjustment to control these symptoms.
3. See Preoperative and Postoperative Care (page 738).	

Prostatectomy

Prostatectomy is a partial or complete removal of the prostate gland. There are four different surgical approaches to a prostatectomy, each with a different outcome:

1. Transurethral resection of the prostate (TURP)
   - abnormal tissue removed via a rectoscope inserted through the urethra
   - no postoperative dressing required
   - a Foley catheter required postoperatively

2. Suprapubic prostatectomy
   - lower abdominal incision made through the bladder neck
   - wound dressing, wound drainage device, Foley catheter, and suprapubic catheter needed postoperatively

3. Retropubic prostatectomy
   - incision made in lower abdomen
   - no incision made in bladder
   - wound dressing, Foley catheter, and wound drainage device needed postoperatively

4. Perineal prostatectomy
   - incision made between scrotum and anus
   - used when radical prostatectomy is required
   - vasectomy is usually performed as prophylaxis against epididymitis
   - bowel preparation required preoperatively (enemas, low-residue diet, and antibiotics)
   - postoperatively a perineal dressing and wound drainage are in place; later, sitz baths are required

   With TURP, suprapubic, and retropubic prostatectomies, potential outcomes can include:

   - temporary urinary incontinence
   - voiding cloudy urine after intercourse and temporary infertility (low sperm count) caused by retrograde ejaculation of semen into the bladder

With perineal prostatectomy, in which a modified lymphadenectomy and nerve sparing radical prostatectomy (cystoprostatectomy) is performed, long-term incontinence, impotence, or infertility are not experienced. However, if this technique was not used, the outcome will be permanent impotence, sterility, and urinary incontinence.

Preoperative preparation is the same for any patient undergoing surgery. Postoperatively, the patient has an IV infusion and a three-way Foley catheter with a 30 mL balloon to provide hemostasis. A sterile irrigating solution may be attached to the Foley catheter for continuous or intermittent bladder irrigation.

If a suprapubic catheter is in place, the Foley catheter is removed first. Residual urine is assessed before removing the suprapubic catheter.

The mean LOS for a DRG of prostatectomy without complications is 4.0 days and 6.9 days with complications (Lorenz, 1991).

Integrative Care Plans

• Immobility
• Cancer if malignancy is present
• Preoperative and postoperative care

Discharge Considerations

• Follow-up care
• Signs and symptoms requiring medical attention
• Activity limitations

THE PREOPERATIVE PERIOD

 # ASSESSMENT DATA BASE

1. History or presence of factors necessitating surgery:
   • benign prostatic hypertrophy (BPH) associated with outflow obstruction
   • cancer of the prostate
2. Check medical record for results of digital rectal examination, which reveal a rock-hard, irregular, nonpliable prostate (malignancy) or firm, enlarged, pliable gland (benign).
3. Ask about voiding difficulties. Look for manifestations of urethral obstruction resulting from the enlarged prostate gland:
   • postvoiding dribbling
   • hesitancy
   • narrowing of urinary stream
   • frequent voiding of small amounts
   • nocturia (most common initial symptom)

Additional symptoms can include:

- low back pain (consistent with malignancy)
- hematuria (caused by rupture of tiny blood vessels from overdistention of the bladder or infection)
- urinary infection (burning with voiding, cloudy urine, foul-smelling urine)

4. Diagnostic studies:

- Biopsy differentiates benign growth from malignant growth.
- Serum acid phosphatase is elevated with malignancy.
- Serum alkaline phosphatase is elevated with malignancy when bone metastasis has occurred.
- Scans (bone, lung, liver) to assess metastasis if biopsy is positive for malignancy.
- X rays of kidney, ureter, bladder can reveal hydroureters, hydronephrosis, pyelonephritis with severe obstructions.
- Urinalysis can show bacteriuria, WBCs, or pus if infection is present.

5. See Preoperative and Postoperative Care (page 738).

THE PREOPERATIVE PERIOD

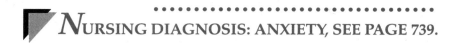

NURSING DIAGNOSIS: ANXIETY, SEE PAGE 739.

INTERVENTIONS	RATIONALE
1. Explain that postvoiding dribbling can occur temporarily after the catheter is removed and that perineal exercises (also called Kegel's exercises) can help strengthen spincter muscle tone to correct this problem. Teach and have the patient practice perineal exercises: • Tighten abdominal and perineal muscles as if trying to stop urine flow. • Hold contraction for ten seconds, then relax.	Practicing postoperative exercises preoperatively helps promote a smoother recovery.

●●●●●●●●●●●●●●●●●●●●●●●●●●●●●●●

◤ NURSING DIAGNOSIS: PAIN

RELATED TO FACTORS: Urethral obstruction secondary to prostate enlargement

DEFINING CHARACTERISTICS: Verbalizes voiding problems, observation of suprapubic distention, reports urge to void but cannot do so, reports frequent voiding of small quantities but still has urge to void

PATIENT OUTCOME (collaborative): Demonstrates relief from discomfort

EVALUATION CRITERIA: Denies pain, relaxed facial expression

●●●●●●●●●●●●●●●●●●●●●●●●●●●●●●●

INTERVENTIONS	RATIONALE
1. Catheterize as ordered for acute urinary retention: frequent voiding in small amounts, suprapubic distention, complaints of the urge to void after voiding, complaints of the urge to void but cannot do so.	Urinary retention predisposes to urinary tract infection, hydroureter, and hydronephrosis.
2. If difficulty is encountered with a straight tip catheter, use a Coudé catheter (a curved tip catheter). If unable to access the bladder with a Coudé catheter, notify physician. **Never** attempt to force the catheter through the urethra.	A urologist uses a special filiform catheter to catheterize the patient. Forceful catheterization can cause severe damage and possible rupture to the urethra. For patients with inoperable cancer of the prostate, a permanent suprapubic catheter is required.

THE POSTOPERATIVE PERIOD

 *A*SSESSMENT DATA BASE

1. See Preoperative and Postoperative Care (page 741).

●●●●●●●●●●●●●●●●●●●●●●●●●●●●●

◤ NURSING DIAGNOSIS: HIGH RISK FOR COMPLICATIONS

RELATED TO FACTORS: Prostatectomy

DEFINING CHARACTERISTICS: May show early manifestations of hemorrhage, infection, voiding abnormalities

PATIENT OUTCOME (collaborative): Demonstrates no complications

EVALUATION CRITERIA: Discharged within LOS for DRG, absence of hemorrhage, infection, and urinary incontinence

• •

INTERVENTIONS	RATIONALE
Hemorrhage:	
1. Monitor: • BP, pulse, and respirations q4h • intake and output q8h • color of urine	Early detection of complications with prompt intervention can prevent permanent tissue damage.
2. Notify physician of persistent bright red, opaque urine. Obtain vital signs and maintain bedrest. Administer aminocaproic acid (Amicar) or prepare for return to surgery as prescribed.	Normally, urinary drainage during the initial 24 hours is a translucent cherry red. It should gradually become lighter, then pink, and eventually clear within a few days. Amicar decreases fibrinolysis.
3. While traction is on the Foley catheter, instruct the patient to refrain from flexing the leg to which the catheter is anchored. Release traction only if ordered by physician.	Traction is often employed after a TURP to provide hemostasis. To apply traction, the urologist pulls the catheter taut and tapes it securely to the patient's thigh.
4. Restrain the patient if he becomes confused and attempts to pull out intrusive devices such as the IV infusion or catheters.	To prevent self-injury.
5. Perform serial urine sampling as ordered after the catheter(s) are removed according to facility protocol and procedures. Teach the patient how to perform this task.	To assess resolution of bleeding. Involving the patient in postoperative care helps foster independence.
6. Provide a high-fiber diet and prescribed stool softeners if the patient has history of constipation.	Straining increases pressure on the prostatic fossa, which could precipitate bleeding.
7. Irrigate the catheter(s) when clots are detected in the tubing.	Clots can obstruct the catheter, causing bladder distention and bleeding.

INTERVENTIONS	RATIONALE
Infection:	

1. Monitor:
   • temperature q4h
   • appearance of wound during dressing changes
   • voiding after removal of catheter(s)
	Early detection of signs of infection with prompt treatment can prevent permanent tissue damage.

2. Administer antibiotic therapy as ordered and evaluate effectiveness.	Antibiotics are needed to prevent and resolve infections.
3. Ensure daily fluid intake of at least 2–3 liters, unless contraindicated.	Fluids aid in the distribution of medication throughout the body. The risk of UTI developing is reduced when a constant dilute flow of urine is maintained through the kidneys.

4. Collect a specimen (urine or wound) for culture and sensitivity studies if signs of infection occur:
   • urine — cloudy, burning, urgency, frequency, foul-smell
   • wound — increased incisional pain, redness, drainage, fever
	A culture provides identification of the infective agent. A sensitivity study identifies the antibiotics that is most effective against the pathogen.

5. Change wound dressings prn as ordered using aseptic technique. Use a "tracheostomy" gauze dressing, which is already fenestrated, to simplify dressing changes with a suprapubic catheter.	With a suprapubic catheter, urine may sometimes saturate the dressing, necessitating frequent dressing changes. Moist dressings provide a good culture medium for bacteria.
6. Provide catheter care twice a day according to facility protocol and procedures.	To reduce risk of infection.
7. If a perineal approach was used, provide a sitz bath after each bowel movement and as ordered. Teach the patient how to perform own sitz bath.	Feces is a source of bacterial contamination.

INTERVENTIONS	RATIONALE
8. Follow universal precautions (handwashing before and after patient care, wearing gloves when contact from blood or body fluid is likely to occur) with all direct patient care procedures.	Caregivers are the most common source of nosocomial infection. Universal precautions protect both the caregiver and patient.
Urinary Incontinence:	
1. Instruct the patient to report postvoiding dribbling. Perform measures to achieve continence based on patient's preference: • Wear a sanitary pad and belt • Void when the urge is felt • Wear a condom catheter • Wear disposable briefs	Incontinence is embarrassing for the patient. Allowing patient involvement in selection of continence control measures helps the patient maintain a sense of control when in a physical uncontrollable situation.

◥ NURSING DIAGNOSIS: PAIN

RELATED TO FACTORS: Bladder spasms and surgical incision secondary to prostatectomy

DEFINING CHARACTERISTICS: Verbalizes discomfort, reports sudden intermittent spurts of urine around Foley catheter with pain, moaning, frowning

PATIENT OUTCOME (collaborative): Demonstrates relief from discomfort

EVALUATION CRITERIA: Denies pain, relaxed facial expression, fewer reports of urine escaping around the catheter

INTERVENTIONS	RATIONALE
For Incisional Pain:	
1. Administer prescribed analgesic prn and evaluate effectiveness.	Analgesics block the pain pathway.
2. When allowed out of bed, do not allow the patient to sit for long periods after an open prostatectomy.	To reduce strain on the incision.

INTERVENTIONS	RATIONALE
3. Assist the patient to assume a position of comfort. Keep head of bed elevated about 30 degrees and knees slightly flexed after open prostatectomy. Splint an abdominal incision when coughing.	To reduce strain on the incision.
For Bladder Spasms: 1. Administer prescribed antispasmodic agent prn, which can be belladonna and opium (B&O) suppositories.	To control bladder spasms.
2. Avoid taking rectal temperatures.	Rectal temperatures trigger bladder spasms.
3. Keep urinary drainage tubes secured to the thigh to prevent excess tension on the bladder. Irrigate the catheter when clots appear in the tubing.	Obstruction of the tubing by clots can cause bladder distention, which trigger spasms.

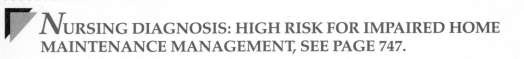

NURSING DIAGNOSIS: HIGH RISK FOR IMPAIRED HOME MAINTENANCE MANAGEMENT, SEE PAGE 747.

INTERVENTIONS	RATIONALE
1. Provide discharge instructions that should include: • Avoid sexual intercourse until approved by physician, usually about six weeks. • Avoid heavy lifting and strenuous physical exertion for about eight weeks. Short walks around the house are permitted but jogging, bicycling, or swimming is not permitted.	Discharge teaching helps ensure a safe postoperative recovery.

INTERVENTIONS	RATIONALE

• Void when the urge occurs.
• Continue with perineal exercises if incontinence persists. Perform these exercises q2h for ten counts. No special position must be assumed to perform perineal exercises.
• Drink at least eight glasses of fluid daily, especially water.
• Notify urologist if signs of infection occur:
  — wound: increased tenderness and redness, drainage, fever
  — urinary: burning and pain with voiding, persistent post-voiding dribbling, cloudy, foul-smelling urine, frequency
• Some passage of urinary blood may occasionally occur. If bleeding is more than slight, lie down and drink a glass of water every hour until the urine clears. If bleeding persists or becomes profuse, contact physician.
• Avoid straining when having a bowel movement. Take a mild laxative or stool softener, as needed, to prevent constipation.	

2. Provide written instructions for home care and follow-up appointment.	Verbal instructions may be easily forgotten.
3. Ensure patient has a prescription for an analgesic if pain is still present.	To ensure continued comfort during recovery.
4. Advise the patient to contact physician if signs of urethral obstruction recur.	Prostate enlargement can recur with partial removal of the gland.

Mastectomy

Mastectomy is removal of all or part of the breast because of stage I or II breast cancer. A combination of chemotherapy, radiation therapy, and hormone therapy are recommended for stage III or IV breast cancer. In premenopausal women with inoperable breast cancer, hormonal therapy can consist of androgens or antiestrogen agents because breast cancer in these women is often estrogen- or testosterone-dependent (Bachman, 1989).

The outcome of breast surgery varies depending on the type of surgery:

1. Following a lumpectomy or a partial mastectomy:
   - breast prosthesis is not needed
   - lymphedema does not occur
   - radiation therapy is often required afterward

2. Following a simple mastectomy or a modified radical mastectomy:
   - a breast prosthesis is required because the entire breast is removed and lymphedema often occurs

Patients are often concerned about disfigurement and the threat of a shortened lifespan with breast cancer. The risk of metastases is always present even with surgical removal of the tumor. Common sites of distant metastases include the bone, lungs, brain, and liver (Bachman, 1989).

Breast reconstruction surgery can be done by a plastic surgeon immediately after the mastectomy to avoid a second hospitalization or after the incision heals and the course of radiation therapy is completed. Breast reconstruction does not interfere with chemotherapy or radiation therapy, nor does it adversely affect the mastectomy.

Preoperative preparation is the same for any patient undergoing surgery. Postoperatively, the patient may return to the medical/surgical unit with:

- IV infusion
- wound drainage device
- pressure dressing over operative area
- arm on operative side elevated on pillows

674

INTERVENTIONS	RATIONALE
8. Review the American Cancer Society's recommendations for breast screening, especially if the patient has daughter(s). Share these recommendations with the patient's daughter(s) or advise the patient to do so: • monthly self-breast examination beginning at age 20 • baseline mammography at age 35–40 for all women • mammography every 1–2 years for high-risk groups: — women over age 50 — women with large pendulous breasts because it is difficult to palpate lumps in very large breasts — women with a positive family history of breast cancer — women who have had a mastectomy	Early detection of breast abnormalities improves chances for a more favorable outcome. Two important screening practices are breast self-examination and mammography.
9. Assist the significant other in learning how to cope with anticipated psychosocial changes that may cause stress in the relationship. Refer the significant other to the local Man-to-Man program provided by the American Cancer Society.	Significant others also will grieve the loss or altered body image in the loved one. The Man-to-Man program is a support group for the spouse of a breast cancer patient.

· ·

▶ NURSING DIAGNOSIS: HIGH RISK FOR IMPAIRED HOME MAINTENANCE MANAGEMENT

RELATED TO FACTORS: Knowledge deficit about self-care on discharge

DEFINING CHARACTERISTICS: Verbalizes lack of understanding, observation of unsafe practices, requests information

PATIENT OUTCOME: Demonstrates willingness to comply with self-care activities on discharge

EVALUATION CRITERIA: Verbalizes understanding of instructions, correct performance of required shoulder exercises

• •

INTERVENTIONS	RATIONALE
1. On discharge, ensure the patient: • has a sufficient supply of dressings for wound care and can perform dressing changes • knows how to perform monthly self-breast examination and knows findings that require medical attention • has a list of shoulder exercises and knows how to perform shoulder exercises. (Encourage use of both arms when doing housework or ADL to ensure adequate exercise). • has the name and address of businesses that supply breast prothesis, if one is required • has a prescription for a mild analgesic	Discharge teaching is essential to make a smooth transition from facility to home. Also, it helps the patient know what to do to maintain health and how to provide safe self-care at home.
2. Teach the patient measures for lifetime protection of the arm on the operative side: • **no** BPs, venipunctures, or injections in the arm on the operative side • avoid: — carrying a handbag on the shoulder of the operative side — gardening without wearing thick gardening gloves — using deodorants on the operative side until approved by physician — lying on the operative side until approved by physician — lifting heavy objects	With lymph node removal, the risk of infection developing in the arm on the operative side is significantly increased.

INTERVENTIONS	RATIONALE
3. Provide the patient with written self-care instructions and a written appointment for follow-up visits.	Verbal instructions may be easily forgotten.
4. Instruct the patient to contact physician if drainage, increased tenderness, and redness of the wound, or fever occur.	These findings indicate infection and a need for antimicrobial therapy.
5. Advise the patient to resume work gradually and to take planned rest periods throughout the day. Explain that a mastectomy is major surgery, which places tremendous stress on the body.	Patient may set unrealistic goals and attempt to resume a full lifestyle as a means of coping with current body image changes.

BIBLIOGRAPHY

Bachman, J.W. (1989). Breast problems. **Primary Care, 15,** 643–663.

Lilly, L. (1991). Impact of radiation on prostate cancer. **Geriatric Nursing, 12,** 174–177.

Lorenz, E.W. (1992). **St. Anthony's DRG Working Guidebook.** Alexandria: St. Anthony's Publishing Company.

Wozniak-Perofsky, J. (1991). BPH: Treating older men's most common problem. **RN, 54,** 32–38.

CHAPTER THIRTEEN

Problems of the Immune System

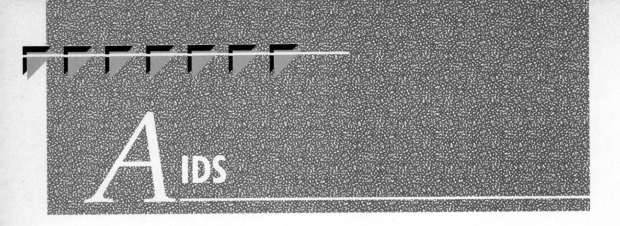

AIDS

AIDS means acquired immune deficiency syndrome. It is caused by the human immun-odeficiency virus (HIV). The only identified routes of transmission are through blood and semen contaminated with the HIV. Transmission can be through sexual contact, exposure to contaminated blood and blood products (transfusions, sharing needles used for illegal IV drugs, accidental needle puncture, broken area on skin directly exposed to contaminated blood), and from pregnant female to unborn child.

When the HIV enters the bloodstream, it attacks the immune system and weakens the person's ability to fight disease. Target cells are the T cells (type of white blood cell called lymphocytes that are produced in the thymus). Although they do not secrete antibodies, T cells are essential for normal immune function. Without them, cell-mediated immunity deteriorates, allowing opportunistic diseases to invade the body. In response to this invasion, the body begins to produce antibodies. Within two weeks to three months after infection, these antibodies can usually be detected by a blood test.

There are three possible outcomes for individuals who become infected with HIV:

- they can remain healthy, asymptomatic carriers of the virus
- they can develop AIDS- related complex (ARC)
- they can develop classic AIDS

Currently, no cure exists for AIDS. All asymptomatic HIV positive persons require periodic T_4 cell tests (also called CD_4 cell count) usually every six months to monitor the status of their immune system. When the CD_4 cell count falls below $500/mm^3$ (normal is $1,000/mm^3$), pharmacotherapy is often initiated, followed by laboratory monitoring of the T_4 cell count every three months (AIDS Guide, 1992). Because of the increased risk of opportunistic infections, additional screening tests include:

- skin tests: purified protein derivative (PPD) to rule out tuberculosis (TB)
- candida, mumps, or tetanus toxoid to evaluate a patient's immune response
- serum studies for hepatitis B antibodies

General Medical Management

* Pharmacotherapy:
  — zidovudine (Retrovir), also called AZT
  — dideoxyinosine (DDI)
  — dideoxycytidine (DDC), also called zalcitabine (pending approval by the Food and Drug Administration [FDA])
  — antibiotics such as co-trimoxazole (sulfamethoxazole) and trimethoprim (Bactrim, Septra), when the CD_4 cell count falls below 200/mm³ to prevent *Pneumocystis carinii* pneumonia (PCP)

Integrative Care Plans

* Loss
* Immobility (when patients reach terminal phase)

Discharge Considerations

* Follow-up care
* Medications to continue at home
* Prevention of infection
* Maintaining adequate nutritional intake

 # ASSESSMENT DATA BASE

1. History or presence of high-risk behaviors:
   * multiple sexual partners
   * male with homosexual or bisexual lifestyle
   * IV drug abuse
   * hemophiliac (receiving clotting factors before 1985)

2. Physical examination based on a general survey (Appendix F) and laboratory examination may reveal:
   a. ARC (defined by first three findings below)
      * lymphadenopathy
      * oral *Candidiasis*
      * CD_4 cell count of 500/mm³ or less
      * intermittent fevers with night sweats (often the first symptom)
      * persistent diarrhea
      * anorexia
      * constant fatigue
      * bruising easily and bleeding (indicative of idiopathic thrombocytopenia purpura)

- weight loss
- skin rashes
- AIDS-related tumors, for example, Hodgkin's disease or cancer of the mouth
- neurologic complications such as psychosis (memory loss, indifference, dementia), seizures, partial paralysis, painful peripheral neuropathy, and loss of coordination

b. AIDS

- opportunistic infections, such as tuberculosis, *Pneumocystis carinii* pneumonia (PCP) evidenced by persistent cough, fever, and shortness of breath
- Kaposi's sarcoma (type of skin cancer) evidenced by multiple purplish blotches and bumps on skin
- CD_4 cell count of 200/mm^3 or less

3. Diagnostic studies:

- HIV infection confirmed by positive serologic tests:
  — enzyme-linked immunosorbent assay (ELISA) test
  — Western blot considered most specific test for HIV infection; performed on the same blood specimen if ELISA test is positive (times two)

4. Assess understanding of condition and emotional response to diagnosis and treatment plan.

NURSING DIAGNOSIS: HIGH RISK FOR INFECTION

RELATED TO FACTORS: Decreased immune response, broken skin

DEFINING CHARACTERISTICS: Positive Western blot, demonstrates manifestations of ARC or AIDS, reports history of frequent hospitalizations for treatment of infections, currently receiving drug(s) to treat HIV infection

PATIENT OUTCOME (collaborative): Demonstrates resolution of current infection

EVALUATION CRITERIA: Temperature and WBC return to normal range, fewer reports of night sweats, absence of coughing, increased dietary intake, achieves timely healing of wounds/lesions

INTERVENTIONS	RATIONALE
1. Monitor: • results of CBC and CD_4 reports • temperature q4h • general status (Appendix F) q8h	Objective data is essential for evaluating effectiveness of therapy.

INTERVENTIONS	RATIONALE
2. Administer prescribed antibiotics and evaluate effectiveness. Ensure daily fluid intake of at least 2–3 liters.	Antibiotics specific to the pathogen are required to resolve an opportunistic infection. Fluids help medication distribution throughout the body.
3. Follow principles of universal blood and body fluid precautions. Use appropriate barrier precautions to prevent contamination of skin and mucous membranes when in contact with blood or body fluids: • Wear gloves when contact with blood or body fluid is likely to occur. • Wash hands before and after patient contact, including before and after wearing gloves. • Place a category specific isolation card on the patient's door. If pulmonary TB is present, wear a mask and advise all household members to be screened for TB. Explain that TB is contagious. A mask is not required for PCP because it is an opportunistic infection caused by the person's normal body flora. • Wear gowns and goggles when splashing is likely to occur. • Avoid recapping needles. Place all sharps in a puncture-proof container for disposal. • Clean blood spills with a facility spill kit or a 1:10 solution of household bleach (sodium hypochlorite). • Do not allow caregivers with exudative lesions or sweeping dermatitis to provide patient care or handle patient care equipment until lesions heal.	To reduce the risk of nosocomial infection and to protect the patient from new infections.
4. Maintain a comfortable room temperature. Keep skin clean and dry.	Night sweats can be a source of discomfort, especially when the sleeping attire is wet and cold from perspiration.

NURSING DIAGNOSIS: ALTERATIONS IN NUTRITION: LESS THAN BODY REQUIREMENTS

RELATED TO FACTORS: Inadequate nutritional intake secondary to AIDS wasting syndrome, painful oral lesions

DEFINING CHARACTERISTICS: Manifestations of AIDS wasting syndrome: weight loss greater than 10% of baseline weight accompanied by nausea, vomiting, profound weakness and fatigue, chronic diarrhea, serum albumin below normal level, negative nitrogen balance; may report difficulty chewing and swallowing; may have whitish plaques in mouth

PATIENT OUTCOME (collaborative): Demonstrates adequate nutritional status

EVALUATION CRITERIA: No further weight loss, laboratory reports reveal a positive nitrogen balance and serum albumin within normal range, fewer reports of fatigue and weakness, verbalizes feeling of well-being

INTERVENTIONS	RATIONALE
1. Monitor: • weight daily • intake and output q8h • serum albumin and BUN studies • percentage of food consumed with each meal	To identify indications of progress toward or deviations from expected outcomes.
2. If profuse watery diarrhea is present: • keep NPO and initiate TPN infusions (page 220) as prescribed. • administer prescribed antidiarrheal and evaluate effectiveness. Gradually resume oral feedings when diarrhea is under control. Advise intake of lactose-free, low-fat, high-soluble fiber in the presence of low-volume diarrhea. Consult physician if diarrhea persists or worsens.	Diarrhea is often caused by a protozoa *(Cryptosporidium)* that invades the epithelial lining, causing increased production of gas and pull of fluids into the intestine. Patients may lose ten liters of fluid daily with diarrhea. Bowel rest is the only effective treatment.
3. Refer to dietitian for assistance in selection and planning meals that meet nutritional needs.	A dietitian is a nutritional specialist who can assist the patient in planning a menu that meets nutritional needs in view of current condition.

◥ NURSING DIAGNOSIS: HIGH RISK FOR INEFFECTIVE INDIVIDUAL COPING

RELATED TO FACTORS: Actual and perceived losses secondary to AIDS

DEFINING CHARACTERISTICS: May report difficulty coping with condition and other people's reaction; may verbalize depression or low self-esteem; may report being shunned by family, friends, coworkers; may verbalize feeling a loss of independence and social identity; may report fear of dying

PATIENT OUTCOME (collaborative): Demonstrates effective coping

EVALUATION CRITERIA: Verbalizes plans to get involved with AIDS community support groups, verbalizes understanding of self-care instructions for maintaining health, reports satisfaction with the home care plan

INTERVENTIONS	RATIONALE
1. See Loss (page 733).	
2. Provide a supportive relationship: • Be where the patient is. • Be aware of own attitudes, thoughts, feelings, and concerns. • Help patient clarify thoughts, feelings, and concerns. • Be honest and project a non-judgmental attitude.	Caregivers' attitudes, thoughts, and feelings influence the quality of a nurse-patient relationship.
3. Refer the patient and significant others to local AIDS community support groups.	Support groups are a source of strength for both the patient and significant other.

◥ NURSING DIAGNOSIS: HIGH RISK FOR IMPAIRED HOME MAINTENANCE MANAGEMENT

RELATED TO FACTORS: Knowledge deficit about condition and measures to control the spread of infection, lack of adequate finances, absence of adequate support system to provide needed assistance

DEFINING CHARACTERISTICS: May verbalize lack of understanding about condition and use of infection control measures at home, may report needs assistance with some aspect of ADL but lacks adequate assistance at home, may verbalize need for financial assistance

PATIENT OUTCOME (collaborative): Demonstrates ability to meet continuing care needs

EVALUATION CRITERIA: Verbalizes satisfaction with home maintenance plans, identifies community resources that provide home care assistance, verbalizes plans for securing financial assistance with medical care as needed, discharged within LOS for DRG

· ·

INTERVENTIONS	RATIONALE
1. Evaluate patient's and significant other's understanding of condition: definition of HIV/AIDS, prognosis, mode of transmission of HIV, ways to prevent spread of HIV, importance of notifying all previous sexual contacts. Correct any misconceptions. Maintain patient confidentiality about a diagnosis of HIV/AIDS.	Compliance is enhanced when patients and significant others understand the condition and their role in controlling the spread of infection. Because of the social stigma attached to HIV infection and AIDS, patient confidentiality is important to establish and maintain a trusting nurse-patient relationship.
2. Evaluate awareness of community resources. Refer to social services or discharge planning department for community resources that focus on care of HIV/AIDS individuals and for help in financing medical needs if financial distress reported.	Social services or discharge planners are specialists who can arrange for continuity of care on discharge by using available community resources to meet identified needs.
3. Review infection control measures for home use: • Use of latex condoms with spermicide for intercourse. • Avoid sharing personal care items that may be contaminated with blood, such as toothbrush, razors. • Wash eating utensils in hot soapy water. There is no need to separate eating utensils or bed linen for washing unless visibly contaminated with fresh blood. Add household bleach when laundering all items stained with blood or body fluid. • Encourage females to practice birth control. Explain that HIV can be transmitted to the unborn fetus.	HIV is a bloodborne virus. Currently, no cure exists for HIV/AIDS. Infected individuals must assume responsibility in controlling the spread of the virus.

INTERVENTIONS	RATIONALE
4. Teach health promotion activities: • Eat well-balanced meals. Include more protein-rich foods as this nutrient is essential for immune function. Confer with a dietitian for assistance in planning meals that meet nutritional needs in view of current health status and economic situation. Discourage fad diets and excess use of vitamin/mineral supplements. Explain that using nutritional supplements should be under the direction of dietitian and physician following a thorough nutritional analysis. • Keep immunizations current to prevent infections: — tetanus booster every ten years. — have hepatitis B antibody level checked. Explain that hepatitis B vaccine (Recombivax HB, Heptavax-B, Engerix-B) is required if no antibodies are present. Let the patient know that hepatitis B vaccines are given in a series of three injections (page 532). • Encourage females to have pelvic examinations and Pap smears at least every six months. Explain that vaginal infections are common and require extensive treatment in HIV/AIDS females. • Reduce sources of stress. Get adequate sleep. Exercise regularly. Stop smoking, consuming alcohol, and using IV illicit drugs if these are habits. Refer to community sources to help resolve these addictions. • Avoid crowded, congested situations in the winter months when the incidence of influenza and colds is high.	Individuals must take an active role in managing their disease.

Cancer

Cancer is a disorder that can affect any organ in the body. It is characterized by the proliferation of abnormal cells. For solid mass producing cancers, the terms tumor and neoplasm are often used.

Tumors are benign or malignant. Benign tumors do not invade surrounding tissue and are nonlethal. Malignant neoplasms spread to surrounding tissue, ultimately interfering with normal function. Malignant cells divide more rapidly than normal cells. Metastases occurs to distant body sites by the bloodstream, lymphatics, or by direct invasion of adjourning organs and tissue. Tumors are named according to the tissue type from which they originate:

- carcinoma—originates in epithelial tissue (skin, lungs, stomach, breast, intestine)
- lymphoma—originates in lymphatics
- leukemia—originates in bone marrow
- sarcoma—originates in connective tissue (bone)

Cancer has a high mortality rate. Early detection allows effective treatment to begin before the cancer metastasizes thus improving the five-year survival rate for most cancers. Early cancer diagnosis is achieved by encouraging persons to:

1. have annual physical examinations

2. seek medical attention if warning signs of cancer occur:
   - change in bowel and bladder patterns
   - sore that does not heal
   - unusual bleeding or discharge
   - lump or thickening of the breast
   - difficulty swallowing
   - persistent dry cough or hoarseness

The course of the disease is characterized by periods of remission and exacerbation (recurrence), rapid deterioration, or steady progress toward cure. The patient with cancer who requires inpatient care is usually kept on an oncology unit. Oncology nurses specialize in the care of patients with cancer.

Tumors are described by both grading and staging definitions. Grading defines the tumor differentiation as well, moderately, or poorly differentiated. Differentiate means the extent to which the cancer cell looks and acts like the tissue of origin.

Staging involves using several diagnostic studies to confirm the location of a tumor, its size, cell type, and extent of metastasis. The carcinoma is labeled as Stage I, II, III, or IV. The higher the stage, the worse the prognosis.

After the cell type and stage have been determined, the physician discusses with the patient the best treatment plan to maximize the possibility of a cure, prognosis, and anticipated complications. The word "cure" in relation to cancer refers to control and remission of symptoms for an extended time.

Tumor response is evaluated by using tumor markers:

* solid tumors
  — size of the palpable mass
  — radiologic studies of tumor
  — bone marrow aspiration
* leukemia
  — blood counts and peripheral smears to examine cell maturity
* other cancers
  — presence or absence of specific serum and urinary paraproteins
  — gonadotropin filters
  — organ function studies
  — disappearance of symptoms
  — absence of CEA (carcinoembryonic antigen)

General Medical Management

* Primary Therapies:
  — chemotherapy
  — radiation therapy
  — surgery
* Investigative Therapies:
  — immunotherapy
  — whole body hyperthermia
  — alpha-interferon therapy
  — intraoperative radiation
  — photodynamic therapy

Integrative Care Plans

* Loss
* Fluid and biochemical imbalances
* Immobility

- Pain
- Radiation therapy
- Chemotherapy

Discharge Considerations

- Hospice care if end-stage
- Follow-up care

ASSESSMENT DATA BASE

1. History or presence of risk factors:
   - lung cancer — cigarette smoking, prolonged exposure to carcinogens in the workplace (asbestos, ionizing radiation, arsenic)
   - colon cancer — lack of adequate intake of dietary fiber
   - skin cancer — prolonged exposure to ultraviolet rays
   - other cancers — positive family history of cancer
2. Assess the patient's and significant other's response to the diagnosis.
3. Physical examination base on a general survey (Appendix F) may reveal manifestations of complications associated with cancer, especially if the patient is in the terminal stage. These complications are due to metastases and the therapies used to treat the cancer:
   - pain
   - bone marrow suppression (anemia, leukemia, thrombocytopenia)
   - fluid and biochemical imbalances
   - symptoms of multiple organ dysfunction as the cancer metastasizes to distant sites (brain, liver, lungs, bone, reproductive organs, peritoneal cavity)
4. Assess the patient's understanding and concerns about the prescribed treatment modalities.
5. Assess the patient's and significant other's need for spiritual support.
6. Assess nutritional status, including weight, appetite, dietary intake, and general condition of the skin and oral mucosa.

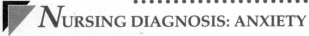

NURSING DIAGNOSIS: ANXIETY

RELATED TO FACTORS: Knowledge deficit about condition and treatments
DEFINING CHARACTERISTICS: Verbalizes lack of understanding, requests information

PATIENT OUTCOME (collaborative): Demonstrates relief from anxiety

EVALUATION CRITERIA: Verbalizes understanding of condition, prognosis, and treatments; reports feeling less anxious

• •

INTERVENTIONS	RATIONALE
1. If the patient has a poor prognosis, discuss with significant others arrangements for care when the patient reaches the terminal phase. Contact social services to arrange for home care or placement in an extended care facility or inpatient hospice, according to the family's preference and needs.	Preplanning helps lessen some stress as the patient approaches death. Hospice is a program providing supportive care for dying patients and their family when patients wish to die at home.
2. Refer the patient and significant others to local support groups such as the American Cancer Society, Hospice, or National Cancer Information Center (The Office of Cancer Communication National Cancer Institute, Building 31, Room 10, A-18, Bethesda, MD, 20982, or telephone 1-800-cancer).	External support systems can be sources of comfort. The National Cancer Information Center provides information about causes of cancer, prevention, symptoms, diagnosis, treatments, nutrition, and current research.
3. Assist the patient in deciding what, how, and when to share the diagnosis with family and friends (if patient is newly diagnosed). Prepare the patient for possible reactions of family members and friends. Emphasize the importance of being honest and open with feelings and concerns.	Preparing the patient to deal with the reactions of significant others also can help the patient cope with the certainty of death.
4. If in remission, help the patient deal realistically with the possibility of recurrences. Keep the patient and significant others informed of test results. As long as the patient is alert and oriented, allow patient to make choices.	To allow the patient to maintain a sense of control over the current situation.

INTERVENTIONS	RATIONALE
5. Convey hope.	To eliminate despair. Hopelessness is the result of an environment in which the patient feels out of control and powerless. Hope can play a significant role in the patient's will to live.
6. Explain the purpose and side effects of prescribed therapy (chemotherapy, radiation). Inform the patient of ways to minimize the side effects. Reassure the patient that most side effects are temporary and usually disappear within a few weeks after therapy is completed. Allow the patient to express feelings about anticipated side effects.	A knowledge of what to expect helps lessen anxiety.

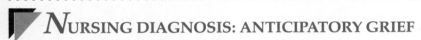

NURSING DIAGNOSIS: ANTICIPATORY GRIEF

RELATED TO FACTORS: Actual and anticipated losses secondary to cancer and its treatment, threat of death

DEFINING CHARACTERISTICS: Verbalizes concerns about dying, may verbalize statements reflecting grief process

PATIENT OUTCOME (collaborative): Demonstrates effective coping

EVALUATION CRITERIA: Verbalizes feelings and concerns openly, verbalizes realistic plans, follows therapeutic program

INTERVENTIONS	RATIONALE
1. See Loss (page 733).	

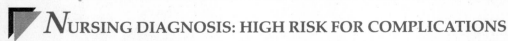

NURSING DIAGNOSIS: HIGH RISK FOR COMPLICATIONS

RELATED TO FACTORS: Metastatic cancer

DEFINING CHARACTERISTICS: May report persistent and severe pain; laboratory reports reflect dehydration, metabolic acidosis, anemia, WBC below normal limits, thrombocytopenia; may report persistent weakness, anorexia, weight loss

PATIENT OUTCOME (collaborative): Demonstrates relief from complications

EVALUATION CRITERIA: Reports decrease in intensity of pain, fewer manifestations of dehydration and bone marrow depression, reports less weakness, stable weight

• •

INTERVENTIONS	RATIONALE
1. See Pain (page 700).	
2. See Fluid and Biochemical Imbalances for dehydration and metabolic acidosis (page 773).	
3. See Anemia (page 436), Leukemia (page 414), and Thrombocytopenia (page 406).	
4. See Immobility (page 725).	
Weight Loss:	
1. Monitor weight weekly and amount of food consumed at each meal.	To evaluate effectiveness of therapy.
2. Encourage intake of a diet high in protein, vitamins, and calories.	Cancer and treatment modalities increase the basal metabolic rate and protein loss. If caloric needs are not met, the body uses its fat and protein stores to generate energy. Over time, muscle and fat deposits are lost; weight declines, and the patient develops an emaciated appearance.
3. If food intake is poor (less than 30%) and progressive weight loss continues: • refer the patient to a dietitian for assistance in planning nutritious meals. • suggest a nutritional supplement between meals. • suggest a calorie count. • suggest TPN (total parenteral nutrition) as a last resort.	A dietitian is a nutritional specialist who can assess the patient's nutritional status and plan a diet to meet nutritional needs. Liquid nutritional supplements can supply the required protein, vitamins, minerals, and calories. A calorie count allows the dietitian to assess the need for nutritional supplements or TPN.

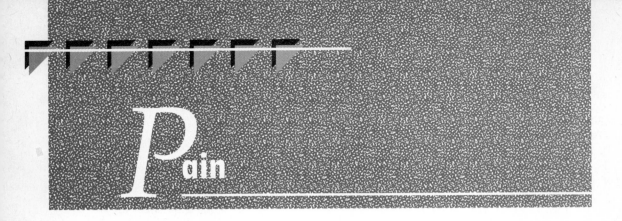

Pain

Pain is a subjective state in which the person demonstrates discomfort, verbally, nonverbally, or both. It may be acute (having a definite duration) or chronic (lasting months to years).

The pain experience consists of two components: perception and reaction. An intact nervous system is required to perceive pain. Pain reaction is what the individual feels, thinks, and does about the perceived pain.

An individual's response to pain is influenced by emotions, level of consciousness, cultural background, past experiences with pain, and meaning of pain. Pain interferes with a person's ability to rest, concentrate, and perform normal activities. Chronic pain often causes feelings of powerlessness and depression.

Potent narcotics can be given orally, parenterally, topically, or intrathecal. The parenteral and intrathecal routes provide rapid relief and are used for severe pain. The parenteral route can include intramuscular (IM), subcutaneous (SC), or IV (using central vascular access devices or lines).

Patient-controlled analgesia (PCA) is a widely used system that allows the patient to self-administer intravenously a prescribed bolus of the prescribed analgesic when needed. Use of the PCA system is recommended only for 72 hours after which the patient should be placed on an oral analgesic.

General Medical Management

- Pharmacotherapy — narcotic or nonnarcotic analgesics
- Ice — applied following musculoskeletal injuries and some orthopedic surgeries for relief of headaches
- Acupuncture, heat, biofeedback, Transcutaneous Electrical Nerve Stimulator (TENS) unit.
- Surgery:
  —cordotomy: severing of pain pathways in spinothalamic tract of spinal cord
  —rhizotomy: severing of posterior nerve roots at spinal cord junction
  —sympathectomy: severing of different nerve fibers to an extremity
- Nerve blocks — injection of a local anesthetic or neurolytic agent into a nerve
- Distraction and relaxation techniques

ASSESSMENT DATA BASE

1. Assess for the presence of factors that cause pain:
   - surgery
   - invasive diagnostic procedures
   - trauma (fractures, burns)
   - prolonged pressure on a body part imposed by immobility
   - chronic disease (cancer, arthritis, herniated intervertebral disc, glaucoma)
   - acute disorders characterized by obstruction of blood flow (pulmonary embolism, myocardial infarction, peripheral vascular disease)
2. Assess the pain in relation to:
   - provoking factors
     — What makes the pain worse?
     — What relieves the pain?
   - quality
     — What does the pain feel like?
     — Is pain sharp, dull, heavy pressure, throbbing, knifelike, choking, burning?
   - region
     — Where is the pain?
     — Does pain radiate or remain in one place?
   - severity
     — How severe is the pain?
     — Is pain mild, moderate, or severe?
   - time
     — How long ago did pain start?
     — Is pain constant or intermittent?
     — Does pain occur suddenly or gradually?
3. Assess for overt manifestations of pain.

NURSING DIAGNOSIS: PAIN

RELATED TO FACTORS: Specify causative factor

DEFINING CHARACTERISTICS: Verbalizes discomfort; rigid body posture; clenching teeth; frowning; moaning; restlessness; crying; guarding painful site; may have increased BP, pulse, and respiration or BP lower than baseline value with severe pain

PATIENT OUTCOME (collaborative): Demonstrates relief from discomfort

EVALUATION CRITERIA: Denies pain, reports pain less intensity, stable vital signs, relaxed facial expression and body posture

INTERVENTIONS	RATIONALE
1. Monitor: • BP, pulse, and respirations q4h • intensity of pain • level of consciousness	To identify indications of progress toward or deviations from expected outcome.
2. Administer prescribed analgesic prn and evaluate effectiveness. Give prescribed analgesic according to pain intensity as described by the patient: • mild pain — oral nonnarcotic analgesic • moderate pain — oral narcotic analgesic or nonsteroidal anti-inflammatory drugs (NSAID) such as Toradol • severe pain — a parenteral narcotic analgesic	Patients are the best judge of pain intensity because pain is a subjective experience. Strong analgesics are required for more severe pain.
3. Notify physician if the pain worsens or does not respond to analgesic intervention within the prescribed interval.	This can indicate a need for a stronger, more potent analgesic or the beginning of complications.
4. Notify physician of adverse effects of narcotic analgesics and intervene appropriately: • respiratory depression — slow, irregular respirations less than 12 per minute — administer naloxone Hcl (Narcan) IV as ordered — administer half the lower dose of the prescribed narcotic for patients not fully recovered from anesthesia. • sedation — if patient is difficult to arouse, reduce amount of analgesic and avoid giving other drugs that cause central nervous system depression (hypnotics, tranquilizers, or phenothiazines) until patient is more alert	Respiratory depression is the major side effect with narcotic analgesics. Narcan is the narcotic antagonist. Excess sedation signals an overdose of the drug. Patients with renal failure, liver disease, and the elderly are especially vulnerable to medication overdoses. Constipation is a problem with chronic use of narcotic analgesics. Urinary retention is more likely to occur with narcotic analgesic control of acute pain.

INTERVENTIONS	RATIONALE

• constipation
   — encourage liberal intake of fluid, high-fiber foods, and stool softener
• urinary retention
   — catheterize as ordered if patient complains of the inability to void but has the urge, accompanied by suprapubic distention	

5. Assist the patient to assume a position of comfort. Elevate painful edematous extremities. Flex knees using a pillow or knee gatch of the bed to relieve strain on abdominal muscles after abdominal surgery or when back pain is present.	Placing the body in a position to relieve pressure and prevent muscle stretching helps relieve discomfort.
6. Apply ice or heat (unless contraindicated). Avoid applying heat to fresh cuts and incisions.	Cold prevents swelling. Heat relaxes muscles and dilates vessels to improve circulation.
7. Teach the patient rhythmic breathing techniques with mild to moderate pain in conjunction with other pain relief interventions: • Instruct the patient to maintain eye contact on an object while inhaling slowly through the mouth and exhaling through pursed lips.	Distraction interferes with the pain stimulus by modifying awareness of pain. Distraction does not alter pain intensity. It is best used for short periods with mild to moderate pain.
8. Provide rest until pain resolves. Reduce noise and bright lights. Keep the patient warm by providing extra blankets.	Rest reduces energy expenditure. Peripheral vasoconstriction occurs with severe pain, causing the patient to feel cold. Usually, intense environmental stimuli intensifies pain perception.

INTERVENTIONS	RATIONALE
9. Instruct the patient to request pain medication **before** the pain reaches a severe level. If oral and IM analgesics are prescribed and providing BP remains within normal range and patient does not become extremely drowsy or confused, alternate the dose for the first 24 hours when pain is severe so patient is receiving an analgesic every two hours.	Pain is best controlled by maintaining a consistent level of the drug in the bloodstream.
10. **Always** use a pump controller with a continuous analgesic drip regardless of the administration route.	Maintaining an accurate rate control is essential to reducing the risk of overmedication.
For Intrathecal (Epidural) Analgesic: 1. Follow facility protocol and procedures about bolus administration if pain not effectively controlled. Use only analgesics free of preservatives and additives such as Duramorph or fentanyl (morphine sulfate injection) citrate injection.	Depending on the facility and because of the danger of spinal cord injury, either a specially trained nurse or anesthesiologist can reinject the catheter with the appropriate bolus of the prescribed analgesic. Normally, with the bolus method, pain control lasts for 12–24 hours. A continuous epidural drip, however, provides more consistent and effective pain relief than the bolus method, especially with chronic intractable pain. Additives and preservatives used in drugs can be neurotoxic when given via the epidural route.
2. Keep the patient attached to an apnea monitor according to facility protocol and procedures. Ensure resuscitative equipment is readily accessible.	A major adverse effect of Duramorph and fentanyl is respiratory depression. Objective and measurable data about a patient's present response provide evidence of whether outcome criteria are achieved.
3. Do **not** give any other type of analgesic or sedative unless approved by the anesthesiologist.	These agents increase the risk of respiratory depression.

INTERVENTIONS	RATIONALE
4. Administer naloxone Hcl (Narcan) if the respiratory rate falls below 12 per minute, if the patient is difficult to arouse, or if severe hypotension occurs. Notify physician immediately. Reassess vital signs after administering Narcan.	Narcan is a narcotic antagonist.
5. Maintain the appropriate flow sheet for documentation according to facility protocol.	To have a permanent record of therapy.
6. Check status of the back dressing q2h. Notify physician if the dressing is wet.	This can indicate catheter dislodgment and a need for it to be discontinued with an alternative route for administering analgesia prescribed.
7. Describe an epidural catheter and explain the reason for frequent assessments: a special catheter inserted into the epidural space in the spinal column between L_3 and L_4 by the anesthesiologist at time of surgery. The tubing is securely taped to the patient's back to prevent dislodgment. It is left in place for about 72 hours and then removed. In some cases it can be used in the management of chronic cancer pain as a continuous analgesic drip.	A knowledge of what to expect helps foster patient cooperation.
8. If a continuous epidural drip is used, provide catheter site care according to facility protocol using sterile technique: wear sterile gloves and a mask with site care, maintain a sterile field and supplies. Do **not** use alcohol at the site.	The epidural catheter provides a direct route entry of bacteria into the spinal canal, which increases the risk for meningitis. Alcohol is a preservative that could be neurotoxic.

INTERVENTIONS	RATIONALE
If PCA Is Used:	
1. Explain how to use the pump. When pain is experienced, instruct the patient to depress the button to deliver a bolus dose of the prescribed agent, which is meperidine HCl (Demerol) or morphine sulfate. Tell the patient that accidental overdosing will not occur because only low doses are given. Also, the machine is automatically preset to lockout when the prescribed amount for a given period has been delivered.	
2. Restart IV site if the patient complains of discomfort at the site or the site appears redden and swollen.	A patent IV site is essential for effective use of a PCA system because the patient self-administers intravenously the prescribed dose of the prescribed analgesic when needed.
3. Maintain appropriate flow sheet for documentation according to facility protocol for PCA.	To have a permanent record of therapy.
4. If respiratory rate falls below 12 per minute or severe hypotension occurs accompanied by a decrease in level of consciousness, stop the infusion immediately, administer Narcan following facilty protocol, and notify the physician. Reassess vital signs after administering Narcan.	Narcan is a narcotic antagonist.

INTERVENTIONS	RATIONALE
Neurotoxicity:	
1. Notify physician if the patient experiences jaw pain, visual disturbances, headaches, numbness, tingling, gait disturbances, persistent constipation, paresthesia, or diminished sensorium.	These findings indicate early nerve damage and a need to discontinue the drug.
Pulmonary Toxicity:	
1. Monitor: • lung sounds q8h • vital signs q4h	To detect early manifestations of pulmonary dysfunction.
2. Notify physician if a persistent dry cough, rales, or dyspnea on exertion occur. Obtain chest x ray and pulmonary function studies as ordered. Administer corticosteroids and discontinue chemotherapy as ordered.	Pneumonitis and pulmonary fibrosis are the major toxic effects. The onset of pulmonary toxicity occurs slowly over several months, with the earliest symptom being increasing dyspnea with exertion. Corticosteroids are given to reduce inflammation.
3. Encourage deep breathing q2h if pulmonary problems are detected or if the patient is restricted to bedrest.	Deep breathing helps expand the alveoli.
Cardiotoxicity:	
1. Monitor vital signs q4h.	To detect early signs of cardiac involvement.
2. Report abnormalities in the pulse rate and rhythm. Obtain an EKG as ordered.	An EKG confirms the cardiac abnormality. The drug is discontinued if cardiac disturbance is confirmed.
Hepatotoxicity:	
1. Monitor results of liver function studies (serum bilirubin, alkaline phosphatase).	To detect early signs of liver involvement.
2. Notify physician if the patient experiences jaundice, dark and smoky urine, clay stools, pruritus, or abdominal pain.	These findings suggest liver damage and a need to discontinue the drug.

INTERVENTIONS	RATIONALE
3. Instruct the patient to avoid intake of alcohol and aspirin while on chemotherapy.	These substances can cause liver damage with long-term use.

Local Tissue Necrosis:

INTERVENTIONS	RATIONALE
1. **Always** check for patency of the venous access device (implanted port, external atrial catheter, or peripheral IV line) before starting chemotherapy infusion. Inspect the infusion site qh for signs of infiltration (swelling, sluggish flow rate). Instruct the patient to signal if pain or burning occurs at the site. Stop the infusing immediately if infiltration occurs. Apply a cold moist compress. Administer Regitine directly into the affected tissue or the antidote prescribed by facility protocol.	Chemotherapy agents are highly toxic to tissue. Burning, pain, and swelling at the site signal infiltration. Regitine is given to counteract drug toxicity. Cold applications help reduce phlebitis and tissue edema. A backflow of blood (also called a flashback) ensures patency and that the vascular access device is in the vessel. Extravasation of agents that are vesicants can cause necrosis and sloughing of tissue. Agents that are irritants can cause phlebitis (less often than tissue necrosis).
2. **Always** use an infusion pump when giving chemotherapy agents by continuous IV drip.	To regulate the flow more accurately, thereby reducing the chance of overload.

NURSING DIAGNOSIS: ALTERATIONS IN NUTRITION: LESS THAN BODY REQUIREMENTS

RELATED TO FACTORS: Nausea and vomiting secondary to chemotherapy, anorexia

DEFINING CHARACTERISTICS: Reports loss of appetite, persistent weight loss, reports decreased food intake, reports gastric discomfort

PATIENT OUTCOME (collaborative): Demonstrates adequate nutritional status

EVALUATION CRITERIA: No further weight loss, dietary intake greater than 50% each meal, fewer reports of nausea and vomiting

INTERVENTIONS	RATIONALE
1. Monitor: • weight weekly • amount of food consumed with each meal • results of serum protein and albumin studies	To evaluate effectiveness of therapy.
2. Administer prescribed antiemetic 30 minutes before chemotherapy, at regular intervals during chemotherapy, and for 2–3 doses after completion of chemotherapy. Suggest combination antiemetic therapy: • lorazepam (Ativan) in combination with dexamethasone (Decadron) or diphenhydramine HCl (Benadryl). • metoclopramide HCl (Reglan) in combination with Decadron or Benadryl.	Nausea causes anorexia. Combination antiemetic therapy is the most effective in controlling nausea.
3. If dietary intake is extremely low, weight continually declines for five days, and nutritional studies reflect a persistent nutrient deficit, suggest total parenteral nutrition (TPN) therapy.	TPN supplies essential protein and calories. Essential fatty acids and vitamins can be given IV as supplements along with TPN solutions. Proteins, carbohydrates, and fats are essential to normal cellular development and functioning.
4. Encourage intake of foods high in protein, vitamins, minerals, and calories.	Chemotherapy and cancer are associated with increased catabolism.
5. Refer the patient to a dietitian for assistance with meal planning.	A dietitian is a nutritional specialist who can assess the patient's nutritional needs and direct the patient in preparing meals to meet nutritional needs.
6. Provide six small meals instead of three large meals.	Small feedings cause less gastric distention thus preventing nausea.
7. Provide nutritional supplements, such as Sustacal or Ensure, with or between meals when food intake is poor.	These supplements provide essential protein, vitamins, minerals, and calories.

INTERVENTIONS	RATIONALE
8. Advise the patient to avoid eating a full meal before chemotherapy. If hungry, encourage intake of crackers or dry toast with 7-Up or ginger ale. Wait 3–4 hours after chemotherapy treatment to consume a regular meal.	Distention of the stomach when the mucosa lining is inflamed triggers vomiting.

NURSING DIAGNOSIS: DISTURBANCE IN SELF-CONCEPT

RELATED TO FACTORS: Actual body image changes secondary to chemotherapy

DEFINING CHARACTERISTICS: May report feeling less attractive because of alopecia, may verbalize low self-esteem or worthlessness because of altered sexual functioning

PATIENT OUTCOME: Demonstrates acceptance of self in current situation

EVALUATION CRITERIA: Verbalizes ways to incorporate physical changes into lifestyle, verbalizes positive statements about self

INTERVENTIONS	RATIONALE
1. Teach the patient about prescribed chemotherapy drugs including name, dose, schedule, purpose, and common side effects.	Knowing what to expect facilitates acceptance of therapy and outcomes.
2. Allow the patient to express feelings and concerns about anticipated side effects.	Verbalizing feelings helps facilitate coping.
3. Inform the patient that hair will regrow when the prescribed chemotherapy is completed. Advise the patient to buy wigs or decorative headscarfs before beginning chemotherapy. Assist or refer the patient to a stylist for help in arranging the headscarf in a fashionable style.	Planning ways to effectively deal with anticipated alterations in body image helps facilitate coping.

INTERVENTIONS	RATIONALE
4. Inform the patient about the effect of chemotherapy on the reproductive organs. Encourage the male patient of childbearing age to discuss sperm banking with his physician before starting chemotherapy.	In males, chemotherapy agents suppress the sperm count, which usually results in permanent sterility. Females experience cessation of menses. Usually, about two months after chemotherapy is stopped menses returns.
5. Advise the female patient against becoming pregnant while taking chemotherapy.	Chemotherapy agents have a teratogenic effect.

NURSING DIAGNOSIS: ALTERATIONS IN BOWEL FUNCTIONING

RELATED TO FACTORS: Adverse effects of chemotherapy

DEFINING CHARACTERISTICS: Reports constipation or diarrhea

PATIENT OUTCOME (collaborative): Demonstrates relief from alterations in bowel function

EVALUATION CRITERIA: Fewer reports of constipation and diarrhea

INTERVENTIONS	RATIONALE
1. Monitor color, consistency, and number of stools.	To identify indications of progress toward or deviations from expected outcome.
2. For constipation: • administer prescribed stool softener. • encourage daily intake of 2–3 liters of fluid. • encourage intake of high-fiber foods (fresh fruits and vegetables, whole grain breads and cereals, prune juice).	To prevent constipation. Fluids and fiber help speed movement of food through the intestines.
3. If no bowel movement occurs in three days, give a laxative. If no results after 24 hours, give an enema.	Cathartic drugs act by increasing the volume of water in feces. Enemas cleanse feces from the bowel.

INTERVENTIONS	RATIONALE
For Diarrhea:	
1. Administer prescribed antidiarrheal agent after each loose stool and evaluate effectiveness.	These agents work by decreasing spasticity of the GI tract.
2. Limit intake of caffeine, high-fiber foods, and milk.	Caffeine is a stimuli that causes increased peristalsis. High-fiber foods create bulk, which causes bowel distention thus stimulating peristalsis. Milk can be gas-forming, which also stimulates peristalsis by bowel distention.
3. Report signs of fluid, bicarbonate, and potassium deficits (see Fluid and Biochemical Imbalances, page 773).	These substances can be rapidly lost in large quantities rapidly with diarrhea.
4. Assist with perineal care after each loose stool. Cleanse with mild soap and water. Apply petroleum jelly or A and D ointment to the anal area, or use Tucks (a commercially prepared wipe containing witch hazel).	These measures promote comfort. Frequent and loose stools are acid that cause anal irritation.
5. Provide a low-residue or liquid diet until diarrhea is under control. Encourage consumption of electrolyte fluids such as Gatorade.	These dietary changes allow the bowel to rest. Gatorade can help replace both fluids and electrolytes lost with persistent diarrhea.
6. Consult physician if diarrhea or constipation persists.	Chemotherapy dosage may need to be reduced.

Radiation Therapy

Radiation is used as a curative or palliative therapy in cancer care. Palliative therapy is done for inoperable tumors to relieve pain and shrink the tumor to relieve compression on adjacent organs.

Radiation therapy can be given internally or externally, depending on the type and site of the cancer. External radiation involves sophisticated machinery to deliver a prescribed voltage of x-ray beam. Megavoltage machines, such as the cobalt-60, which emits gamma rays, and the linear accelerator, which emits electron beams, are widely used.

When the decision to treat the cancer with radiation therapy has been made, the radiation oncologist uses a simulator to accurately define the treatment area when external radiation is used. The area to be treated is then outlined with India ink, leaving a visible mark on the patient's skin.

Radiation can interfere with wound healing. For this reason, it may be done before or after surgery with a recovery period between the two interventions. Internal radiotherapy requires hospitalization. Patients receiving external radiotherapy may be treated on an outpatient basis.

Internal radiation therapy involves the placement of sealed radioactive material within or near the tumor. The radioactive isotope may be implanted by the radiation oncologist in the form of wires, ribbons, tubes, needles, seeds, or capsules depending on the tumor size and location. Internal radiotherapy often is used in the treatment of cancers of the head, neck, cervix, and bladder.

Integrative Care Plans

• Cancer

Discharge Considerations

• Follow-up care
• Skin care for external radiotherapy

ASSESSMENT DATA BASE

1. Perform a general survey (Appendix F) to establish baseline values. An ongoing assessment should look for radiotherapy side effects. Systemic side effects can occur regardless of the area irradiated and include anorexia, nausea, vomiting, malaise, and fatigue. Local side effects are caused by irradiation of tissue and organs that lie within the treatment field.

2. Assess the patient's understanding, concerns, and anxiety level about having radiation therapy.

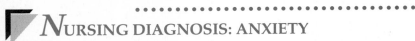

NURSING DIAGNOSIS: ANXIETY

RELATED TO FACTORS: Knowledge deficit about radiation therapy, fear of some aspect of treatment

DEFINING CHARACTERISTICS: May verbalize feelings of nervousness, repetitive questioning, verbalizes lack of understanding, may report fear of some aspect of treatment

PATIENT OUTCOME: Demonstrates relief from anxiety

EVALUATION CRITERIA: Relaxed body posture, reports feeling less nervous about treatment, verbalizes understanding of anticipated side effects

INTERVENTIONS	RATIONALE
1. Provide instructions about radiation therapy including: a. how radiation therapy works. b. anticipated general and specific side effects for the particular area to be irradiated and when side effects are expected to disappear. c. simulation process before initiation of therapy. d. avoid attempting to wash the ink markings between treatments.	A knowledge of what to expect helps lessen anxiety.
2. If possible, arrange for a visit to the radiation department so the patient can see the equipment and meet the staff who will be providing treatment. Assure the patient that he or she will not be radioactive.	To provide feelings of stability and comfort.

INTERVENTIONS	RATIONALE
3. Allow the patient and significant others to express their feelings and concerns about radiation therapy. Clarify any misconceptions.	Verbalizing feelings helps facilitate coping.
4. Encourage rest after treatments.	Malaise and fatigue are anticipated due to bone marrow suppression during therapy.
5. If internal radiation therapy is planned, explain safety precautions that are effective throughout the treatment period (Table 13–2).	

◣ NURSING DIAGNOSIS: HIGH RISK FOR ALTERATIONS IN SKIN INTEGRITY

RELATED TO FACTORS: Radiation therapy

DEFINING CHARACTERISTICS: Erythema with possibly dry or moist desquamation, hair loss and decreased sweating in the irradiated area

PATIENT OUTCOME: Demonstrates no permanent skin damage

EVALUATION CRITERIA: Absence of skin breakdown, healing of damaged areas

INTERVENTIONS	RATIONALE
1. Teach proper skin care. Instructions should include: • Wear loose fitting clothing over the irradiated area. Explain that clothing rubbing against irradiated skin can cause irritation. • Avoid applying lotions containing alcohol to irradiated skin because they have a drying effect. • Remove lotions, creams, and deodorant from the skin **before** radiation treatments to reduce severity of skin irritation.	Teaching self-care measures promotes patient involvement in self-care.

INTERVENTIONS	RATIONALE
• Protect the skin from prolonged exposure to direct sunlight, chlorinated pools, and heat appliances during treatment and for one month after therapy completion because these can dry the skin. • Use a light dusting of cornstarch to treat moist desquamation because it will absorb moisture. Use A and D ointment covered with a nonadherent dressing to treat moist pruritus.	
2. Avoid applying tape to the irradiated area.	To prevent irritation.
3. Avoid use of the term "radiation burn" when explaining a skin reaction. Instead, tell the patient that a "skin reaction," such as redness, may occur.	Use of the term burn implies accidental damage.

. . . .

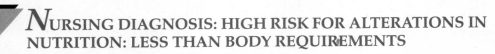

Nursing Diagnosis: High Risk for Alterations in Nutrition: Less Than Body Requirements

RELATED TO FACTORS: Gastric disturbances secondary to radiotherapy

DEFINING CHARACTERISTICS: Reports anorexia; reports altered sense of taste; may report nausea, dyspepsia, dysphagia, or stomach pain following irradiation of neck or abdomen

PATIENT OUTCOME (collaborative): Nutritional status remains stable

EVALUATION CRITERIA: No further weight loss, increased dietary intake, fewer complaints of gastric discomfort

. . . .

INTERVENTIONS	RATIONALE
1. Monitor: • weight weekly • amount of food consumed with each meal	To identify indications of progress toward or deviations from expected outcome.
For Esophagitis:	
1. Encourage use of Viscous Xylocaine about 5–10 minutes before meals. Place the solution in the back of the throat to prevent unnecessary numbing of the tongue and mouth.	Viscous Xylocaine is a topical anesthetic that helps reduce pain and makes swallowing more comfortable.
2. Provide liquid nutritional supplements between meals such as Ensure or Sustacal if oral intake is less than 30%.	These supplements can supply all essential nutrients.
3. Provide a bland, soft or pureed diet high in protein, vitamins, and calories. Instruct the patient to use a blender to convert regularly prepared meals at home to a pureed consistency.	Pureed foods cause less irritation and are easier to swallow. Spicy foods irritate the gastric lining. Proteins and vitamin C are essential for tissue repair.
4. Advise the patient to sit erect when eating.	To prevent gastric reflux into the esophagus.
5. Administer prescribed antacid 30 minutes before or after meals and prn	Antacids neutralize gastric acids.
6. Guaiac coffee-ground emesis and black tarry stools. Notify physician if guaiac is positive.	These findings indicate gastrointestinal bleeding.
For Dysphagia: 1. Instruct the patient to place small amounts of food at the back of the throat and remain erect when eating.	To facilitate swallowing.

INTERVENTIONS	RATIONALE
2. Reassure the patient that esophagitis and dysphagia are temporary and will resolve after therapy is completed.	A knowledge of what to expect helps lessen anxiety. Anxiety can heighten dysphagia.

▶ **N**URSING DIAGNOSIS: HIGH RISK FOR ALTERATIONS IN ORAL MUCOSA: STOMATITIS (SEE PAGE 709)

▶ **N**URSING DIAGNOSIS: HIGH RISK FOR ALTERATIONS IN BOWEL ELIMINATION (SEE PAGE 717)

▶ **N**URSING DIAGNOSIS: HIGH RISK FOR IMPAIRED GAS EXCHANGE

RELATED TO FACTORS: Pneumonitis (see page 713)

▶ **N**URSING DIAGNOSIS: HIGH RISK FOR DISTURBANCE IN SELF-CONCEPT

RELATED TO FACTORS: Alopecia and altered sexual functioning (see page 716)

▶ **N**URSING DIAGNOSIS: PAIN

RELATED TO FACTORS: Cystitis (see page 712)

Immobility

Immobility means total inability or limited ability to move the whole body or a body part. When movement of the whole body is limited or impaired, adverse effects can occur, which affect almost every system in the body.

ASSESSMENT DATA BASE

1. Presence of conditions commonly associated with immobility:
   - bedrest
   - mechanical devices (traction, cast, restraints)
   - amputation of an extremity
   - generalized weakness caused by impaired cardiopulmonary functioning
   - degenerative neuromuscular diseases (multiple sclerosis, myasthenia gravis)
   - intractable pain due to chronic degenerative, inflammatory, or infectious process of bones or joints (arthritis, osteomyelitis)
   - paralysis caused by impaired sensorimotor transmission (spinal cord injury, brain tumor)

2. Assess functional ability. Rate activities of daily living (ADL) from dependence to independence: bathing, feeding self, dressing, getting in and out of bed, moving self in bed, control of bowel and bladder, toileting, walking, hygienic care.

NURSING DIAGNOSIS: HIGH RISK FOR COMPLICATIONS: DISUSE OSTEOPOROSIS, JOINT STIFFNESS, MUSCLE ATROPHY, CONTRACTURES, CONSTIPATION, HYPOSTATIC PNEUMONIA, ORTHOSTATIC HYPOTENSION, VENOUS THROMBOSIS, RENAL CALCULI, SKIN BREAKDOWN

RELATED TO FACTORS: Impaired physical mobility secondary to (specify deficit).

DEFINING CHARACTERISTICS: Observation of limited range-of-motion, impaired coordination, prescribed bedrest, reports inability to move extremity

PATIENT OUTCOME (collaborative): Demonstrates no complications from impaired physical mobility

EVALUATION CRITERIA: Observation of joint flexibility, passage of a soft formed stool, clear lung sounds, absence of falls, absence of manifestations of venous thrombosis, denies void discomfort, intact skin

• •

INTERVENTIONS	RATIONALE
General:	
1. Monitor general status (Appendix F) q8h.	To identify indications of progress toward or deviations from expected outcome.
Disuse Osteoporosis, Joint Stiffness, Muscle Atrophy, Contractures:	
1. Provide passive range-of-motion (ROM) exercises q2h if the patient is unable to perform active ROM. Encourage the patient to use the unaffected extremity to exercise the affected extremity. Remove restraints q2h to exercise limbs and to inspect the skin for signs of irritation.	Passive ROM helps maintain joint flexibility. Active ROM exercises help maintain joint flexibility and muscle tone.
2. Allow the patient to do as much as possible for self.	Performing self-care helps exercise joints and muscles and maintains sense of independence.
3. Refer the patient to physical therapy for gait training or a planned exercise program as ordered.	A physical therapist is a rehabilitation specialist in musculoskeletal deficits and can plan an exercise program that reflects the patient's potential for recovery.
4. When ambulation is allowed, provide assistance as needed. If the patient has an order to be out of bed, ensure the patient gets out of bed.	Bone needs the stress and strain of weight bearing to stimulate calcium uptake. Demineralization of bone occurs with disuse that predisposes bones to fracture. Increasing calcium intake in the diet or using calcium supplements does not prevent demineralization from immobility.

INTERVENTIONS	RATIONALE
5. Maintain affected extremity in proper alignment. Use splints as needed. Use a footboard to prevent foot-drop, especially with paralysis or traction of the lower extremity.	Muscle strain is reduced when body parts are kept in proper alignment. Disuse coupled with overstretching of muscles contributes to muscle weakness.
6. Administer prescribed analgesic before activity as needed.	Pain further limits movement.
7. Plan rest periods throughout the day if chronic fatigue limits movement.	Rest allows the body to replenish energy stores.

Constipation:

1. Monitor daily for passage and consistency of stool.	To identify indications of progress toward or deviations from expected outcome.
2. Administer prescribed laxative if no bowel movement occurs in three days. If no bowel movement results from laxative in 24 hours, administer prescribed enema. Suggest a daily stool softener if persistent passage of a hard stool that requires straining occurs.	Decreased activity promotes parasympathetic stimulation, resulting in decreased gastric motility and peristalsis that contributes to anorexia and constipation. Laxatives, enemas, and stool softeners help promote bowel evacuation.
3. Provide a diet high in fiber (prune juice, fresh fruits and vegetables, bran cereals and breads). Consult a dietitian for appropriate meal selection.	Fiber promotes bulk, which helps stimulate bowel evacuation. A dietitian is a nutritional specialist who can assist the patient in planning meals to meet nutritional needs in view of current health status.
4. Encourage daily intake of 2–3 liters of fluid if no history of heart failure or coexisting fluid retention problem.	Fluids help keep the stool soft.

Hypostatic Pneumonia:

1. Encourage use of the incentive spirometer q2h. When possible, place the patient in an upright position for deep breathing, exercises.	An incentive spirometer promotes deep breathing, which helps to prevent atelectasis. An upright position allows fuller lung expansion.

INTERVENTIONS	RATIONALE
2. Reposition q2h.	To allow fuller lung expansion in dependent areas and prevent stasis in one part of the lung.
3. Suction prn if the patient has moist, gurgling respirations coupled with an ineffective cough and depressed level of consciousness.	To clear the airway.

Orthostatic Hypotension:

INTERVENTIONS	RATIONALE
1. Monitor for manifestations of fainting, dizziness, and light-headedness when assisting with ambulation for the first time following prolonged immobility. Allow to dangle and encourage slow deep breathing **before** beginning ambulation.	These findings represent orthostatic hypotension. Changing position slowly prevents the sudden gravitational pooling of blood in the lower extremities that occurs subsequent to a weak vasomotor tone caused by immobility.
2. Elevate head of the bed at least q4h if not contraindicated.	Periodic elevation helps maintain an even distribution of blood.
3. Consult physician if manifestations of orthostatic hypotension persist or worsen.	This can indicate hypovolemia or anemia and a need for further medical evaluation.

Venous Thrombosis:

INTERVENTIONS	RATIONALE
1. Monitor peripheral vascular status (Appendix E) q8h.	To identify indications of progress toward or deviations from expected outcome.
2. Apply antiembolism stockings as ordered. Remove daily to inspect the skin and provide skin care.	These stockings promote venous return by compressing blood vessels in the legs. Stasis of blood in the lower extremities occurs subsequent to decreased vasomotor tone.
3. Encourage active ROM to tolerance.	Venous blood flow is enhanced by contraction of muscles.
4. Ensure daily intake of at least 2–3 liters of fluid.	Dehydration contributes to venous stasis.

INTERVENTIONS	RATIONALE
5. Notify physician if manifestations of thrombophlebitis (page 381) occur. Administer aspirin or low-dose heparin as ordered. Evaluate effectiveness of anticoagulant therapy.	Prophylactic anticoagulant therapy is especially beneficial to persons at risk for thrombus formation (history of heart disease, peripheral vascular disease, long bone fractures). Aspirin prevents platelet adhesion. Heparin prevents formation of fibrin.
Renal Calculi (stones):	
1. Monitor urinalysis report, especially the pH.	To detect the presence of factors that predispose patient to stone formation (crystals, alkaline pH).
2. Encourage a daily fluid intake of at least 2–3 liters if not contraindicated. Reposition q2h. Keep the urine acid by giving cranberry juice daily.	Changing positions prevents pooling of urine in the renal pelvis that promotes crystalization, especially in the presence of increased renal excretion of calcium. Fluids help flush the kidneys. Cranberry juice promotes an acid urine, reducing the risk of stone formation.
Skin Breakdown:	
1. Evaluate condition of skin, especially bony prominences. Determine stage of skin breakdown, if present, according to facility protocol and procedures: • Stage I — reddened area • Stage II — blister, skin break • Stage III — skin break exposing subcutaneous tissue • Stage IV — skin break exposing muscle and bone	Redness indicates impaired circulation. Constant pressure to the skin obstructs blood vessels, which can causes tissue hypoxia. Bony prominences experience the most pressure. Skin care measures vary depending on the stage of skin breakdown.
2. Implement measures following facility protocol and procedures to prevent skin breakdown that can include: • repositioning and providing ROM exercises q2h • massaging redden areas and applying a skin protector (extra padding)	Changing positions relieves pressure on dependent areas. Exercise and massage promote circulation. Special pressure relieving mattresses allow the weight of the patient's body to be redistributed.

INTERVENTIONS	RATIONALE
• applying a pressure relieving mattress to the bed (water mattress, air mattress, eggcrate mattress), or using a special flotation bed such as the Clinitron or RotoRest bed, especially for paralysis of the lower extremities	
3. Provide an adequate dietary intake of foods high in protein and vitamins.	Protein and vitamin C are essential for tissue repair.
4. Keep the skin clean and dry. Apply a moisturizer to excessively dry skin areas.	Clean, dry, supple skin is less likely to breakdown.

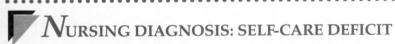

NURSING DIAGNOSIS: SELF-CARE DEFICIT

RELATED TO FACTORS: Impaired physical mobility

DEFINING CHARACTERISTICS: Requests assistance with activities of daily living (ADL), observation of poor hygiene

PATIENT OUTCOME: Demonstrates lifestyle changes to meet ADL

EVALUATION CRITERIA: Participates in self-care within context of physical capabilities, requests assistance when needed, observation of a well-groomed appearance, verbalizes ADL are being met

INTERVENTIONS	RATIONALE
1. Ensure call bell is always within the patient's reach. Arrange requested items on the bedside table for easy access.	To ensure patient safety.
2. Assist with ADL as needed. Encourage the patient to do as much as possible for self.	Self-care helps maintain self-esteem and promotes return to independent living.

INTERVENTIONS	RATIONALE
3. Refer to occupational therapy department if permanent or long-term physical impairments are likely.	An occupational therapist is a specialist who can assist the patient in learning how to adapt lifestyle to accommodate physical limitations and who can determine appropriate assistive devices if needed.
4. Consult social services or discharge planning department to arrange for home care services or placement in an extended care facility as needed.	To provide continuity of care in the presence of a chronic or permanent physical impairment.
5. Offer praise for accomplishments and progress.	To motivate the patient to continually comply with the prescribed rehabilitation program.

NURSING DIAGNOSIS: DIVERSIONAL ACTIVITY DEFICIT

RELATED TO FACTORS: Impaired physical mobility

DEFINING CHARACTERISTICS: Verbalizes boredom, makes requests for something to do to pass time

PATIENT OUTCOME: Demonstrates relief from decreased stimulation

EVALUATION CRITERIA: Fewer reports of feeling bored, initiates appropriate coping measures

INTERVENTIONS	RATIONALE
1. Plan diversional activities based on the patient's preference and physical limitations (painting, reading, needle work, television, radio, puzzles, crafts).	Sensory deprivation occurs when the environment lacks sufficient stimuli to maintain psychological well-being.
2. Encourage visits from family and friends.	To promote social interaction.

INTERVENTIONS	RATIONALE
3. Provide a clock and calendar.	To maintain orientation.
4. When possible, allow patient to assist in planning daily activities.	To promote a sense of control over self.
5. If possible, provide a change of scenery (place patient near a window, transport to day room).	A variety of activities helps promote sensory stimulation.
6. Allow the patient to express feelings about limitations imposed by condition.	Verbalizing feelings helps promote coping.

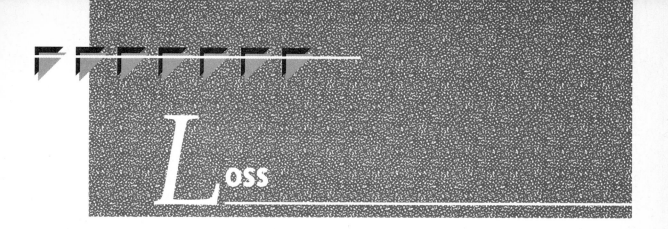

LOSS

The concept of loss refers to something that an individual had in the past. It may be actual or perceived. Grief is a normal reaction to loss. Because people invest emotions in their body and its well-being, internal or external changes that prevent individuals from pursuing their normal or usual activities often evoke emotional and behavioral manifestations of grief. Changes in personal, professional, and social relationships also precipitate grief.

Psychological movement through the grief process allows individuals to reintegrate the new body image and self-concept. Often with loss caused by altered body image (mastectomy, amputation, stoma, hysterectomy), the reality of the situation may not be apparent to the individual until after the surgery. When loss occurs, both the patient and significant others grieve the loss. Each may be at a different phase and progress through the grief process at different rates.

ASSESSMENT DATA BASE

1. Determine the source of loss:
   - death
   - chronic illness requiring lifestyle changes
   - surgical removal of an external body part
   - changes in body function caused by surgical removal of an internal meaningful body organ
   - permanent change in mental acuity

2. Assess patient's and significant others response to the loss. Look for clues reflecting the phase of the grief process:
   - Shock and confusion — may report difficulty concentrating, verbal statements such as "No, this can't be true," "No, this can't be happening to me."
   - Denial — avoids talking about the illness, verbalizes disability, displays a superficial cheerful attitude, noncompliant with prescribed therapeutic plan, may refuse to look at or touch surgical site, uses inappropriate terms to address illness or altered body image.
   - Depression — crying, sadness, verbal statements of guilt or embarrassment, indecisiveness, impaired concentration, irritability, mood swings from cheerfulness to crying to

constant complaining and demanding, withdrawal from social activities, self-disparagement characterized by statements such as "I'm not good enough.", lack of involvement in self-care.

- Bargaining — verbalizes "If only I could have."
- Dependency — reports inability do simple tasks or make decisions.
- Anger — verbalizes "Why me?"
- Acceptance — verbalizes statements reflecting realistic plans, begins to show interest in people and self, acknowledges chronic illness or physical limitations, talks about the effect of current condition on lifestyle and relationships with significant others, uses appropriate terms to refer to condition ("cancer," "tumor," or "stoma").

3. Inquire about the need for spiritual support.

4. Assess for factors that may prevent the patient from directing own life (inadequate support systems, decreased physical endurance, financial constraints, impaired mobility). Ask the patient, "What has your current condition prevented you from doing? Were you able to do those things before you developed the current health problem?"

▶ NURSING DIAGNOSIS: DISTURBANCE IN SELF-CONCEPT

RELATED TO FACTORS: Actual or perceived loss (specify)

DEFINING CHARACTERISTICS: May verbalize fear of death, incapacitation, pain, abandonment, loss of self-esteem, or disturbance in family relationships; may report shame, worthlessness; may verbalize suicidal ideation

PATIENT OUTCOME: Demonstrates acceptance of self in current situation

EVALUATION CRITERIA: Increased participation in self-care, verbalizes realistic lifestyle plans that incorporate present lifestyle changes, verbalizes positive statements about self

INTERVENTIONS	RATIONALE
1. Allow the patient and significant others to express feelings.	Verbalizing feelings facilitates coping and also allows the caregiver to identify which phase of the grief process the patient is experiencing.
2. If condition is terminal and approaching end-stage, discuss hospice care.	Hospice is a program of care aimed at meeting the social, emotional, physical, and spiritual needs of dying patients and their families. A multidisciplinary team of healthcare workers and community volunteers are involved in hospice care.

INTERVENTIONS	RATIONALE
3. Avoid bombarding the patient with information during early phases of the grief process. Answer specific questions. Include additional information and instructions as the patient begins to show readiness to learn self-care measures. Use a "one-day-at-a-time" approach.	Therapeutic interaction can help move the individual to acceptance. Information overload can further increase anxiety that can cause frustration and depression.
4. For alterations in body image that affect a person's ability to resume previous work, refer to a vocational counselor for assistance in exploring other employment training options.	Emotional responses to a chronic illness or altered body image often inhibit the individual from exploring all possible career options.
5. Provide the patient and family with a telephone number of a person to contact for support on discharge. Help the patient's family deal with the patient's grief response. Inform them of behavioral reactions that commonly occur in response to grief. Tell family members that it is not unusual for them to feel threatened or inadequate in handling the patient's reactions to loss. Remind them that the patient now sees and experiences the world from a different perspective. Tell family that they must accept the patient as he/she presents self now.	A strong support system such as the family is essential to helping the patient progress through the grief process. The family that understands grief reactions and knows how to respond appropriately can assist the patient in accepting the condition and outcomes.
6. Inform the patient and significant others that their feelings are normal and that it takes time to accept and live with the outcomes of a chronic illness or altered body image. Avoid analyzing or criticizing the patient's behavior. Inform the patient that you are available to talk when needed.	During the grief process, patients generally react but do not understand why they feel and act as they do. Moreover, the patient's feelings are influenced by immediate caregivers and significant others.

INTERVENTIONS	RATIONALE
7. When the patient is in denial, accept this without reinforcing denial. Refrain from arguing with the patient and overloading patient with reality. Gradually raise questions or reply with a doubtful voice to convey reality.	This approach shows acceptance of the patient and opens the door for the patient to feel comfortable in honest expression of feelings.
8. During the anger and bargaining phase of grief: • **DO NOT:** — argue with patient — moralize — force your values and beliefs on patient — take patient's reactions personally • **DO:** — listen to patient without becoming defensive — allow patient to express anger — provide honest answers but avoid giving false reassurance — be patient	A calm, accepting attitude from caregivers helps diffuse anger and shows support.
9. Offer praise for expressing feelings. Direct the patient to community support groups as indicated.	Continued support is essential to promote progress toward acceptance.
10. When the patient begins to ask questions about treatments and asks to assist in self-care, provide more instructions and information about self-care activities to prepare for discharge home. Repeat instructions as often as opportunity arises.	This indicates acceptance and that the patient is ready to learn. Repetition facilitates learning.
11. Assist the patient with planning ways to overcome self-perceived obstacles by focusing on health strengths. Begin by identifying areas of self-control.	Adaptation to a loss can be facilitated by capitalizing on health strengths rather than focusing on weaknesses.

INTERVENTIONS	RATIONALE
12. Keep the family informed about the patient's progress. Involve the family frequently in the patient's care throughout hospitalization not only on discharge.	To help the patient reintegrate the new body image.
13. Encourage the patient to do as much as possible for self in view of current health status. Offer praise for each successfully completed task.	To facilitate adaptation to health status and to promote independence.
14. When possible allow the patient to make choices in self-care, routines in hygienic care, or sequence of care.	To promote a sense of self-control.
15. Following disclosure of a terminal diagnosis by the physician, remain with the patient and show acceptance of the patient's feelings and reactions. Encourage the patient to express feelings by using simple statements such as "This must be a very hard time for you now," or "What are some of your concerns right now."	A diagnosis of an incurable illness creates feelings of isolation, helplessness, and fear. Remaining with the patient shows support and concern.
16. Help the patient view the chronic illness or altered body image as a challenge for growth rather than an impossible situation. Use the term "physically challenged" rather than disability. If a terminal illness exits, emphasize that research for a cure is continual. Avoid giving false reassurance.	False reassurance thwarts the individual's need for expression of feelings. Exploring the positive outcomes of the situation helps foster hope.
17. Initiate a psychiatric referral as ordered if necessary.	Professional help may be necessary to help the patient who shows maladaptation, such as prolonged denial, social withdrawal, regression, neurosis, psychosis.

Preoperative and Postoperative Care

During the preoperative period, the focus is on ensuring the patient is physiologically and psychologically stable to withstand the stress of surgery. Routine preoperative laboratory assessments include CBC, urinalysis, EKG (if over age 40), and coagulation studies (if potential for bleeding is high). Because considerable blood loss sometimes occurs, type and crossmatch studies also can be done. As prevention against postoperative infection, IV antibiotics can be given just before surgery.

General preoperative preparation can include:

- giving preanesthetic medication to provide sedation and facilitate relaxation and induction.
- showering with an antimicrobial solution, such as povidone-iodine (Betadine), the evening of and the morning of surgery to reduce the number of transient bacteria on the skin.
- allowing nothing by mouth (NPO) after midnight the evening of surgery to reduce the risk of vomiting and aspiration while under anesthesia.
- shaving the operative area, which can be done in holding area.
- initiating IV therapy to provide vascular access for administration of medications or anesthesia, which can be done in the holding area.
- applying antiembolism stockings as a prophylaxis against thrombophlebitis, especially for extensive surgical procedures.

Postoperatively, the patient is kept in the recovery area until stable, usually for about 1–2 hours, depending on the extent of surgery. The patient returns to the medical/surgical unit with:

- IV solution
- wound dressing
- possibly wound drainage device, e.g. Jackson-Pratt, Hemovac, or Portovac

The patient remains NPO until peristalsis returns. When peristalsis returns, a clear liquid diet is allowed and is later advanced to a regular diet, according to the patient's tolerance. Prophylactic IV antibiotics are often prescribed for a few days. Ambulation begins the first postoperative day. The wound drainage device is removed when drainage is scant. Daily dressing changes are then started. Deep breathing using an incentive spirometer is usually initiated in the recovery room.

Integrative Care Plans

- IV Therapy
- Pain
- Fluid and biochemical imbalances

Discharge Considerations

- Follow-up care
- Wound care
- Signs and symptoms requiring medical attention
- Measures to prevent constipation
- Activity restrictions
- Medications for home use

THE PREOPERATIVE PERIOD

ASSESSMENT DATA BASE

1. Assess understanding of operative procedure and its outcomes using a simple statement such as "What has your physician told you about the surgery?"
2. Physical examination based on a general survey (Appendix F) to establish baseline values.
3. Assess the patient's feelings and concerns about the surgery using simple statements such as, "How do you feel about having surgery?" or "What concerns do you have about your surgery?"
4. Check results of preoperative laboratory studies.
5. Inquire about the availability of support system at home to provide assistance after discharge.

NURSING DIAGNOSIS: ANXIETY

RELATED TO FACTORS: Knowledge deficit about preoperative and postoperative events, fear of some aspect of surgery

DEFINING CHARACTERISTICS: May verbalize fear of some aspect of surgery, requests information, reports feeling nervous or anxious, tense body posture and facial expression, may talk excessively

PATIENT OUTCOME: Demonstrates relief from anxiety

EVALUATION CRITERIA: Verbalizes understanding of preoperative and postoperative events, fewer reports of feeling anxious or nervous, relaxed facial expression, less talkative

INTERVENTIONS	RATIONALE
1. Explain what happens during the preoperative and postoperative periods, including preoperative laboratory tests, skin preparation, reason for NPO status, preoperative medication, holding area activities, recovery room stay, and postoperative course. Inform the patient that pain medication is available as needed to control pain. Advise the patient to request pain medication before pain becomes severe.	A knowledge of what to expect helps lessen anxiety and promotes patient cooperation during recovery. Maintaining a consistent blood level of the analgesic provides the best pain control.
2. Teach and have the patient practice: • deep breathing • turning • getting out of bed • splinting the surgical site when coughing If available use an audiovisual program for the specific surgery.	To promote patient involvement in self-care.
3. Allow the patient and significant others to express feelings about the surgical experience. Correct any misconceptions. Refer specific questions about the surgery to the surgeon.	Expressing feelings helps promote coping and allows the caregiver to identify misconceptions that can be the source of the fear. Significant others are a support system for the individual. To be effective, a support system must have strong coping mechanisms.
4. Complete activities on the preoperative checklist (Appendix K). Notify physician of abnormalities in preoperative laboratory test results.	A checklist ensures all required activities are completed. These activities are designed to ensure the patient is physiologically prepared for surgery thus reducing the risk of delayed recovery.
5. Reinforce the physician's explanation.	Repetition enhances learning.
6. If patient is currently taking routine medications, consult physician to determine medications that should be withheld.	

THE POSTOPERATIVE PERIOD

 ## ASSESSMENT DATA BASE

1. On receiving the patient:
   - perform a routine postoperative assessment (Appendix L)

• •

 ## NURSING DIAGNOSIS: PAIN

RELATED TO FACTORS: Surgery

DEFINING CHARACTERISTICS: Verbalizes discomfort, moaning, frowning, tense body posture

PATIENT OUTCOME (collaborative): Demonstrates relief from discomfort.

EVALUATION CRITERIA: Denies pain, relaxed body posture, absence of moaning

• •

INTERVENTIONS	RATIONALE
1. See Pain (page 700).	
2. If intramuscular analgesic is prescribed, administer the analgesic on a routine basis during the first 24 hours instead of waiting for the patient to request it.	Maintaining a consistent blood level of the analgesic provides the best pain control.
3. Notify physician if the analgesic fails to provide sufficient pain relief.	This can indicate the need to change the dosage, interval, or type of analgesic. Also, it can indicate a complication, such as bleeding into the operative site.

• •

 ## NURSING DIAGNOSIS: HIGH RISK FOR COMPLICATIONS: ATELECTASIS, PARALYTIC ILEUS, DEHISCENCE, INFECTION, FLUID AND BIOCHEMICAL DEFICITS, THROMBOPHLEBITIS

RELATED TO FACTORS: Surgery

DEFINING CHARACTERISTICS: May show early manifestations of complications, observation of postsurgical incision

PATIENT OUTCOME (collaborative): Demonstrates no complications

EVALUATION CRITERIA: Absence of infection, clear breath sounds, absence of hemorrhage, wound heals, discharged within LOS for DRG

INTERVENTIONS	RATIONALE
Atelectasis: 1. Monitor lung sounds q4h x 24 hours then q8h, especially among persons at risk for postoperative atelectasis (smokers, the elderly, and persons with chronic lung disease).	To identify indications of progress toward or deviations from expected outcome.
2. Encourage use of the incentive spirometer q2h. If adventitious lung sounds are detected, increase frequency of use to qh. Ensure patient uses the device properly. Explain purpose of the device.	The incentive spirometer promotes deep breathing that helps expand alveoli thus preventing atelectasis.
3. Reposition q2h. Allow the patient to do as much as possible. Ambulate as ordered.	Activity stimulates deep breathing.
4. Ensure pain is controlled.	Individuals resort to shallow rapid respirations when experiencing severe pain, which in turn restricts full expansion of the alveoli.
Paralytic Ileus: 1. Monitor: • nasogastric (N/G) tube drainage (color and amount) q8h if N/G tube is present • abdominal status (auscultate bowel sounds, inquire about passage of flatus) q8h	To identify indications of progress toward or deviations from expected outcomes.

INTERVENTIONS	RATIONALE
2. Notify physician if cessation of bowel sounds accompanied by progressive abdominal distention, nausea, vomiting, or increased discomfort occur. Keep the patient NPO. Obtain abdominal x ray as ordered. Insert an N/G tube and connect to intermittent suction as ordered. Maintain tube patency by irrigating prn or allow ice chips by mouth sparingly.	These findings indicate paralytic ileus caused by interference with neuromuscular stimulation as a result of manipulation of the intestines (following abdominal surgery) or a side effect of anesthesia and analgesia. An abdominal x ray confirms a paralytic ileus. Gastric decompression with an N/G tube allows the bowel to rest.
3. Measure and record abdominal circumference q8h if abdominal distention is suspected.	To obtain objective data.
4. Resume oral feedings when bowel sounds return, flatus is passed, and abdominal distention lessens.	These findings indicate return of peristalsis and normal bowel function.

Dehiscence:

INTERVENTIONS	RATIONALE
1. Monitor appearance of wound edges during each dressing change.	To identify indications of progress toward or deviations from expected outcome.
2. Have the patient splint the abdominal incision when coughing.	To prevent strain on the suture line.
3. If dehiscence (wound separation) occurs, cover the incision with a sterile dressing moistened with a saline solution to protect the area. Notify physician.	Moisture protects the tissue from drying.
4. Provide wound care as ordered, using strict aseptic technique.	Wound infection is the most common cause of dehiscence.

Infection:

INTERVENTIONS	RATIONALE
1. Monitor: • temperature q4h • appearance of wound when performing wound care • results of CBC reports, particularly leukocyte count (WBC)	To identify indications of progress toward or deviations from expected outcome.

INTERVENTIONS	RATIONALE
2. If temperature rises to 99°F within 48 hours, initiate aggressive pulmonary toileting qh and increase oral fluid intake, if not contraindicated. Notify physician if temperature rises above 101°F.	A temperature above normal within the first 48 hours indicates the beginning of atelectasis, whereas after the fifth postoperative day it indicates a wound infection or infection somewhere else. Fever is a temperature of 101°F or greater.
3. Administer prescribed antibiotics. Provide at least two liters of fluid daily while on antibiotic therapy.	Antibiotic therapy is required to prevent and resolve an infection. Fluids help distribute medication to body tissue.
4. Change dressing prn as ordered, using aseptic technique.	A moist dressing provides a culture medium for bacterial growth. Following aseptic technique reduces the risk of bacterial contamination.
5. Notify physician of the following findings: wound appears red with purulent drainage, separation of wound edges, wound extremely tender, and leukocyte count above normal. Obtain a wound specimen for culture and sensitivity (C&S) test.	These findings indicate wound infection. A culture helps identify the infective organism so appropriate antibiotic therapy can be prescribed. A senstivity report identifies which antibiotics are most effective in destroying the causative organism.
6. Administer prescribed antipyretic if fever exists.	Antipyretic agents reset the thermostatic mechanism in the brain to resolve fever.
7. Provide perineal care twice a day according to facility protocol and procedures while the Foley catheter is in place. After the catheter is removed, report any problems with voiding (burning, pain, dribbling, urgency, frequency with small quantities).	Cleansing the genitalia helps reduce the number of transient bacteria. Damage to the urinary sphincter and infection are the major problems associated with an indwelling bladder catheter.
8. If frequent dressing changes are required, use Montgomery straps.	To prevent skin irritation from frequent tape removal.
9. Follow universal precautions (good handwashing before and after patient care, wearing gloves when contact with blood or body fluid is likely to occur) when providing patient care.	Surgical patients are at risk for infection because the stress of surgery weakens their immune system. Special protective measures help reduce the risk of a nosocomial infection. Caregivers are the most common source of nosocomial infections. These precautions protect patients and caregivers.

INTERVENTIONS	RATIONALE
Fluid and Biochemical Deficits:	
1. See Fluid and Biochemical Imbalances (page 773).	Antibiotic therapy is required to prevent and resolve an infection. Fluids help distribute of medication to body tissue.
2. Keep intake and output on all patients x 48 hours and on all patients receiving IV fluid. If no Foley catheter is in place, ensure the patient voids. Notify physician of complaints of the inability to void despite the urge, suprapubic distention, or not voiding within 6–8 hours with adequate fluid intake. Catheterize as ordered.	A comparison of intake and output provides objective data about fluid status and kidney function. These findings indicate acute urinary retention. Nerves used in voiding can be inhibited by narcotic analgesics and general anesthesia in postoperative patients. Catheterization allows the bladder to empty.
Thrombophlebitis:	
1. Monitor circulation in the lower extremities q8h until ambulation begins: pedal pulses, Homan's sign, calf tenderness, capillary refill, color, and temperature.	To identify indications of progress toward or deviations from expected outcome.
2. Apply antiembolism stockings as ordered. Remove twice daily to inspect skin and apply lotion.	These stockings promote venous return, preventing venous stasis.
3. Encourage range-of-motion exercises while in bed q2h. When ambulation begins, ensure the patient engages in progressive ambulation at least three times daily (t.i.d.).	Exercise stimulates circulation.
Hemorrhage:	
1. Monitor: • BP, pulse, and respiration q4h • output from the wound drainage device, if present, q8h • general status (Appendix F) q8h	To identify indications of progress toward or deviations from expected outcome.
2. Reapply suction to the wound drainage device after emptying.	This device helps prevent hematoma formation.

INTERVENTIONS	RATIONALE
3. Notify physician if wound drainage is bright red and continually increases.	Normally, wound drainage is between 50–100 mL per 24 hours and is dark serosanguineous. It should gradually decrease.
4. If wound dressing becomes saturated often with bright red drainage, reinforce dressing, keep patient on bedrest, and notify physician.	This can indicate hemorrhage, especially in the absence of a penrose drain.

◢ NURSING DIAGNOSIS: SELF-CARE DEFICIT (SPECIFY)

RELATED TO FACTORS: Limited physical mobility secondary to surgery.

DEFINING CHARACTERISTICS: Requests assistance with some aspect of ADL (feeding, bathing dressing, grooming, toileting, ambulating)

PATIENT OUTCOME: Demonstrates that ADL needs are met

EVALUATION CRITERIA: Identifies areas of need, verbalizes ADL are met

INTERVENTIONS	RATIONALE
1. Determine degree of assistance needed. Provide assistance with ADL as needed. Allow the patient to do as much as possible for self.	To promote independence.
2. Allow sufficient time for the patient to accomplish the activity.	Rushing the patient through an activity causes frustration.
3. Instruct the patient in necessary adaptations to accomplish ADL. Begin with a familiar task that is easily accomplished and then progress to more difficult ones. Offer praise for each accomplishment.	To promote independence. Praise motivates for continued learning.
4. Keep call bell within reach.	To promote safety.

NURSING DIAGNOSIS: HIGH RISK FOR IMPAIRED HOME MAINTENANCE MANAGEMENT

RELATED TO FACTORS: Knowledge deficit about self-care on discharge

DEFINING CHARACTERISTICS: Verbalizes lack of understanding, requests information, observation of inability to perform required self-care procedures, reports lack of support system at home

PATIENT OUTCOME: Demonstrates willingness to comply with self-care activities on discharge

EVALUATION CRITERIA: Verbalizes understanding of instructions, correctly performs required self-care skills, identifies areas of need

INTERVENTIONS	RATIONALE
1. Ensure the patient has written instructions for self-care and a written appointment for follow-up visits.	Verbal instructions may be easily forgotten.
2. Teach and have the patient practice wound care if dressing changes will be required at home. Stress the importance of handwashing before and after wound care.	Practice helps patient develop confidence in self-care. Also, it allows the caregiver an opportunity to evaluate the patient's ability to perform the skill independently and to determine if assistance will be required. Measures to prevent infection must be continued until the wound completely heals.
3. Evaluate needs for home care assistance and availability of an adequate support system to provide needed assistance. Contact the social services discharge planning or department to arrange for home care assistance if the patient requires assistance with a required skill but has no support system at home.	Social services or discharge planners serve as a vital link for patient transition to the home environment or extended care facility to ensure continued recovery or rehabilitation.
4. Instruct the patient to notify physician if wound infection occurs: redness, increased tenderness, drainage, fever.	Antibiotic therapy is required to resolve infections.

INTERVENTIONS	RATIONALE
5. Ensure the patient has sufficient supplies for wound care and a prescription for analgesic.	Preparation is essential to reduce anxiety commonly associated with discharge, especially when continued care is required. An analgesic ensures comfort and promotes sleep.
6. Instruct the patient to rest throughout the day, to gradually resume activities to tolerance, and to avoid heavy lifting and overexertion.	Surgery is a stressor.

TABLE 13–1. Protective Care Measures
For Decreased WBC (1,000/mm³ or less)

1. Wear a mask when in contact with the patient.

2. Wash hands before and after patient care contact.

3. Restrict number of visitors.

4. Place in a private room with door closed.

5. Change bed linen daily.

6. Monitor:
   - temperature q4h
   - results of CBC reports
   - lung sounds q8h
   - oral cavity for inflammation daily

7. Give antipyretic as ordered. Use acetaminophen instead of aspirin.

8. Avoid rectal temperatures and IM injections if possible.

9. Change IV sites at the earliest signs of phlebitis.

10. Administer prescribed prophylactic antibiotics.

11. Provide a bath daily and perineal care twice daily to decrease transient bacteria on the skin.

12. Administer granulocyte or leukocyte transfusions as ordered.

13. Post a "Protective Care" sign on door.

TABLE 13–2. Precautions For Internal Radiation Source

Three major factors in radiation protection are time, distance, and shielding. Precautions to observe based on these three factors are:

1. Avoid being assigned to more than one patient with an internal radioactive source.

2. Plan nursing care to spend as little time as possible in close contact with patient.

3. Wear a film badge obtained from radiology department.

4. Post a radiation warning sign on patient's door.

5. Place patient in a private room with doors closed.

6. Eliminate bed bath until radioactive source is removed.

7. Ensure patient has an electric self-adjusting bed.

8. Work quickly to accomplish necessary bedside activities.

9. Avoid being assigned to care for patients with internal radiation if pregnant.

10. Always keep long-handled forceps and a shielded transport container (obtained from the radiology department) in patient's room to use if implant becomes dislodged.

11. Allow no visitors or housekeeping personnel in room.

12. Prepare the meal tray outside patient's room.

13. Plan diversional activities **before** the implant (reading, television).

14. Keep bed linen in room until implant is removed.

15. Notify radiation safety officer if implant becomes dislodged. Avoid touching implant.

BIBLIOGRAPHY

AIDS Guide For Health Care Workers. (1992). Atlanta: American Health Consultants Inc.

Anastasi, J.K., & Rivera, J.L. (1991). AIDS drug update: DDI and DDC. **RN, 54,** 41–43.

Baker, W.L. (1990). Postoperative problems: Current nursing management. **Critical Care Nursing Clinics of North America, 2,** xvii–610.

Barrick, B. (1988). Caring for AIDS patients. **Nursing 88,** 18, 50–59.

Blair, K.A. (1990). Aging: Physiological aspects and clinical implications. **Nurse Practitioner, 15,** 14–16, 18, 23, 26–28.

Campbell, A., & Johnston, C.A. (1991). OR/PACU reports: What they should tell you about your postoperative patient. **Nursing, 21,** 49–51.

Cawley, M.M. (1990). Recent advances in chemotherapy: Administration and nursing implications. **Nursing Clinics of North America, 25,** 377–391.

Camp-Sorrell, D. (1991). How to control chemotherapy adverse effects. **Nursing 91,** 21, 34–41.

Curry, L.C., & Stone, J.G. (1991). The grief process: A preparation for death. **Clinical Nurse Specialist, 5,** 17–22.

Gudlatte, M. (1989). Managing an implanted infusion device. **RN, 52,** 45–49.

Katzin, L. (1990). Chronic illness and sexuality. **American Journal of Nursing, 90,** 54–59.

Kelly, P. (1992). Counseling patients with HIV. **RN, 55,** 54–58.

Lorenz, E.W. (1991). **St. Anthony's DRG Working Guidebook,** Alexandria: St. Anthony's Publishing Company.

Michels, K.A. (1991). Centers for Disease Control release new AIDS guidelines. **AANAJ, 59,** 305–308.

Olson, E.V. (1990h. The hazards of immobility. **American Journal of Nursing, 90,** 43, 46–48.

Sallstrom, J.F. (1991). Psychosocial considerations in adult cancer patients. **Physician Assistant, 15,** 27–28, 37–38, 40.

C

HAPTER FOURTEEN
Problems of the Integumentary System

Burns
IV Therapy
Shock
Fluid and Biochemical Imbalance
References

B urns

Burns disrupt skin integrity, predisposing a person to a multitude of problems especially if the burn is extensive. The American Burn Association recommends inpatient treatment for all burns except:

• superficial burns

• adults with partial thickness burns less than 15% body surface area (BSA) involvement

• children and the elderly with partial thickness burns less than 5% BSA involvement

• persons with full thickness burns less than 2% BSA involvement

Flame burns of the head, neck, and thorax are always treated on an inpatient basis regardless of the BSA involvement because of the risk of inhalation injury.

Major complications associated with extensive burn injury are septicemia, contractures, hypertrophic scarring, protein-calorie deficits, and cardiopulmonary and renal failure.

General Medical Management

1. The first priority in treating burns is to stop the burning process. This involves first-aid intervention at the scene:

   • For thermal (flame) burns, "stop, drop, and roll." Cover the person with a blanket and roll to smother the flames. Apply cool water to reduce the temperature of the wound. (Ice or cold water causes further injury to the compromised tissue.)

   • For chemical (liquid) burns, flush with copious amounts of water to remove the chemical from the skin. For chemical (powder) burns, brush powdered chemical from the skin then flush with water.

   • For electrical burns, turn off the electrical source first before attempting to remove the victim from the hazard.

2. The second priority is establishing a patent airway. For patients with suspected inhalation injury, administer 100 % humidified oxygen at 10 L/min via mask. Use nasotracheal intubation and place on a mechanical ventilator if arterial blood gases show severe hypoxia or hypercapnia despite supplemental oxygen.

3. The third priority is aggressive fluid resuscitation to restore lost plasma volume. Essentially, half of the estimated fluid volume is given the first eight hours postburn, and the other one half is given during the next 16 hours. Types of fluids used include crystalloids, such as lactated Ringer's solution and/or colloids such as albumin or plasma.

4. The fourth priority is burn wound care:

   • daily cleansing and application of a topical antimicrobial cream such as silver sulfadiazine (Silvadene).

   • use of various types of synthetic dressings or biological dressings (skin grafts) especially with full thickness burns.

Integrative Care Plans

• Fluid and biochemical imbalance
• Loss with extensive full thickness burns

Discharge Considerations

• Follow-up care
• Skin care
• Exercises to prevent contracture
• Signs and symptoms requiring medical attention

 # ASSESSMENT DATA BASE

1. Obtain a burn history. Inquire about:

   • cause of the burn — chemical, thermal, or electrical

   • time of burn — important because fluid resuscitation needs are calculated from time of burn injury, not from arrival time at hospital

   • place where injury occurred — open or closed area

   • presence of current medical problems

   • allergies, especially to sulfa since many topical antimicrobials contain sulfa

   • date of last tetanus immunization

   • medications currently taken

2. Perform a general assessment (Appendix F). Obtain a baseline weight.

3. Perform a burn assessment:

   • extent of wound (percentage) using facility method, which may be the Lund and Browder chart or the Rule of Nines

   • depth of wound, which can be:

     a. superficial partial thickness—involves epidermis; characterized by tenderness, slight swelling, and erythema that blanches with pressure

    b. partial thickness — involves epidermis and dermis; characterized by erythema, dry or moist painful wound, edema, and blister formation.

    c. full thickness — involves all skin layers often extending to subcutaneous tissue and muscle; characterized by dry, hard, painless, leathery wounds that are white or black

- Inspect exit wound for electrical burns. These burns have both an entry and exit wound, with the exit wound often more severe than the entry wound.

4. Assess for smoke inhalation injury with flame burns to the face, head, neck, or chest. Look for:

- singed nasal and facial hair
- red buccal mucosa
- pulmonary rales

5. Check results of laboratory studies:

- CBC assesses for hemoconcentration.
- Serum electrolytes detect fluid and biochemical imbalance. It is particularly important to check the potassium for elevations in the initial 24 hours because elevated potassium can cause cardiac arrest.
- Arterial blood gases (ABG) and chest x ray assess pulmonary function, especially with smoke inhalation injury.
- BUN and creatinine assess kidney function.
- Urinalysis reveals myoglobin and hemochromogens signaling muscle damage with extensive full thickness burns.
- Bronchoscopy helps confirm smoke inhalation injury.
- Coagulation studies are clotting factors that may be depleted with massive burns.
- Serum carbon monoxide level is elevated with smoke inhalation injury.

6. Assess the patient's and significant others understanding of treatments, concerns, and feelings about the injury.

Nursing Diagnosis: Alterations in Fluid Volume: Deficit

RELATED TO FACTORS: Extensive burns

DEFINING CHARACTERISTICS: Low BP accompanied by tachycardia and tachypnea, decreased urinary output, thirst, serum hematocrit and sodium above normal range

PATIENT OUTCOME (collaborative): Demonstrates improved fluid and biochemical status

EVALUATION CRITERIA: Absence of manifestations of dehydration, resolution of edema, serum electrolytes within normal range, urine output above 30 mL/hr

INTERVENTIONS	RATIONALE

1. Monitor:
   • vital signs qh during emergent period, q2h during acute period, and q4h during rehabilitation period
   • color of urine
   • intake and output qh during emergent period, q4h during acute period, and q8h during rehabilitation period
   • results of CBC and electrolyte reports
   • weight daily
   • CVP (central venous pressure) qh if required
   • general status (Appendix F) q8h
	To identify indications of progress toward or deviations from expected outcome. The emergent period (initial 48 hours postburn) is a critical period characterized by hypovolemia predisposing a person to inadequate tissue and renal perfusion. Complications are most likely to occur during the acute period, which characterizes the healing phase. The rehabilitative period begins on hospital admission and continues until reentry into society.

2. On admission to the hospital, remove all clothing and jewelry from the burned areas.	For adequate inspection of the wound.
3. Initiate prescribed IV therapy with a large-bore (18-gauge) needle, preferably through skin that has not been burned. If the patient has severe extensive burns and shows symptoms of hypovolemic shock, assist physician with insertion of a central venous catheter for monitoring central venous pressure (CVP).	Rapid fluid replacement is essential to prevent renal failure. Significant fluid loss occurs through burned tissue with extensive burns. Measuring central venous pressure provides objective data about the status of intravascular fluid volume.
4. Notify physician of the following: urine output less than 30 mL/hr, thirst, tachycardia, CVP less than 6 mm Hg, serum bicarbonate below normal range, serum sodium above normal range, restlessness, BP below normal range, dark burgundy or dark amber urine.	These findings indicate hypovolemia and a need for increased fluids. With extensive burns, fluid shifts from the intravascular space to interstitial space, leading to hypovolemia. Also, large amounts of fluid and potassium chloride are lost during the diuretic phase as fluid shifts from interstitial to intravascular spaces. A dark burgundy urine indicates myoglobinuria or hemoglobinuria. A dark amber urine indicates concentrated urine.

INTERVENTIONS	RATIONALE
5. Consult physician if manifestations of fluid excess (page 778) occur.	Patients are susceptible to intravascular volume overload during the recovery period when fluid shifts from the interstitial compartment to the intravascular compartment.
6. Guaiac coffee-ground emesis or black tarry stools. Report positive findings.	A guaiac positive finding indicates GI bleeding. GI bleeding is a sign of stress ulcer (also termed Curling's ulcer).
7. Administer prescribed antacid or histamine receptor antagonist such as cimetidine (Tagamet).	To prevent GI bleeding. Extensive burns predispose patient to stress ulcers caused by increased secretion of adrenal hormones and hydrochloric acid by the stomach.

◤ NURSING DIAGNOSIS: HIGH RISK FOR IMPAIRED GAS EXCHANGE

RELATED TO FACTORS: Smoke inhalation injury or thoracic compartment syndrome secondary to circumferential burns of chest or neck

DEFINING CHARACTERISTICS: Observation of signs of smoke inhalation injury, dyspnea, hypoxia accompanied by hypercapnia

PATIENT OUTCOME (collaborative): Demonstrates adequate oxygenation

EVALUATION CRITERIA: Respiratory rate 12-24 per minute, normal skin color, ABG within normal range, clear breath sounds, denies breathing difficulties

INTERVENTIONS	RATIONALE
For Smoke Inhalation Injury:	
1. Monitor ABG reports and serum carbon monoxide levels.	To identify indications of progress toward or deviations from expected outcome. Smoke inhalation can damage the alveoli, interfering with gas exchange at the capillary-alveoli membrane.

INTERVENTIONS	RATIONALE
2. Administer supplemental oxygen at prescribed level. Insert or assist with endotracheal tube and place patient on a mechanical ventilator as ordered if respiratory insufficiency develops (evidenced by hypoxia, hypercapnia, rales, tachypnea, and change in sensorium).	Supplemental oxygen increases the amount of oxygen available to tissue. Mechanical ventilation is needed to support respiration until the patient can do so independently. Endotracheal intubation is performed by persons with advanced cardiac life support (ACLS) certification, a respiratory therapist, nurse anesthetist, or anesthesiologist.
3. Encourage deep breathing with use of incentive spirometer q2h while on bedrest.	Deep breathing expands the alveoli, reducing risk of atelectasis.
4. Maintain a semi-Fowler's position, if hypotension is not present.	To facilitate ventilation by reducing abdominal pressure against the diaphragm.
5. For a circumferential thoracic burn, notify physician if dyspnea accompanied by tachypnea occurs. Prepare the patient for surgery — escharotomy as ordered.	Circumferential thoracic burns can restrict chest expansion. Slits in the skin (escharotomy) allow for chest expansion.

 NURSING DIAGNOSIS: HIGH RISK FOR INFECTION

RELATED TO FACTORS: Loss of skin integrity caused by burns

DEFINING CHARACTERISTICS: Observation of loss of skin and possibly subcutaneous tissue and muscle

PATIENT OUTCOME (collaborative): Remains free of infection

EVALUATION CRITERIA: Absence of fever, formation of granulation tissue, discharged within LOS for DRG

INTERVENTIONS	RATIONALE
1. Monitor: • appearance of wounds (burned areas, donor site and status of dressing over graft site if skin graft performed) q8h	To identify indications of progress toward or deviations from expected outcome.

INTERVENTIONS	RATIONALE
• temperature q4h • amount of food consumed at each meal	
2. Cleanse the burned areas daily and remove necrotic tissue (debridement) as ordered. Provide a whirlpool bath as ordered. Implement prescribed care for donor site, which can be covered with a Vaseline dressing or Op site.	Cleansing and removing necrotic tissue promote granulation formation.
3. Remove old cream from the wound before applying fresh cream. Wear sterile gloves and apply the prescribed topical antimicrobial cream to the burned areas with fingertips. Apply the cream generously to completely cover the wound.	Topical antimicrobials help prevent infection. Following aseptic principles protects the patient from infection. Denuded skin provides a good culture medium for bacterial growth.
4. Notify physician if fever, purulent drainage or foul odor from the burned areas, donor site, or graft site dressing occur. Obtain a wound culture and administer prescribed IV antibiotics.	These findings indicate infection. A culture helps identify the causative pathogen so appropriate antibiotic therapy can be prescribed. Since the graft site dressing is only changed every 5–10 days, this site provides a good culture medium for bacterial growth.
5. Place the patient in a private room and initiate "Reverse Protective Care" precautions for extensive burns covering a large area of the body. Use sterile bed linens, towels, and gowns for the patient. Wear sterile gown, gloves, and a cap with mask when providing patient care. Place a radio or television in the patient's room to alleviate boredom.	Skin is the body's first line of defense against infection. Sterile technique and other reverse protective care measures protect the patient against infection. Lack of varied external stimuli and freedom of movement predispose patient to boredom.
6. If immunization history is inadequate, administer tetanus immune human globulin (Hyper-Tet®) as ordered.	To protect against tetanus.

INTERVENTIONS	RATIONALE
7. Initiate a referral to the dietitian. Provide a high-protein, high-calorie diet. Give nutritional supplements such as Ensure or Sustacal with or between meals if food intake is less than 50%. Suggest TPN (total parenteral nutrition) or enteral feedings if the patient cannot take food orally.	A dietitian is a nutritional specialist who can best evaluate a patient's nutritional status and plan a diet to meet nutritional needs in view of current health situation. Adequate nutrition (proteins, carbohydrates, and vitamins) is essential for wound healing and for meeting energy needs. Metabolism is increased with severe burns.

NURSING DIAGNOSIS: HIGH RISK FOR DISTURBANCE IN SELF-CONCEPT

RELATED TO FACTORS: Disfigurement, possible contractures secondary to full thickness burns

DEFINING CHARACTERISTICS: May verbalize suicide ideation, verbalizes low self-esteem and embarrassment

PATIENT OUTCOME (collaborative): Demonstrates acceptance of self in current situation

EVALUATION CRITERIA: Verbalizes realistic expectations from treatments, verbalizes positive statements about self

INTERVENTIONS	RATIONALE
1. Allow time for the patient and significant other to express feelings. Inform the patient about expected outcomes for the depth of burned areas: some depigmentation occurs with partial thickness burns; scarring occurs with full thickness burns; superficial partial thickness burns heal completely within one week without scarring. Ensure the patient understands that full thickness burns require autografting to heal.	Expressing feelings helps facilitate coping. An accurate knowledge of expected outcomes helps facilitate transition through the grief process.
2. See Loss (page 733).	

INTERVENTIONS	RATIONALE
3. Encourage active range-of-motion exercises q2h. Position burned parts in functional body alignment. With extensive burn injury to extremities, refer to a physical therapist for evaluation of the need for splints, traction, or other prescribed devices.	To prevent progressive tightening of scar tissue and contractures. A physical therapist is a rehabilitative specialist who can evaluate a patient's recovery potential and plan an exercise program to maximize the patient's recovery. Active exercise helps maintain joint flexibility and muscle tone and promotes circulation.
4. Encourage the patient to do ADL (activities of daily living). Assist as needed.	Performing ADL provides active exercise, facilitating the maintenance of joint flexibility and muscle tone. Also, it promotes circulation thus wound healing.

 # Nursing Diagnosis: PAIN

RELATED TO FACTORS: Burn injury

DEFINING CHARACTERISTICS: Verbalizes discomfort, moaning, frowning, tense body posture

PATIENT OUTCOME (collaborative): Demonstrates relief from discomfort

EVALUATION CRITERIA: Denies pain, reports feeling comfortable, relaxed facial expression and body posture

INTERVENTIONS	RATIONALE
1. Administer prescribed narcotic analgesic prn and at least 30 minutes before wound care procedures. Evaluate effectiveness. Suggest IV analgesic if burn wounds are extensive.	Narcotic analgesic is required to block pain pathways with severe pain. Absorption of IM medications is poor in patients with extensive burns caused by plasma shifting to interstitial associated with increased capillary permeability.
2. Keep room door closed, increase room temperature, and provide extra blankets to provide warmth.	Heat and water are lost through burn tissue, causing hypothermia. These external measures help conserve heat loss.

INTERVENTIONS	RATIONALE
3. Apply an overbed cradle if needed.	To reduce pain by keeping the weight of the bed linen off the wounds and to reduce exposure of nerve endings to air currents.
4. Assist with repositioning q2h if needed. Obtain additional assistance as needed, especially if patient cannot assist with turning self.	To relieve pressure on dependent bony prominences. Adequate support to burned areas during movement helps minimize discomfort.

◤ NURSING DIAGNOSIS: HIGH RISK FOR IMPAIRED TISSUE PERFUSION

RELATED TO FACTORS: Circumferential burns of the extremity or deep electrical burns

DEFINING CHARACTERISTICS: Observation of some neurovascular deficits such as decreased sensation, and edema

PATIENT OUTCOME (collaborative): Circulation remains adequate

EVALUATION CRITERIA: Normal skin color, denies numbness and tingling, palpable peripheral pulses

INTERVENTIONS	RATIONALE
1. For circumferential burns of the extremity or electrical burns, monitor neurovascular status (Appendix D) of the affected extremity q2h.	To identify indications of progress toward or deviations from expected outcome.
2. Keep swollen extremities elevated.	To enhance venous return and reduce swelling.
3. Notify physician immediately if diminished pulse, poor capillary refill, cyanosis, coldness, numbness and tingling, or diminished sensation occur. Prepare for surgery— escharotomy— as ordered.	These findings indicate impaired distal circulation. Physician can assess tissue pressure to determine the need for surgical intervention. An escharotomy (slits into the eschar) or fasciotomy may be required to restore adequate circulation.

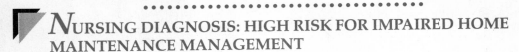

NURSING DIAGNOSIS: HIGH RISK FOR IMPAIRED HOME MAINTENANCE MANAGEMENT

RELATED TO FACTORS: Knowledge deficit about self-care activities on discharge, absence or lack of adequate support system to assist with home care therapy

DEFINING CHARACTERISTICS: Verbalizes lack of understanding, requests information, may report lack of access of a support system to assist with home care needs

PATIENT OUTCOME (collaborative): Demonstrates willingness to comply with recommended home management activities

EVALUATION CRITERIA: Verbalizes understanding of instructions, correctly performs skin care activities, verbalizes satisfaction with home care plan, identifies resources for providing home care assistance if needed

INTERVENTIONS	RATIONALE
1. Evaluate continuing care needs and ability to meet those needs independently. If assistance is needed, determine availability and adequacy of support system. Refer to social services or discharge planning department if help is needed to meet continuing care needs because of lack of a support system or adequate finances.	A social worker or discharge planner is a specialist who can use community resources to meet the patient's continuing care needs on discharge.
2. Teach the patient proper care of the burned areas until completely healed. Instructions should include: • Wash burned areas with mild soap and apply a lanolin-based moisturizer daily. • Protect the burned areas from extended exposure to direct sunlight: apply a sunscreen or wear long sleeve clothing and a hat. • Avoid vigorous rubbing of the areas. • Continue with range-of-motion exercises as instructed by physical therapist.	Health teaching is essential for safety in self-care at home.

INTERVENTIONS	RATIONALE
3. If a pressure garment is prescribed (such as the Jobst pressure garment), explain its purpose and encourage the patient to wear the garment as prescribed. Explain that the garment helps minimize hypertrophic scarring, it is custom made to fit, and must be worn for one year.	A knowledge of what to expect helps promote compliance.
4. Instruct the patient to inspect the wound (burned areas, graft site, and donor site) daily. Report increased warmth and tenderness, redness, purulent drainage, fever, or foul odor to physician.	These findings indicate infection and a need for antimicrobial therapy.
5. Provide home care instructions and appointment for follow-up visit in writing.	Verbal instructions may be easily forgotten.

Intravenous Therapy

Intravenous (IV) therapy is essential for the treatment of many illnesses. It is used to correct or stabilize the body's fluid environment or to administer medications. The patient receiving IV therapy is subjected to many hazards but most can be avoided by prudent nursing care.

IV solutions are:

- isotonic such as ringer's lactated, 0.9% normal saline, or D–5–W
- hypertonic such as 5% dextrose in 0.45% saline, or 5% dextrose in normal saline, or 5% dextrose in lactated Ringer's
- hypotonic such as 0.45% saline, 0.33% saline, or 2.5% dextrose in water

Hypotonic solutions allow fluid to be pulled into the cell to relieve fluid deficits. With isotonic solutions, water does not enter or leave the cell because the osmotic pressure inside and outside the cell is the same. Isotonic fluids are beneficial when replacement of intravascular fluid loss is needed. With hypertonic solutions, the osmotic pressure is greater outside the cell than inside, so water is pulled out of the cell causing it to shrink. These solutions are useful when diuresis or additional calories are desired.

ASSESSMENT DATA BASE

1. Perform a general survey (Appendix F) to establish baseline values.

NURSING DIAGNOSIS: HIGH RISK FOR COMPLICATIONS

RELATED TO FACTORS: IV therapy

DEFINING CHARACTERISTICS: May show manifestations of phlebitis, infiltration, or fluid overload

PATIENT OUTCOME: Demonstrates no permanent tissue damage

EVALUATION CRITERIA: Observation of IV solution infusion at prescribed rate, venous access site with signs of phlebitis or infiltration, absence of signs of fluid overload

INTERVENTIONS	RATIONALE

1. Monitor:
  • IV infusion qh: flow rate (if no IV pump used), insertion site
  • intake and output q8h
	To identify indications of progress toward or deviations from expected outcome.

2. Explain reason for initiating IV therapy: to administer medication, provide vascular access in the event medications are urgently needed to correct a health threat, or to replace lost fluids. Instruct the patient to signal for help if discomfort is felt at the venous access site.	Patients are more likely to comply with therapy when they understand why it is necessary.

3. Stop the IV infusion and change the site if the following occur:
  • infiltration — sluggish or cessation of flow, swelling at site, cool temperature where swollen, absence of backflow of blood in the tubing when IV bag is held below body level or tubing proximal to insertion site is pinched
  • phlebitis — heat, redness, and tenderness at insertion site, painful infusion
	Infiltration indicates the needle or catheter is not in the vein. The risk of vein inflammation increases with infusions of medications or when the patient is allergic to the venipuncture material.

4. Reduce the IV flow rate to KVO (keep vein open) rate and notify physician immediately if hypertension, rales, daily weight gain, urinary output significantly lower than fluid intake, or tachycardia occur. Administer prescribed diuretic and evaluate effectiveness.	These findings indicate fluid overload. Infusing IV fluids too rapidly places sudden strain on the heart and kidneys, especially if these organs are diseased. A diuretic rids the body of excess fluid. A therapeutic response to a diuretic is resolution of manifestations of fluid overload.
5. Change the IV site and tubing every 72 hours and prn.	To prevent phlebitis and a systemic pyrogenic reaction.

INTERVENTIONS	RATIONALE
6. Use an infusion pump for patients with a history of heart failure, renal failure, the elderly, and for continuous infusion medications.	For better control of flow rate. Efficient pumping action of the heart is essential for continuous movement of fluid throughout the circulatory system. Excess fluid is excreted by the kidney to maintain fluid balance. The elderly are less capable of adapting to sudden fluid volume changes because of the normal physiologic changes that occur with aging (decrease in number of renal nephrons, narrowing of blood vessels).
7. **Always** use a filter when infusing IV solutions, unless contraindicated. Consult pharmacy about using a filter when infusing any prescribed medications.	Filters help reduce particulate and bacterial contamination linked to IV infusions and medications.
8. Prime IV tubing before connection to the vascular access device.	To prevent air embolus.
9. Use a catheter-over-needle venipuncture device to start the IV infusion.	When vascular access is ensured, the needle is removed leaving only the catheter in place. This reduces the possibility of infiltration from incidental perforation of the vein.
10. Do **not** place the venous access device over a joint. Tape the venipuncture device securely to prevent it from moving in the vein. Use a venipuncture device with a large diameter when giving viscous solutions such as blood.	To reduce the likelihood of incidental infiltration. The diameter of the venous access device affects the IV solution flow rate.

Shock

    Shock is a clinical syndrome characterized by decreased tissue perfusion. When systemic circulation is impaired, catecholamines (epinephrine and norepinephrine) and glucocorticosteroids are released as a compensatory attempt by the body to maintain adequate circulatory volume. Vasoconstriction of blood vessels in the skin, kidneys, and intestines allows redirection of blood to vital organs (brain, liver, heart) where vasodilation occurs. When these compensatory mechanisms are exhausted, tissue ischemia occurs resulting in multiple organ failure if circulation is not restored promptly.

    Shock has been classified by the primary mechanisms involved:

1. **neurogenic shock** — caused by spinal cord injury or diseases that impair transmission of sympathetic nerve impulses to peripheral blood vessels. Extensive vasodilation occurs because of sympathetic input loss. Consequently, there is pooling of blood, diminished venous return to the heart, and diminished cardiac output (Dolan, 1991). These changes ultimately cause decreased tissue perfusion.

2. **septic shock** — caused mostly by gram-negative pathogens. May also be caused by gram-positive pathogens. Endotoxins released from the bacteria cell wall cause vasodilation, eventually leading to decreased circulatory volume. The most common causes are perforation of a segment of the GI tract, burns, or chemotherapy (Wall, 1989).

3. **cardiogenic shock** —caused by severe heart disease that results in loss of functioning cardiac muscle, especially the left ventricle; can occur as a complication of myocardial infarction, valvular heart disease, or rupture of the septum or papillary muscle (Gunnar, 1989).

4. **hypovolemic shock** — caused by extensive loss of blood or plasma subsequent to surgery or trauma. Internal loss of large amounts of intravascular fluid occurs when fluid shifts to interstitial space in conditions such as massive burns, peritonitis, or intestinal obstruction. External loss occurs with prolonged vomiting, diarrhea, GI bleeding, diabetic ketoacidosis, or hemorrhage from other sites.

5. **anaphylactic shock** — is an acute hypersensitivity reaction resulting from exposure to an allergen. This antigen-antibody reaction causes histamine release, which leads to vasodilation. It may be caused by drugs, pollen, insect stings, or administration of blood or blood products.

    Major complications associated with shock are disseminated intravascular coagulation (DIC), renal failure, and respiratory distress syndrome. If untreated, shock can cause lactic acidosis, multiple organ failure, and death. Cardiogenic shock has the highest mortality rate because of the coexistence of impaired functioning of the heart muscle (Gunnar, 1989).

General Medical Management

1. Placement in an ICU with continuous ECG monitoring.

2. Insertion of a Foley catheter to monitor hourly urinary output.

3. Insertion of an intra-arterial catheter for continuous monitoring of BP and for obtaining blood samples for arterial blood gases (ABG).

4. IV administration of vasoactive drugs:
   - inotropic agents, such as dopamine HCL (Intropin, Dopastat), dobutamine, or epinephrine
   - vasodilators such as nitroprusside sodium (Nipride) or nitroglycerin enhance cardiac output after adequate systolic pressure is achieved

5. IV infusion of crystalloids (lactated Ringer's) or colloids (plasma protein fractions, dextran, hetastarch, serum albumin) to maintain intravascular volume.

6. Oxygen therapy to increase oxygen available to the tissue. If respiratory distress occurs, insert endotracheal tube and place on a mechanical ventilator with PEEP (positive end-expiratory pressure).

   A transcutaneous oximetry clip can be applied to the earlobe or finger to monitor oxygen tension continuously.

7. Insertion of a central venous catheter to monitor central venous pressure (CVP).
   - **For Septic Shock:**
     — IV administration of broad-spectrum antibiotics such as aminoglycosides, penicillin derivatives, or cephalosporins
   - **For Cardiogenic Shock:**
     — Insertion of a Swan-Ganz catheter to monitor pulmonary artery pressure (PAP), CVP, pulmonary wedge pressure (PWP), and cardiac output (CO)
     — Use of intra-aortic balloon counterpulsation. A cylindrical-shaped helium balloon is inserted through the femoral artery and advanced to the thoracic aorta just below the arch. The balloon inflates during diastole, pushing blood into coronary arteries, and deflates during systole. The balloon is attached to a machine that synchronizes the inflation and deflation of the balloon in relation to the QRS complex on the ECG. This device increases coronary blood flow and cardiac output, reduces myocardial oxygen demand, and decreases left ventricular pressure.
   - **For Anaphylactic Shock:**
     — IV administration of corticosteroids, antihistamines, and bronchodilators
   - **For Hypovolemic Shock:**
     — Surgery if caused by postoperative hemorrhage
     — Transfusions of blood or blood products to restore clotting factors or blood cell components

Integrative Care Plans

- IV therapy
- Fluid and biochemical imbalances

ASSESSMENT DATA BASE

1. Physical examination based on a general survey (Appendix F) may reveal classical manifestations of shock: hypotension, tachycardia, tachypnea, pallor, cold clammy skin, peripheral cyanosis, low urinary output, restlessness, alterations in sensorium (delirium, confusion, agitation, lethargy, obtundation, coma).

In addition, look for manifestations specific to the type of shock:

- **septic shock** — characterized by two phases:
  a. "warm shock phase" occurs initially and usually lasts less than 24 hours: fever, tachypnea, warm dry skin, and flushed appearance (caused by arterial vasodilation and compensatory increased cardiac output, stroke volume, and pulse pressure)
  b. "cold shock phase" develops as compensatory mechanisms are exhausted; manifested by classical symptoms of shock.
- **cardiogenic shock** —severe pulmonary congestion (dyspnea, rales, left ventricular S3 gallop), distended neck veins, elevated CVP, and diaphoresis in combination with classical manifestations of shock. Persistent chest pain also can occur caused by increasing myocardial ischemia
- **anaphylactic shock** — severe wheezing and dyspnea; diaphoresis; edema of lips, pharynx, and extremities; diffuse red rash
- **hypovolemic shock** — extreme thirst, flat or collapsed neck veins
- **neurogenic shock** — hypotension with a warm flushed appearance; reflex sympathetic reactions typical of shock do not occur, such as tachycardia and tachypnea

2. Diagnostic studies:
- ABG reveal metabolic acidosis and hypoxia. Anaerobic metabolism occurs with hypoxia, which results in lactic acid accumulation.
- Serum electrolytes reveal fluid and electrolyte deficits.
- CBC reveals deficits in blood components with hypovolemic shock and elevated WBC with anaphylactic and septic shock.
- Coagulation studies such as the PT and PTT are useful to rule out a clotting disorder with hemorrhagic hypovolemic shock.
- EKG determines the source of myocardial damage with cardiogenic shock.
- Chest x ray reveals pulmonary venous congestion or interstitial edema initially with cardiogenic or anaphylactic shock.

••••••••••••••••••••••••••••••••

NURSING DIAGNOSIS: ALTERATIONS IN TISSUE PERFUSION

RELATED TO FACTORS: Diminished cardiac output secondary to (specify type of shock)

DEFINING CHARACTERISTICS: Observation of classical manifestations of shock

PATIENT OUTCOME (collaborative): Demonstrates improved tissue perfusion

EVALUATION CRITERIA: Vital signs within normal range, urinary output above 30 mL/hr, alert and oriented mental status, normal skin color, warm and dry skin

•••••••••••••••••••••••••••••••••

INTERVENTIONS	RATIONALE
1. Monitor: • BP, pulse and respiration rates qh and temperature q4h • hemodynamic readings q1–2h • results of ABG reports • general status (pedal pulses, lung sounds, heart sounds, skin color and temperature, level of consciousness, neck veins, and bowel sounds) q2h • ECG tracings frequently	To identify indications of progress toward or deviations from expected outcome.
2. Act promptly when symptoms of shock are detected: • Place the patient in a modified Trendelenburg position (flat with feet elevated). • Notify physician immediately. Start an IV of 5% dextrose in water (if not diabetic) or 0.9% sodium chloride (if diabetic) until a specific IV order is obtained. Have someone remain with the patient. • Start nasal oxygen at 2 L/min if history of COPD, otherwise 6 L/min until ABG results are available. • Arrange for transfer to ICU to closely monitor cardiopulmonary status.	A modified Trendelenburg position enhances venous return. Supplemental oxygen helps increase the oxygen available to tissue. Prompt intervention is aimed at supporting cardiopulmonary circulatory function. If untreated, shock can lead to death.

INTERVENTIONS	RATIONALE
3. Assist physician with insertion of hemodynamic monitoring devices (arterial line, CVC, Swan-Ganz catheter).	These devices provide for direct monitoring of cardiovascular functioning.
4. Administer prescribed medications to combat shock and evaluate effectiveness. Always use IV pump to administer medications prescribed for continuous infusion. Implement appropriate actions while IV therapy is in place to prevent complications (page 764).	Specific medications can improve cardiac output, renal perfusion, and produce selective vasoconstriction and vasodilation. An IV pump ensures accurate control of flow rate.
5. Notify physician if manifestations of shock persist or worsen.	This indicates a need for further testing to identify any type of secondary factors that may contribute to shock, to consider alternative drug therapy, or to increase the dosage of the drugs currently used.
6. Attach to ECG monitor. Place a strip of the ECG tracing on the chart q8h and prn if an arrhythmia is detected. Treat arrhythmias following facility protocol or ACLS protocol.	ECG recordings allow for continuous monitoring of cardiac pattern since arrhythmias can occur with severe shock as a result of decreased myocardial perfusion. Persistent arrhythmias further impair cardiac output.
7. Notify physician if persistent rales, neck vein distention, insufficient urinary output despite large fluid intake, hypertension, or CVP above 10 mm Hg occur.	These findings indicate fluid overload and a need to reduce fluid intake or to administer diuretic therapy.
8. Keep NPO if level of consciousness is depressed. Give oral care q2h. Apply petroleum ointment to lips prn.	Aspiration can easily occur if one attempts to give oral feedings to patients whose sensorium is diminished. Lubrication prevents drying of the mucosa.
9. Notify the physician if bowel sounds are absent and distention occurs. Insert an N/G tube and connect to intermittent suction as ordered.	Peristalsis diminishes with severe shock resulting from decreased mesenteric blood flow. Gastric decompression is needed until peristalsis returns, evidenced by bowel sounds and passage of flatus.

INTERVENTIONS	RATIONALE
10. Maintain complete bedrest until vital signs return to normal and the patient is alert.	Bedrest reduces oxygen tissue demands.
11. Suction prn if patient is unconscious.	To remove secretions to keep airway patent.
12. Insert (if ACLS certified) or assist with endotracheal tube and placement of a mechanical ventilator as ordered if respiratory distress syndrome (page 2) occurs.	Respiratory distress is a major complication associated with shock. Insertion of an endotracheal tube requires special training and is performed by persons with ACLS certification, a respiratory therapist, anesthesiologist, or nurse anesthetist. Mechanical ventilation supports breathing until the patient can do so independently.
13. Keep the patient warm.	Hypothermia reduces tissue oxygenation.
14. While on bedrest, q2h: • reposition • keep the skin dry and clean • provide passive exercises	Bedrest increases the risk for skin breakdown, especially over bony prominences as a result of diminished blood flow and increased pressure on the tissue. Measures to relieve pressure and maintain circulation reduce the risk of skin breakdown.

Fluid and Biochemical Imbalance

Maintaining fluid and biochemical balance is a dynamic process because the body's metabolic needs are constantly changing in response to physiological and environmental stressors. Fluids and biochemicals (electrolytes, acids, and bases) are interrelated. Isolated imbalances rarely occur. Often an imbalance in one component causes an alteration in another component. This secondary alteration is the body's way of compensating for the primary imbalance. Imbalances are in the form of an excess or deficit.

Electrolytes are present in all fluid compartments (intracellular and extracellular) in varying quantities. The intracellular compartment is the largest fluid compartment.

With mild imbalances, the patient remains asymptomatic except by laboratory determination because the body's chemical buffer system can adequately compensate for minor changes. When the buffer system is exhausted and if the disorder causing the imbalance is not corrected, the patient becomes symptomatic.

Potassium, the most abundant intracellular cation, is essential for transmission of nerve impulses, uptake of glucose in the cell, and regeneration of cardiac rhythm. Sodium, the major extracellular cation, plays an important role in regulating extracellular fluid volume. When sodium loss occurs water loss occurs, and vice versa. Bicarbonate imbalances are primarily manifested by changes consistent with an acid-base imbalance. Chloride imbalances occur in combination with a sodium and potassium imbalance.

Acid-base balance is regulated by three body systems: chemical buffer systems (phosphates, proteins, and bicarbonate), respiratory system, and renal system. These systems interdependently operate to maintain the hydrogen (H^+) ion concentration within a normal range. Acidosis (hydrogen ion excess) and alkalosis (hydrogen ion deficit) are the two acid-base imbalances. The primary source of the imbalance is respiratory or metabolic.

The elderly patient is especially prone to fluid and biochemical disturbances during an illness because of the normal physiologic changes that occur with aging (narrowing of blood vessels, reduced nerve conduction time, reduced subcutaneous fat, decreased lung tissue compliance, decrease in renal nephrons, and decreased hormone production (Blair, 1990).

General Medical Management (measures to correct underlying pathology)

- **For Metabolic Acidosis:**
  - sodium bicarbonate
  - insulin and potassium chloride if diabetic ketoacidosis is the underlying pathology

- **For Metabolic Alkalosis:**
  — carbonic anhydrase inhibitors to increase renal excretion of bicarbonate.
  — potassium-sparing diuretics to prevent potassium loss
- **For Respiratory Acidosis:**
  — adequate ventilation (suction if needed), supplemental oxygen or mechanical ventilation if respiratory failure occurs
- **For Respiratory Alkalosis:**
  — breathing into a paper bag to raise the carbon dioxide level
  — use of a rebreathing mask with supplemental oxygen
  — relaxation techniques to relieve severe anxiety
  — adjusting settings on the mechanical ventilator if due to overventilation
- Electrolyte supplements to correct the primary electrolyte deficit

Integrative Care Plans

- IV therapy

Discharge Considerations

- Follow-up care if chronic illness exists

 # ASSESSMENT DATA BASE

1. Assess for manifestations of an imbalance.
   - **For Acid-Base Disturbances:**
     — altered patterns of respiration: hyperventilation (with metabolic acidosis) and hypoventilation (with metabolic alkalosis) (these are reversed with respiratory acidosis and alkalosis)
     — altered level of consciousness: confusion, restlessness, disorientation, lethargy, and eventually unconsciousness
     — tetany syndrome with alkalosis (positive Trousseau's and Chvostek's signs, leg cramps, numbness of lips and fingers, hyperactive deep tendon reflexes)
   - **For Sodium Imbalances — Fluid Volume Changes:**
     — hypernatremia (serum sodium greater than 145 mEq/L): dehydration (thirst, dry skin and mucous membranes, poor skin turgor, rapid weak pulse, orthostatic hypotension, decreased urinary output, muscle weakness, and diminished sensorium, serum sodium above normal range)
     — hyponatremia (serum sodium less than 135 mEq/L): if caused by fluid volume excess: elevated BP, distended neck veins, edema, weight gain, bounding pulse, rales, tachycardia, serum sodium below normal range. If caused by sodium deficit: headache, fatigue, muscle weakness, postural hypotension, abdominal cramps, weight loss, rapid thready weak pulse, flat neck veins.

- **For potassium imbalances — heart and skeletal muscle changes:**
  - hypokalemia: U-waves or inverted T waves on ECG tracing, muscle weakness, and serum potassium less than 3.5 mEq/L
  - hyperkalemia: peaked T wave on ECG tracing and serum potassium greater than 5.5 mEq/L

2. Diagnostic studies:
  - Serum electrolyte values (sodium, potassium, chloride, and bicarbonate) are above normal range, reflecting an excess (hyper-), or below normal range, reflecting a deficit (hypo-).
  - ABG report:
    - respiratory acidosis (uncompensated) reflects $PaCO_2$ above normal range, bicarbonate in normal range, and a pH below normal range.
    - respiratory alkalosis (uncompensated) reflects pH above normal range, $PaCO_2$ below normal range, bicarbonate in normal range.

      (**NOTE:** In respiratory disorders a shift in the bicarbonate level in the opposite direction of the primary imbalance reflects compensation).
    - metabolic acidosis (uncompensated) reflects pH and bicarbonate below normal range, $PaCO_2$ in normal range.
    - metabolic alkalosis (uncompensated) reflects pH and bicarbonate above normal range, $PaCO_2$ in normal range.

      (**NOTE:** In metabolic disorders a shift in the $PaCO_2$ level in the opposite direction of the primary imbalance reflects compensation).

◤ NURSING DIAGNOSIS: HIGH RISK FOR INJURY

RELATED TO FACTORS: Altered sensorium secondary to (specify specific imbalance), muscle weakness, cardiac disturbances

DEFINING CHARACTERISTICS: Reports weakness, observation of confusion, restlessness, disorientation, lethargy, abnormal serum electrolyte report, abnormal ECG recordings

PATIENT OUTCOME (collaborative): Remains free of injury

EVALUATION CRITERIA: Denies falls, absence of bruises on extremities, serum electrolyte report reflects values within normal range, ECG reflects normal sinus rhythm

INTERVENTIONS	RATIONALE
1. Monitor: • level of consciousness (LOC) q8h, more often if LOC diminished • results of serum electrolyte reports, especially potassium level • EKG reports • BP, pulse, and respiration q4h	To identify indications of progress toward or deviations from expected outcome.
2. Provide help with activities of daily living as needed. Encourage the patient to do as much as possible for self.	To promote joint flexibility and maintain muscle tone as well as self-esteem.
3. Keep siderails up and call bell within the patient's reach. If weakness is present, instruct the patient to signal for help as needed when getting out of bed.	To avoid falls.
4. If confused apply restraints. Explain purpose of restraints. Remove restraints q2h to check condition of skin and to provide exercises. Document patient's behavior supporting the need for continued use of restraints according to facility protocol, which may be q2–4h.	Restraints help protect the patient from self-injury. Proper documentation is essential to prevent liability against false imprisonment.
5. If hypokalemia exists, administer prescribed potassium supplement and evaluate effectiveness: resolution of manifestations of hypokalemia, serum potassium returns to normal range.	Potassium imbalances must be corrected to prevent disruption of the electrical activity of the heart. Cardiac dysrhythmia can cause reduced cardiac output that can further depress sensorium, thus increasing the risk for physical injury. Potassium supplements are given to correct a potassium deficit.

INTERVENTIONS	RATIONALE
6. If hyperkalemia exists: • avoid medications containing potassium • administer calcium gluconate, as ordered • give loop diuretics as ordered • administer sodium polystyrene sulfonate (Kayexalate) with Sorbitol as ordered Evaluate effectiveness of pharmacotherapy: resolution of manifestations of hyperkalemia, serum potassium within normal range.	To prevent further elevations of potassium level. Calcium gluconate reverses membrane effects of potassium. In the absence of dehydration, loop diuretics enhance renal excretion of potassium. Kayexalate removes potassium from the body by exchanging sodium ions for potassium ions in the intestine. The potassium containing resin is then expelled in the stool. Sorbitol is a mild laxative that helps prevent constipation, a common side effect of Kayexalate therapy.
7. If hyperkalemia is caused by diabetic ketoacidosis, administer sodium bicarbonate and regular insulin IV as ordered.	Insulin facilitates movement of potassium back into the cell as it pushes glucose into the cell. Sodium bicarbonate corrects acidosis. When acidosis occurs, potassium moves out of the cell in exchange for hydrogen ions. This is the body's compensatory attempt to reduce acidity.
8. If hyperkalemia is linked to renal failure, prepare for hemodialysis as ordered.	Hemodialysis rids the blood of nitrogenous waste products, which are normally filtered through the kidneys.
9. Notify physician if hyperkalemia or hypokalemia or muscle weakness persists.	This can indicate worsening of the primary pathology.

NURSING DIAGNOSIS: ALTERATION IN FLUID VOLUME: DEFICIT.

RELATED TO FACTORS: (specify causative factor)

DEFINING CHARACTERISTICS: Manifestations of dehydration

PATIENT OUTCOME (collaborative): Demonstrates adequate fluid balance

EVALUATION CRITERIA: Absence of manifestations of dehydration, serum electrolyte report reflects values within normal range

INTERVENTIONS	RATIONALE
1. Monitor: • intake and output q8h • results of serum electrolyte reports, especially sodium • vital signs q4h • general status (Appendix F) q8h	To identify indications of progress toward or deviations from expected outcome.
2. Provide fluids. Initiate IV therapy as ordered and perform measures to prevent problems associated with IV therapy (page 764). Consult physician if manifestations of dehydration persist despite a high fluid intake (low concentrated urinary output, low BP, elevated serum sodium, rapid pulse).	These findings reflect inadequate fluid replacement.

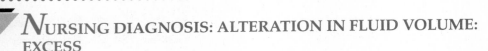

◤ NURSING DIAGNOSIS: ALTERATION IN FLUID VOLUME: EXCESS

RELATED TO FACTORS: (specify causative factor)
DEFINING CHARACTERISTICS: Shows manifestations of fluid volume excess
PATIENT OUTCOME (collaborative): Demonstrates adequate fluid balance
EVALUATION CRITERIA: Absence of manifestations of fluid volume excess

INTERVENTIONS	RATIONALE
1. Monitor: • weight daily • intake and output q8h • results of serum electrolyte reports, especially serum sodium • vital signs q4h • general status (Appendix F) q8h	To identify indications of progress toward or deviations from expected outcome.

INTERVENTIONS	RATIONALE
2. Perform prescribed therapy to resolve fluid retention: • sodium restricted diet • restrict fluid intake • diuretic therapy Evaluate effectiveness of therapy: resolution of manifestations of fluid volume excess, serum sodium returns to normal range.	Sodium attracts water. Diuretics help rid the body of excess water.
3. Notify physician if fluid retention persists or worsens (edema, rales, distended neck veins, daily weight gain, rising BP, low serum sodium).	These findings indicate a need for further testing to rule out another cause of fluid retention.

• •

◣ NURSING DIAGNOSIS: ACTIVITY INTOLERANCE

RELATED TO FACTORS: Ineffective breathing pattern secondary to acidosis or alkalosis

DEFINING CHARACTERISTICS: Observation of hyperventilation or hypoventilation, reports fatigue with minimal physical exertion, tachycardia and tachypnea with minimal exertion

PATIENT OUTCOME (collaborative): Demonstrates improved tolerance to activities

EVALUATION CRITERIA: Denies fatigue with performance of activities of daily living, absence of tachypnea and tachycardia with minimal exertion

• •

INTERVENTIONS	RATIONALE
1. Monitor: • vital signs q4h • results of ABG reports (Table 14–1)	To identify indications of progress toward or deviations from expected outcome.
2. Suction prn if secretions are present, the patient's sensorium is depressed, and patient cannot cough effectively.	To remove secretions thus maintaining a patent airway.

INTERVENTIONS	RATIONALE
3. Maintain a semi-Fowler's position.	A sitting position allows fuller lung expansion by reducing pressure abdominal contents against the diaphragm.
4. Administer prescribed therapy for the specific acid-base imbalance and evaluate effectiveness: resolution of manifestations of the acid-base disturbance, ABG and serum electrolyte values return to normal range or in the presence of chronic disorders ABG reflect compensation.	To resolve the underlying pathology and to support ventilation until the acid-base imbalance is corrected.
5. If sensorium is already depressed, avoid giving medication that depresses respirations.	To prevent respiratory arrest.
6. If signs of respiratory failure (page 2) occur, transfer the patient to ICU for endotracheal as ordered. Intubation and placement on a mechanical ventilator.	Mechanical ventilation supports breathing until the patient can do so independently. Nurses specialized in the care of patients with life-threatening, acute conditions work in the ICU.

● ●

◤ NURSING DIAGNOSIS: HIGH RISK FOR ALTERATIONS IN HOME MAINTENANCE MANAGEMENT

RELATED TO FACTORS: Knowledge deficit about self-care at home, knowledge deficit about primary pathology

DEFINING CHARACTERISTICS: Verbalizes lack of understanding, requests information, history of noncompliance with chronic illness

PATIENT OUTCOME: Demonstrates willingness to comply with self-care measures to maintain fluid and biochemical balance

EVALUATION CRITERIA: Verbalizes understanding of instructions, reports satisfaction with therapeutic plan

● ●

INTERVENTIONS	RATIONALE
1. Teach the patient about medications prescribed for home use, including name, dosage, schedule, purpose, and reportable side effects.	To ensure safe self-medication administration on discharge.
2. Encourage the patient to follow prescribed therapy for the underlying disease process if a chronic illness exists.	Fluid and biochemical imbalances reflect lack of control in the presence of a chronic illness.
3. Ensure the patient has a written appointment for follow-up care and written instructions for self-care on discharge. Explain the importance of follow-up care when a chronic illness is present.	Verbal instructions may be easily forgotten.
4. If chronic illness is the source of the imbalance, review the nature of the illness in relation to the fluid and biochemical imbalance and current medical treatments. Evaluate patient's feelings and concerns about having a chronic illness, especially if history of noncompliance exists.	Cooperation with the therapeutic plan is enhanced when patients understand condition and treatments.

TABLE 14–1. Interpretation of Arterial Blood Gases

Arterial blood gases (ABG) report reflects:

Element	Normal Range	Below Normal	Above Normal
PaO$_2$	greater than 80 mm Hg	hypoxemia	
PaCO$_2$	38 – 42 mm Hg	alkalosis	acidosis
HCO$_3$	22 – 26	acidosis	alkalosis
pH	7.38 – 7.42	acidosis	alkalosis

Step 1. Determine the primary imbalance by examining each component. The PaCO$_2$ reflects the respiratory component. Is it showing alkalosis, acidosis, or within normal range? The HCO$_3$ reflects the metabolic component. Is it showing alkalosis, acidosis, or within normal range? The pH moves in the direction of the primary imbalance. Is it showing alkalosis, acidosis, or within normal range?

Step 2. Determine if the body is compensating for the primary imbalance. The body shows compensation when the metabolic and respiratory components move in the opposite directions. Full compensation exists when the pH moves to a normal range.

BIBLIOGRAPHY

Blair, K.A. (1990). Aging: Physiological aspects and clinical implications. **Nurse Practitioner,** **15,** 14–16, 18, 23, 26–28.

Dolan, J. (1991). **Critical Care Nursing Management,** Philadelphia: F.A. Davis Company.

Duncan, D.J., & Driscoll, D.M. (1991). Burn wound management. **Critical Care Nursing Clinics of North America, 3,** overall xvii–267.

Gunnar, R.M. (1989). Managing cardiogenic shock. **Patient Care, 23,** 59–77.

Lorenz, E.W. (1991). **St. Anthony's DRG Working Guidebook.** Alexandria: St. Anthony's Publishing Company.

Rice, V. (1991). Shock, a clinical syndrome: An update, part I. **Critical Care Nurse, 11,** 20–27.

Shoemaker, W.C., Ayers, S., Grenvik, A., et al (1989). **Textbook of Critical Care.** 2nd ed. Philadelphia: W.B. Saunders Company.

Wall, S.C. (1989). Septic shock: How to detect it early. **Nursing 89, 19,** 52–59.

RESPIRATORY ASSESSMENT

1. Assess respiratory rate and rhythm.

2. Inspect skin color and color of mucous membranes.

3. Auscultate lung sounds.

4. Ascertain if patient uses accessory muscles when breathing:
   - lifting shoulders with inspiration
   - retraction of abdominal muscles with respiration
   - flaring of nostrils

5. Assess if chest expansion is symmetrical or asymmetrical.

6. Assess if chest pain occurs with breathing.

7. Assess cough. If present assess if productive or nonproductive. If productive, determine color of sputum.

8. Determine if patient is experiencing:
   - dyspnea with exertion
   - orthopnea

9. Assess level of consciousness.

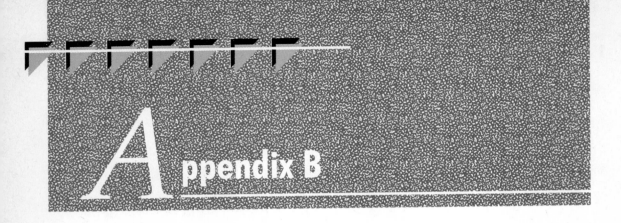

Appendix B

ABDOMINAL ASSESSMENT

1. Inspect size and contour of abdomen.

2. Auscultate bowel sounds in all four quadrants.

3. Palpate for tenderness and masses.

4. Inquire about unusual change in bowel pattern, color, and consistency of stools.

5. Inquire about abdominal discomfort:
   • How is it relieved?
   • What aggravates it?

6. Inquire about sudden changes in weight and appetite.

Appendix C

ASSESSMENT OF MUSCULOSKELETAL FUNCTION

1. Inquire about discomfort with movement (pain, muscle spasms, stiffness).

2. Assess muscle strength:
   - Can patient turn self in bed without assistance?
   - Does patient complain of weakness?
   - Can patient maintain counter-resistance to a force (pulling against examiner's pull)?

3. Inspect joints for any swelling or deformity.

4. Observe patient's gait:
   - Is it normal or altered?

5. Assess range-of-motion (ROM) of joints in which discomfort is experienced.

6. Observe patient's posture.

Appendix D

NEUROVASCULAR ASSESSMENT OF EXTREMITIES

1. Palpate peripheral pulses for equality and strength:
   - femoral and dorsalis pedis if leg is involved
   - radial if arm is involved
   - use a Doppler if pulse is nonpalpable

2. Inquire about any numbness or tingling in the affected extremity.

3. Assess mobility (ask patient to flex and extend fingers, toes, or both).

4. Assess status of skin:
   - color
   - temperature (warm, cold)
   - any swelling
   - character (dry, moist)

5. Assess capillary refill. Use dorsum of fingers/toes since nailbeds can be discolored or too thick to detect blanching or color changes.

PERIPHERAL VASCULAR ASSESSMENT

1. Palpate peripheral pulses for quality and strength:
   - femoral and dorsalis pedis or posterior tibialis if legs are affected
   - radial if arm is affected
   - use a Doppler if pulse is nonpalpable

2. Assess status of the skin:
   - color
   - temperature (warm, cold)
   - hair distribution
   - any swelling
   - character (dry, moist)

3. Assess capillary refill. Use dorsum of toes/fingers since nailbeds can be discolored or too thick to detect blanching or color changes.

4. Palpate calf area for tenderness.

5. Assess for pain. If pain is present, ask patient:
   - Where does pain occur?
   - How is pain relieved: resting, elevation, or placing extremity in dependent position?
   - When does pain occur: with ambulation, after ambulating a short distance, or at rest?
   - How far can you walk before pain occurs? (This is called claudication distance.)
   - Does pain occur at night?

6. Assess for the Homan's sign by dorsiflexing the patient's foot. A negative Homan's sign is indicated by absence of pain in calf when the foot is dorsiflexed. A positive Homan's is indicated by presence of pain in calf when foot is dorsiflexed.

Assess both extremities for comparison.

Appendix F

GENERAL SURVEY

1. Assess level of consciousness. Is patient:
   - alert
   - disoriented
   - oriented
   - stuporus
   - lethargic
   - comatose
   - semiconscious
   - confused

2. Inspect color of skin and note any swelling.

3. Feel skin for temperature changes and moisture. Is it warm, dry, cold, or moist?

4. Auscultate breath sounds.

5. Auscultate heart sounds. Is there a murmur?

6. Auscultate bowel sounds.

7. Obtain vital signs.

8. Palpate peripheral pulses (femoral, pedal). Are the pulses present and equal in strength or nonpalpable? Use a Doppler probe if unable to palpate pulses.

9. Inspect contour of abdomen. Is it round, flat, or distended?

10. When was last bowel movement? Any voiding difficulties?

11. Assess patient's need for assistance with activities of daily living (bathing, eating, toileting, dressing, turning in bed, getting out of bed, ambulating).

A ppendix G

CARDIOVASCULAR ASSESSMENT

1. Obtain vital signs.

2. Auscultate heart sounds.

3. Auscultate breath sounds.

4. Palpate peripheral pulses (femoral, pedal). Use a Doppler probe if pulses are nonpalpable.

5. Assess capillary refill.

6. Inspect for neck vein distention. With patient in erect or semi-Fowler's position, inspect neck for distention of jugular veins. Normally, there is no distention of neck veins when in erect position.

7. Assess skin color, temperature, and moisture.

8. Inspect extremities for swelling.

9. Obtain weight.

10. Assess for activity intolerance (fatigue, palpitations, or syncope when engaging in any activities of daily living).

Appendix H

GENERAL ASSESSMENT OF EYE

1. Inspect external eye structures:
   - Are eyelids symmetrical?
   - Are eyebrows and eyelashes present?
   - Are sclera and cornea clear?

   Normally, external eyelids are symmetrical, eyebrows and eyelashes are present, sclera is white, and cornea is clear. In the elderly, a whitish ring encircling the periphery of the iris (arcus senilis) is a normal finding.

2. Assess the pupil:
   - Are pupils round and equal in size and shape?
   - Do pupils constrict when exposed to a light source?

   Normally, the pupils are round, equal in size and shape, and constrict symmetrically when exposed to a light source.

3. Assess movement of the eyeballs and eyelids:
   - Is there symmetrical movement?

   Normally, blinking of the eyelids is symmetrical, and the eyeballs move in the same direction (conjugate movement).

4. Inspect the irides (colored portion of eye).
   - Are irides equal in size, shape, and color?

   Normally, the irides are round and equal in size, shape, and color.

5. Inquire about visual acuity:
   - Does the patient wear glasses or contact lens?

6. Are there subjective/objective manifestations of an eye problem?

Subjective Manifestations:

a. Complaints of discomfort in the eye:

- pain
- foreign body sensation
- photophobia (hypersensitivity to light)
- itching or irritation
- fatigue

b. Complaints of visual disturbances:

- floaters or spots
- loss of vision (partial or complete)
- loss of peripheral vision (tunnel vision)
- flashes of light
- halos around lights
- blurred vision
- double vision (diplopia)
- curtain or veil over visual field
- difficulty with color discrimination

Objective Manifestations:

- redness
- swelling
- drainage
- tearing
- squinting when attempting to read printed material
- crusting of eyelashes

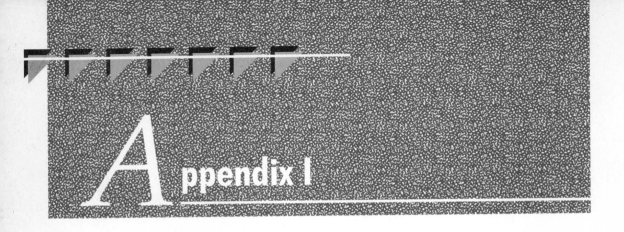

ASSESSMENT OF AUDITORY STATUS

1. Inspect for drainage.

2. Inquire about:
   - feeling of fullness
   - unusual sounds: popping or cracking sounds when yawning or swallowing, heart beating in ear, tinnitus
   - earache
   - ear pain when subjected to loud noise
   - vertigo

3. Inquire about use of a hearing aid.

4. Assess hearing acuity:
   - Is there difficulty hearing in one ear or both?
   - Does patient show behaviors consistent with diminished hearing such as turning head and leaning closer when spoken to, asking for statements to be repeated consistently?

5. If severe hearing deficit exists, inquire about ability to lip-read.

6. Inquire about use of medications that are ototoxic (salicylates, quinine, aminoglycosides).

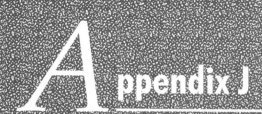

Appendix J

RAPID NEUROLOGICAL ASSESSMENT

1. LOC (based on Glasgow Coma Scale)

Eyes Open	Spontaneously
	To speech
	To pain
	No response
Best Verbal Response	Oriented
	Confused
	Inappropriate
	Incomprehensible
	No response
Best Motor Response	Obeys commands
	Movement to pain
	No response
2. Vital Signs	Temperature
	Pulse
	Respiration
	Blood pressure

3. Pupil Response (CN III)	Reacts to light	R
	=, S (sluggish)	L
	0 (no response)	
	Size in mm	R
		L

1 2 3 4 5 6 7

4. Strength	Hand grips:	
	=, R>L, L>R	
	Bends knees to resistance	
	=, R>L, R>L	

5. Movement of Extremities	F (abnormal rigid flexion)	R upper
		L upper
	E (abnormal rigid extension)	R lower
		L lower
	N (normal)	

6. Babinski Reflex	(+) or (-)

7. Cranial Nerves (+) (-)	Swallows (CN X)
	Protrudes and moves tongue
	Laterally (CN XII)
	Smiles symmetrically (CN VII)
	Moves eyes up/down and side to side
	Blinks eyes (CN V)
	Able to smell (CN I)
	Able to see (CN II)
	Able to hear (CN VIII)
	Turns head and shrugs
	Shoulders to resistance (CN XI)

A ppendix K

PREOPERATIVE CHECKLIST

Patient Sticker

| Allergies _____ |
| Deaf _____ **Mental Status** |
| Blind _____ Alert _____ |
| Hard of Hearing _____ Confused _____ |

OR DATE _____

	Complete	Lab Work	Complete	**For GI Lab only**	
					Complete
Consent(s)* (see Note Below)	____	CBC (over 10 grms & within 7 days)	___	Signed consent	____
ID Band on	___	U/A	___	Addressography plate	___
H&P	___	Coag Profile (if ordered)	___	All lab on chart	___
Consult note	___			V.S. charted	___
Addressography plate	___	Type & cross and blood ready	___	Dentures, glasses, contact lenses and all jewelry removed	___
MAR/Int. Summ.	___	EKG**	___		
V.S. taken & charted	___	Chest X-ray	___	Hospital gown only	
Voided or catheterized	___			Pre-med given (if ordered)	___
I&O charted	___				
Dentures, glasses, contact lenses, and jewelry removed	___			I.V. or Heparin lock in place (if ordered)	___
Hospital Gown on	___				
Elastic Hose	___				
Pre-op med given	___				

Special Comments _____
_____
_____

796

Signatures of Nurses Completing form

3-11_____R.N.

11-7_____R.N.

7-3_____R.N.

To O.R. at_____

HOLDING AREA
I.V. FLUID _____
Needle size and site _____
I.V. Meds _____
_____
_____R.N.

*Note—Consents should be signed and filled in completely. Special forms are needed for amputations, sterilizations, and Refusal of blood transfusion.
**EKG must be done on all operative pts. over 40 or if any signs or symptoms of cardiac disease.
(Courtesy of Halifax Medical Center, Daytona Beach, Florida)

Appendix L

ROUTINE POSTOPERATIVE ASSESSMENT

1. Assess level of consciousness:
   - alert
   - oriented
   - confused
   - disoriented
   - lethargic
   - responding appropriately to verbal commands
   - unresponsive

2. Obtain vital signs.

3. Auscultate breath sounds.

4. Assess skin:
   - color
   - swelling
   - temperature (warm, dry, cold, moist)

5. Inspect status of dressings.

6. Assess for pain or nausea.

7. Assess status of intrusive devices:
   a. Intravenous infusions
      - type of fluid
      - flow rate
      - infusion site for signs of infiltration or phlebitis
   b. Wound drainage devices (Hemovac, Jackson-Pratt pouch). Ensure device is fully compressed to ensure proper suctioning.

    c. Foley catheter
- tubing free of kinks
- color and amount of urine
- tubing anchored to thigh or abdomen (for males)

    d. N/G tube to suction
- color and amount of drainage

    e. Chest tubes

8. Check recovery room report for:
- any medication given
- fluid intake and output
- any special problems
- estimated blood loss

9. Palpate pedal pulses bilaterally.

10. Evaluate return of gag reflex.

11. Check operative report for type of anesthesia given and length of time under anesthesia.

STANDARDS OF PERFORMANCE FOR THE ADULT PATIENT (COMPETENCY STATEMENT)

Competency Statement

Provides nursing care for adult patients experiencing alterations in health status.

Criteria

1. Uses techniques of interviewing to collect data about the patient's psychosocial responses to an altered health state and outcomes of surgical interventions.

2. Performs a rapid physical examination of the body system exhibiting an alteration in function using appropriate techniques of inspection, palpation, percussion, and auscultation.

3. Identifies signs and symptoms of an alteration in function of a given body system (respiratory, cardiovascular, hematologic, musculoskeletal, endocrine, reproduction, neurological, immune, peripheral vascular, GI, renal).

4. Anticipates diagnostic studies commonly performed to establish a diagnosis of the altered body system function.

5. Correlates the results of diagnostic studies with data collected by physical examination.

6. Establishes a nursing diagnosis based on findings from assessments.

7. Establishes a written plan of care that reflects nursing diagnoses, patient outcomes, and strategies to achieve outcomes.

8. Incorporates diagnostic studies into monitoring and evaluating the effectiveness of therapeutic interventions.

9. Differentiates between signs and symptoms indicative of a therapeutic versus nontherapeutic response to a treatment modality, which is medical or surgical.

10. Takes appropriate actions in a timely manner to prevent untoward outcomes when a complication of a treatment modality is detected or suspected.

11. Demonstrates knowledge and skills essential to safe administration of medications specific for the altered body system:
    - Identifies generic and trade name, action, contraindications, recommended dosage range, common adverse reactions, therapeutic response, and laboratory studies used to monitor and evaluate therapeutic levels of prescribed medications.
    - Administers prescribed medications correctly by the appropriate routes such as IM, SC, intradermal, oral, topical, vaginal, rectal, IV.

12. Consults appropriate ancillary healthcare discipline to increase probability of achieving established patient outcomes (primary physician, dietitian, pharmacist, respiratory therapist, physical therapist, occupational therapist, social worker, discharge coordinator, religious leader, local community agency or support group, and so on).

13. Coordinates multidisciplinary referrals as appropriate.

14. Provides assistance as needed with a prescribed therapeutic or bedside diagnostic procedure:
    - Anticipates and obtains equipment/supplies as appropriate.
    - Explains procedure.
    - Obtains written consent following facility protocol and procedures.
    - Obtains baseline assessment before procedure.
    - Monitors patient response during and after procedure.
    - Ensures patient comfort, which can include positioning and administering an analgesic or sedative before and/or after procedure.
    - Labels and sends specimen to appropriate ancillary department.

15. Documents assessment findings, interventions, and patient response to interventions using appropriate medical and nursing terminology.

16. Always maintains a safe environment for the patient and self according to facility protocol and procedures:
    - Use of restraints and bedrails when needed.
    - Infection control measures, for example, handwashing, proper disposal of sharps, use of protective clothing, use of aseptic or sterile technique.
    - Monitoring invasive devices (tubes or drains placed in a body part to infuse or drain fluid).

17. Teaches self-care activities for posthospital management:
    - Recognizes patients and significant others need for information/instructions.
    - Identifies readiness for learning.
    - Identifies existing factors that can interfere with learning.
    - Uses instructional strategies and terminology appropriate for patients and significant others level.
    - Evaluates and documents teaching.

18. Recognizes patients need for assistance with posthospital care and initiates appropriate referrals as needed.

19. Assists patients and significant others in coping with illness and outcomes of therapies:
    - Shares plan of care.
    - Recognizes ineffective coping behaviors.
    - Uses therapeutic communication techniques.
    - Encourages patients and significant others to express feelings.
    - Initiates counseling or group support referrals as needed.

20. Demonstrates knowledge and skills in using equipment/supplies commonly used with alteration in body system function, including purpose, procedure for insertion or application, troubleshooting for malfunctions, maintenance procedures, and removal procedure:

a. Cardiovascular — hemodynamic monitoring devices, pacemaker (permanent and temporary), ECG monitoring, CPR, defibrillation, cardioversion

b. Respiratory — mechanical ventilation, artificial airways, chest drainage systems, suctioning, pulse oximetry

c. Sensory — Snellen chart, ophthalmoscope, otoscope

d. Urinary — catheterization, urostomy care, hemodialysis access devices, peritoneal dialysis, condom catheter

e. Immune — wound care, venipuncture, IV infusion pumps, dressing changes, central vascular access devices for IV infusions, blood transfusions, use of autologous blood collection devices, use of leukocyte-poor blood or platelet filters, epidural catheters for analgesic control, PCA pumps

f. Gastrointestinal — N/G tube suctioning, enteral feedings via N/G or gastrostomy tubes, enemas, ostomy care, rectal tube, guaiac stools

g. Musculoskeletal — traction, cast care, support devices for the back (corsets, braces), CPM machine, use of assistive devices for ambulation (cane, walker, crutches)

h. Peripheral Vascular — antiembolism stockings, use of Doppler probe, use of a Dinamapp

Index